*4th Edition*

*Board of Registry Study Guide*

# Clinical Laboratory
# Certification Examinations

*4th Edition*

## *Board of Registry Study Guide*

# Clinical Laboratory
# Certification Examinations

**Edited by ASCP Board of Registry Staff**

*Barbara M. Castleberry, PhD, MT(ASCP)*
*Mary E. Lunz, PhD*
*Bradford L. Sahl, MT(ASCP)*

American Society of Clinical Pathologists
Chicago

**Library of Congress Cataloging-in-Publication Data**

Board of Registry study guide for clinical laboratory certification examinations / edited by ASCP Board of Registry staff,
    Barbara M. Castleberry, Mary E. Lunz, Bradford L. Sahl.—4th ed.

        p.   cm.
    Includes bibliographical references.
    ISBN 0-89189-416-0
    1. Medical laboratory technology—Examinations, questions, etc.
I. Castleberry, Barbara M. II. Lunz, Mary E. III. Sahl, Bradford L. IV. American Society of Clinical Pathologists. Board of Registry.
[DNLM: 1. Pathology, Clinical—examination questions. 2. Allied Health Personnel—examination questions.
3. Specialty Boards—examination questions. QY 18.2 B662 1996]
RB38.B63  1996
616.07'5'076—dc20
DNLM/DLC
for Library of Congress

*NWST*
*TAHF9068*
*AHW1195*

96-2826
CIP

Printed in the United States of America

00  99  98  97  96    5  4  3  2  1

# Contents

# To the Examinee

You have taken an important first step in your professional career by deciding to become certified. I wish you success as you prepare for these examinations.

*Joel M. Schilling, MD*

Joel M. Schilling, MD
Chairman, Board of Registry

# Introduction

Examination applicants have often expressed a need for a guide to help them prepare for the certification examinations. To respond to this need, the Board of Registry of the American Society of Clinical Pathologists (ASCP) and ASCP Press have produced this study guide for aspiring medical laboratory technicians and medical technologists. This guide contains background on the Board of Registry; guidelines for preparing and taking the test; information on the development, content, structure, and scoring of the examinations; practice questions and answers in the content areas covered by the examinations; and a computer disk that can be used for self-assessment or practice testing.

The practice questions are constructed in a format and style comparable to those on the Board of Registry certification examinations. The practice questions were developed from previously published materials, including Continuing Education Update Examinations, Professional Self-Assessment Examinations Series III, Update/Educate, Audio-Visual Seminar Series in Immunology, and Tech Sample, which were prepared by the committees of the ASCP Commission on Continuing Education and the ASCP Associate Member Section. None of the questions will appear in future Board of Registry examinations.

Taking the computer-administered examinations and answering the practice questions should help you prepare for the actual examinations. Use of this book, however, does not ensure a passing score on the examinations. The Board of Registry's evaluation and credentialing process are entirely independent of this study guide.

For faculty, officials of clinical laboratory education programs, and examinees, this book provides information on how Board of Registry certification examinations are structured and scored. The technical summaries on these topics are designed to briefly explain the pertinent evaluation topics. Further information concerning evaluation techniques can be obtained from the books and articles noted in the education section of the reading list.

# Question Reviewers

*Our thanks to the following individuals who reviewed questions contained in this book.*

## Blood Bank

*Chris Barrasso, MT(ASCP)SBB*
The Johns Hopkins Hospital - Transfusion Medicine
Baltimore, Maryland

*Laurine T. Charles, MHS, MT(ASCP)SBB*
Medical University of South Carolina
Charleston, South Carolina

*Patricia Ellinger, MT(ASCP)SBB*
Hennepin County Medical Center
Maple Grove, Minnesota

*Vicky Clark, MS, MT(ASCP)SBB*
Grady Health System - Blood Bank
Atlanta, Georgia

*Fay Weirich, MT(ASCP)SBB*
Yale New Haven Hospital
West Haven, Connecticut

## Body Fluids

*Pam Crider, MBA, MT(ASCP)*
Baptist Medical Centers
Birmingham, Alabama

*Sue Strassinger, DA, MT(ASCP)*
Orange Beach, Alabama

## Chemistry

*Polly Cathcart, MMSc, MT(ASCP)SC*
Emory University Hospital
Atlanta, Georgia

*Vicky Freeman, PhD, MT(ASCP)SC*
Medical Center, Division of Medical Technology
Omaha, Nebraska

*Linda Kasper, MD, MT(ASCP)SC*
Indiana University
Indianapolis, Indiana

*Cheryl M. Haskins, MS, MT(ASCP)SC*
SUNY Health Science Center at Syracuse
Syracuse, New York

*Trina M. Radich, MT(ASCP)SC*
St. Vincent's Hospital
Portland, Oregon

## Hematology

*Ellen Boswell, MBA, MT(ASCP)SH*
University of Virginia
Charlottesville, Virginia

*Karen Brown, MS, MT(ASCP)*
University of Utah
Salt Lake City, Utah

*Cynthia S. Johns, MT(ASCP)SH*
Lakeland Regional Medical Center
Lakeland, Florida

*Louann Lawrence, DrPH, MT(ASCP)SH*
Louisiana State University
New Orleans, Louisiana

*Theresa O'Laughlin, MT(ASCP)SH*
The Moses H. Cone Memorial Hospital
Greensboro, North Carolina

## Immunology

*Linda Fell, MT(ASCP)*
University of Nebraska Medical Center
Omaha, Nebraska

*Cynthia Karr*
Medical University of South Carolina
Charleston, South Carolina

*Linda E. Miller, PhD, MI(ASCP)SI*
SUNY Health Science Center at Syracuse
Syracuse, New York

*Fred Rodriguez, Jr, MD*
VA Medical Center
New Orleans, Louisiana

*Denise Zito, MT(ASCP)SI*
University of Virginia
Charlottesville, Virginia

## Management

*Jo Anne Edwards, MEd, MT(ASCP)*
Community College of Southern Nevada
Las Vegas, Nevada

*Michael W. Morris, MS, SH(ASCP)DLM*
SUNY Health Science Center at Syracuse
Syracuse, New York

## Microbiology

*Vivi-Anne Griffey, MS, MT(ASCP)*
Villa Julie College
Stevenson, Maryland

*Marilyn S. Held, SpM, MT(ASCP)DLM*
St. John Hospital
Detroit, Michigan

*Susan Sharp, PhD, MT(ASCP)*
Mt. Sinai Medical Center
Miami Beach, Florida

*James Vossler, MS, MT(ASCP)SM, CLS(NCAMLP)*
SUNY Health Science Center at Syracuse
Syracuse, New York

*Dawn Taylor, MLT(ASCP)*
St. John Hospital and Medical Center
Warren, Michigan

# CHAPTER 1

# *Certification*

## The Importance of Certification

The practice of modern medicine would be impossible without the tests performed in the clinical laboratory. A medical team of pathologists, specialists, technologists, and technicians works together to determine the presence, extent, or absence of disease and provides data needed to evaluate the effectiveness of treatment.

Laboratory procedures require an array of complex precision instruments and a variety of automated and electronic equipment. However, men and women interested in helping others are the foundation of a successful laboratory. They must be accurate and reliable, have an interest in science, and be able to recognize their responsibility for human lives.

A critical part of high-quality health care is the assurance that individuals performing laboratory tests are able to carry out their responsibilities in a proficient manner. Therefore, laboratory personnel of demonstrated competence are of prime importance.

Certification is the process by which a nongovernmental agency or association grants recognition of competency to an individual who has met certain predetermined qualifications, as specified by that agency or association. Certification affirms that an individual has demonstrated that he or she possesses the knowledge and skills to perform essential tasks in the medical laboratory. The Board of Registry certifies individuals upon completion of academic prerequisites, clinical laboratory education or experience, and successful performance on a competency-based examination.

## Role of the ASCP Board of Registry

Founded in 1928 by the American Society of Clinical Pathologists (ASCP), the Board of Registry, as the preeminent certification agency in the field of laboratory medicine, promotes the health and safety of the public. Composed of representatives of professional organizations and the public, the Board's mission is to:

1. Certify the competency of laboratory personnel.
2. Set the standard for quality examination development and administration.
3. Assist educational programs in evaluating their effectiveness.
4. Perform research and develop methods of competency evaluation.
5. Provide study materials for examination preparation.
6. Maintain a registry of certified individuals.

The keystone of the Board of Registry is the team of approximately 100 volunteer technologists and technicians, laboratory scientists, physicians, and professional researchers in education, evaluation, and psychometrics who make up the Board of Governors, the Research and Development Committee, and the examination committees. These individuals contribute their time and expertise to achieve the goal of excellence in the certification process for medical laboratory personnel.

The Board of Governors is the policy-making body for the Board of Registry and is composed of twenty-one members. These twenty-one members include technologists, technicians, and pathologists nominated by the ASCP and representatives from the general public and the following societies: American Academy of Microbiology, American Association of Blood Banks, American Society of Cytopathology, American Society of Hematology, Clinical Laboratory Management Association, National Registry in Clinical Chemistry, and the National Society for Histotechnology.

The Research and Development Committee's activities include the review of current methods and research related to competency definition, test development, validity and reliability assessment, examination performance, and standard setting.

The examination committees include technicians, technologists, laboratory scientists, and physicians. These committees are responsible for planning, development, and review of the examinations; determining the accuracy and relevancy of the examinations; and confirming the standard for each examination.


## After Certification

Registration is the process by which names of individuals certified by the Board of Registry are identified on an annual basis as being currently registered. Annual reregistration benefits include an identification card, registration seal, one-year subscription to *Laboratory Medicine*, eligibility for insurance programs, and verification of certification.

Certification in a given category means that an individual has met all criteria for career entry in that category. As they continue on in their careers, many individuals who are certified at one professional level may work to obtain certification at a higher level to reflect their continued growth and development. Thus, a technician may move to the technologist level and even to the specialist level in a specific discipline.

The clinical laboratory sciences are among the fastest changing segments of the health care field. Therefore, each certificant should embrace a philosophy of lifelong learning to remain current in a chosen discipline. This may be accomplished through formal course work, professional continuing education exercises, and individual regimens of journal reading and subscription to professional self-assessment examinations.

# CHAPTER 2

# *Technician and Technologist Certification*

The Board of Registry's professional levels of practice were first compiled in 1982 (*Laboratory Medicine*, 13:312-313, 1982). These professional levels were updated in 1993 under the auspices of the Research and Development Committee. Board of Registry certifications that may be attained include technician and technologist. These professional levels define in a general sense the skills and abilities that an individual is expected to have at career entry. The professional levels are considered hierarchical; that is, each level encompasses the knowledge and skill of the preceding level.

There are several aspects of these definitions that should be noted. First, the roles are defined in a general sense. For example, technologist describes the role of technologists in all general medical technology categories, ie, chemistry, hematology, blood banking, immunology, microbiology, cytotechnology, and histotechnology. Second, the roles refer to skills and abilities that the individual is expected to have at career entry, not those that may be acquired with subsequent experience. Career entry is defined as the point in time when the individual meets all educational and/or experience requirements and is therefore eligible for Board certification. Thus, while supervision, management, and teaching skills are attributes that technicians may possess and apply in the laboratory, they are not skills that the technician is expected to have learned prior to a career-entry examination.

## Technician

### Knowledge
The technician has a working comprehension of the technical and procedural aspects of laboratory tests. The technician maintains an awareness and complies with safety procedures and ethical standards of practice. The technician correlates laboratory tests with disease processes and understands basic physiology, recognizing appropriate test selection and abnormal test results.

### Technical Skills
The technician comprehends and follows procedural guidelines in performance of laboratory tests to include (1) quality assurance monitoring, (2) computer applications, (3) instrumentation troubleshooting, and (4) specimen collection and processing requirements.

## Judgment and Decision Making

The technician recognizes the existence of procedural and technical problems and takes corrective action according to predetermined criteria. The technician prioritizes test requests to maintain standard patient care and maximal efficiency. Technical decisions related to testing are supervised by a technologist, supervisor, or laboratory director.

## Communication

The technician communicates test results, reference ranges, and specimen requirements to authorized sources. The technician prepares drafts of procedures for laboratory tests according to a standardized format.

## Teaching and Training Responsibilities

The technician trains new technicians, provides information to the patient and public as needed, participates in continuing education lectures and conferences for departmental personnel, and demonstrates technical laboratory skills to students and new employees.

# Technologist

## Knowledge

The technologist has an understanding of the underlying scientific principles of laboratory testing as well as of the technical, procedural, and problem-solving aspects. The technologist has a general comprehension of the many factors that affect health and disease, and recognizes the importance of proper test selection, the numerous causes of discrepant test results (patient and laboratory derived), deviations in test results, and ethics including result confidentiality. The technologist correlates abnormal laboratory data with pathologic states, determines validity of test results, and weighs the need for additional tests. The technologist understands and enforces safety regulations, uses statistical methods, and applies business and economic data in decision making. The technologist has an appreciation of the roles and interrelationships of paramedical and other health-related fields and follows the ethical code of conduct for the profession.

## Technical Skills

The technologist is capable of performing and interpreting standard, complex, and specialized tests. The technologist has an understanding of quality assurance sufficient to implement and monitor quality control programs. The technologist is able to participate in the introduction, investigation, and implementation of new procedures and the evaluation of new instruments. The technologist evaluates computer-generated data and software and troubleshoots computer/interface problems. The technologist understands and uses troubleshooting, validation, statistical, computer, and preventative maintenance techniques to ensure proper laboratory operation.

## Judgment and Decision Making

The technologist has the ability to exercise initiative and independent judgment in dealing with the broad scope of procedural and technical problems. The technologist is able to participate in, and may be delegated the responsibility for, decisions involving quality control/quality assurance programs, instrument and methodology selection, preventative maintenance, safety procedures, reagent purchases, test selection/utilization, research procedures, and computer/statistical data.

**Communication**

The technologist communicates pertinent technical information to medical, paramedical, or lay individuals through lectures, conferences, work group interaction, memberships, publications, legislative activities, and continuing education. The technologist develops acceptable criteria, laboratory manuals, reports, guidelines, and research protocols.

**Teaching and Training Responsibilities**

The technologist provides instruction in theory, technical skills, safety protocols, and application of laboratory test procedures. The technologist provides continuing education and professional development for laboratory personnel. The technologist may participate in the evaluation of the effectiveness of educational programs.

**Supervision and Management**

The technologist has an understanding of management theory, economic impact, and management functions. The technologist participates in and takes responsibility for establishing technical and administrative procedures, quality control/quality assurance, standards of practice, safety and waste management procedures, information management, and cost-effective measures. The technologist supervises laboratory personnel.

# CHAPTER 3

## *Applying for the Certification Examination*

The Board of Registry offers computerized adaptive testing in four examination cycles. These cycles are on a recurring quarterly basis: January-March, April-June, July-September, and October-December.

Approximately one year before the date you wish to take the examination, you should contact the Board of Registry to obtain a current application packet. In addition to the application form, the application packet includes the *Procedures for Examination and Certification*. This booklet contains the application deadlines and examination dates, the examination eligibility requirements, and a list of test centers. Since the examination requirements as well as other information included in the application packet are periodically revised, be sure you have the most recent application packet available from the Board of Registry office. Once you have obtained these materials, it is important to review them to make sure that you have adequate time to obtain any required documents prior to the application deadline. Please contact the Board of Registry office at P.O. Box 12277, Chicago, Illinois 60612, for application forms and general information.

### Application Deadlines

Your application and fee must be postmarked no later than January 2 (for the April-June exam cycle), April 1 (for the July-September exam cycle), July 1 (for the October-December exam cycle), or October 1 (for the January-March exam cycle for the following year).

### Examination Eligibility

To be eligible to take the examination, you must:

1. Meet the *current* stated minimum requirements for a particular category or level of certification.
2. Submit a formal application form and pay the appropriate application fee.

The minimum requirements for each examination are summarized in the table. For detailed information, refer to the current Board of Registry eligibility requirements.

| Certification | Requirements |
|---|---|
| Medical Technologist (MT) | Baccalaureate degree and one of the following:<br>• Completion of NAACLS accredited MT program<br>• MLT(ASCP) certification and 3 years' experience<br>• 5 years' experience |
| Medical Laboratory Technician (MLT) | Associate degree or equivalent and one of the following:<br>• Completion of NAACLS accredited MLT program or CLA(ASCP) certification<br>• Completion of 50-week military Medical Laboratory Specialist program<br>• 3 years' experience |
| Histologic Technician (HT) | High school diploma and one of the following:<br>• Completion of NAACLS accredited HT program<br>• Associate degree or equivalent and 1 year's experience<br>• 2 years' experience |
| Histotechnologist (HTL) | Baccalaureate degree and one of the following:<br>• Completion of NAACLS accredited HT program<br>• 1 year's experience |
| Categorical Certification (BB, C, H, I, M) | Baccalaureate degree and 1 to 2 years' experience |
| Cytotechnologist (CT) | Baccalaureate degree and one of the following:<br>• Completion of CAAHEP accredited CT program<br>• 5 years' experience |
| Specialist in Cytotechnology (SCT) | One of the following:<br>• Baccalaureate degree, CT(ASCP) certification, and 5 years' experience<br>• Master's degree, CT(ASCP) certification, and 4 years' experience<br>• Doctorate degree, CT(ASCP) certification, and 3 years' experience |
| Specialist in Blood Banking (SBB) | One of the following:<br>• Baccalaureate degree and completion of CAAHEP accredited SBB program<br>• Baccalaureate degree, MT(ASCP) or BB(ASCP) certification, and 5 years' experience<br>• Master's or doctorate degree and 3 years' experience |
| Specialist Certification (SC, SH, SI, SM) | One of the following:<br>• Baccalaureate degree, Technologist certification, and 5 years' experience<br>• Master's degree and 4 years' experience<br>• Doctorate degree and 2 years' experience |
| Diplomate in Laboratory Management (DLM) | Baccalaureate, master's, or doctorate degree and appropriate laboratory management education and experience |
| Phlebotomy Technician (PBT) | High school graduation (or equivalent) and one of the following:<br>• Completion of NAACLS approved phlebotomy program<br>• Completion of acceptable phlebotomy program at a regionally accredited college/university or accredited laboratory<br>• 1 year of full-time experience in an accredited laboratory |
| Hemapheresis Practitioner (HP) | One of the following:<br>• RN and 3 years' experience<br>• MT(ASCP), BB(ASCP), or SBB(ASCP) certification and 3 years' experience<br>• Baccalaureate degree and 5 years' experience |

# CHAPTER 4

## *Preparing to Take the Examination*

Begin early to prepare for the certification examination. Because of the broad range of knowledge and skills tested by the examination, even applicants with a great deal of college training and professional experience will probably find that some review is necessary, although the amount will vary from applicant to applicant. Generally, last-minute cramming is the least effective method for preparing for the examination. The earlier that you begin, the more time you will have to prepare; and the more you prepare, the better your chance of doing well on the examination.

### Diagnose Your Strengths and Weaknesses Using the Computerized Tests

Chapter 16 provides instructions for using the IBM-compatible computer disk, which constructs computerized tests. The computerized tests may be very useful for continuous self-assessment as you prepare for the examination.

The computer will administer practice tests of 50 questions. The distribution of questions across content areas will be comparable to BOR content guidelines. Upon completion of a computer-administered test, you will have the option to review the questions in your 50-item test. The questions will be displayed on the screen along with the correct answer.

You will be able to take the computer practice tests as often as you wish. Unique questions will be presented until all questions in the bank have been presented. At that time you will be notified on the computer screen and questions will be reused for additional tests.

When you take a computer-constructed test, try to take it under conditions similar to actual testing conditions. Use a computer that is located in a quiet place, allow approximately 2 hours, and do not use reference materials.

You can use the information from your performance on the computer practice tests and other information to diagnose your strengths and weaknesses. For example, if you currently work in the laboratory and do hematology tests, you may want to study the other laboratory areas more thoroughly. If you are a student and your lowest grades were in clinical chemistry, you may want to spend more time on that subject than others. After you have diagnosed your weaknesses from several sources, such as the practice tests, course grades, class tests, and laboratory experience, you are ready to begin studying.

## Study for the Test

Plan a course of study that allows more time for your weaker areas. Although it is important to study your areas of weakness, be sure to allow enough time to review all areas.

It is better to spend a short time studying every day than to spend several hours every week or two. A regular time and special place to study will help, because study will then become part of your daily routine.

Several resources can be used to help you to study. The reading lists at the end of this book identify many useful books by subject area. The practice questions in this book provide an extensive overview of the content of medical technology. They can be used to test your knowledge in each subject area or they may be used to acquire experience in answering multiple-choice questions. You may also wish to consider the following:

*Standard Textbooks:* Textbooks tend to cover a broad range of knowledge in a given field and thus help you survey an entire field. An added benefit is that textbooks frequently have questions at the end of the chapters that you can use to test yourself.

*Competency Statements and Content Guidelines:* The Board of Registry has developed the competency statements and content guidelines to delineate the content and tasks included in the test. Content guidelines for the MLT and MT appear in Chapter 7, "Examination Content Guidelines."

*Current Publications:* It will be helpful to scan major journals to keep up with innovations in the field. Textbooks may be updated only every few years, whereas new questions are added to the examinations every examination cycle. Therefore, it is possible that questions will be asked on content that is not yet in textbooks but has been added to the literature via journals and other periodicals.

## Get Enough Rest Before the Examination

Ease up on your studying before the examination. Try to get plenty of rest, and eat before going to take the examination. The MT and MLT examinations are scheduled for a 2.5-hour period.

## Locate the Test Center

The authorization slip will have the location of the examination test center, the phone number, and the address. Plan to arrive at the test site a half hour before your scheduled appointment to check in and familiarize yourself with the area. You must present a photo ID and the schedule letter before you will be admitted to the test.

# CHAPTER 5

## Taking the Examination by Computer

### Introduction

The Board of Registry has studied assessments done solely by computerized adaptive testing. Results of this in-depth evaluation demonstrate clearly that computerized adaptive tests are as reliable as traditional written tests in measuring ability and reaching a pass-fail decision for certification. Candidates have the same opportunity to demonstrate the required level of knowledge and skill to achieve certification on a computerized test as on a written examination.

### Advantages

Computerized adaptive testing offers many advantages over written examinations:

1. Testing is by individual appointment in a comfortable computer carrel, which affords quiet and privacy for the candidate.
2. Candidates are required to answer fewer questions.
3. Less time is required to take the test.
4. It is easier to enter answers on the computer keyboard than to record answers on a separate answer sheet.
5. Score reporting requires a shorter time (10 working days).

Prior knowledge of computers is not required. The candidate answers each question by either pressing the number key (1, 2, 3, or 4) or using the mouse to "click" on the answer selected. Moving to the next question records the candidate's response. During the examination a "HELP" screen is always available for the candidate to review the instructions for entering responses and moving through the exam.

The total time allowed for the exam is 2.5 hours. Both the MT and the MLT exams consist of 100 questions.

## Test Center Procedures

1. Scratch paper will be provided for you. No books, dictionaries, or paper may be taken into the examination room.
2. The Board of Registry allows the use of nonprogrammable calculators during the test. They must be brought in without carrying cases.
3. You must bring a photo ID and the schedule letter (sent to you after your examination eligibility has been determined) to the test center.
4. You will be required to acknowledge the following statement: "I have read the Examination Instructions. I understand that if an applicant is caught cheating on a certifying examination, his/her results will be held until such time as the applicant appeals to the Board of Registry, at which time the Board will decide each individual case. I certify that I am the candidate whose social security # appeared on the first screen. I also certify that, because of the confidential nature of these copyright materials, I will not retain or copy any examination materials and I will not otherwise reveal the content of these materials." By using the NEXT question box, you have agreed to the above statement and your examination will begin.

## Irregularities

If an examinee is discovered engaging in inappropriate conduct during the examination, such as looking at notes or otherwise giving or obtaining unauthorized information or aid, the test center personnel will notify the Board of Registry office in writing, immediately. Inappropriate conduct by an examinee may result in invalidation of the examinee's test results, as well as revocation of current certification and a bar of admission to Board of Registry–sponsored examinations in the future. Other appropriate action may also be taken against the examinee.

## Suggestions for Taking the Test

1. Read the instructions carefully before beginning. A "HELP" screen that reviews the instructions is available at any time during the test.
2. Read the questions carefully looking for words such as *best*, *most* likely, *least* likely, and *not*.
3. Read all of the answer choices before answering. Sometimes what initially appears to be a correct answer may not be the *best* answer.
4. Budget your time so you can answer each question. Do not spend a large amount of time on any one question.
5. Answer each question to the best of your ability when it is presented. There is no extra penalty for guessing on Board of Registry examinations. In other words, if you have some knowledge about the content of the question, select the best response. The computer requires that you answer the question presented before you can proceed to another question.
6. You may change your answer as often as you wish before moving to the next question.
7. Try to stay relaxed so that you can think clearly and logically through the problems presented on the examination.

8. You may review your answers for some or all questions at the end of the test. The response previously selected appears highlighted. You may choose to change the response by pressing the key for a different response or by using the mouse to "click" on a different answer. By moving to the next question, you are recording your newly selected response. Think carefully before altering a response.

## Commonly Asked Questions About Computerized Testing

Q. *Do I need prior knowledge of how to operate a computer to take the test?*
A. No.

Q. *How many questions will be on the test?*
A. 100 questions.

Q. *What is the content distribution on the test?*
A. BB=20%; Chem=20%; Hema=20%; Immu=10%; Micr=20%; and UA=10%.

Q. *How long will I have to take the test?*
A. 2.5 hours.

Q. *What type of questions will be presented?*
A. Multiple choice.

Q. *How do I enter my answers?*
A. By pressing the number key of your choice or using the mouse to "click" on your answer choice.

Q. *May I review and change my answers?*
A. Yes, after you have seen all 100 questions, directions for reviewing the test and changing answers will appear on the screen.

Q. *Where will visual material be presented?*
A. On the computer screen with the question.

Q. *May nonprogrammable calculators be used?*
A. Yes.

Q. *Will scrap paper be provided?*
A. Scrap paper is provided and collected at the end of the exam.

Q. *How do I check the remaining time during my exam?*
A. There is TIME function on the screen that can be accessed at any time by the candidate.

Q. *What happens when the allotted test time is over?*
A. The test stops automatically when time has run out.

Q. *How is the test scored?*
A. Points are awarded for correct answers.

Q. *When will I receive my test results?*
A. Within 10 working days after the test.

Q. *How will scores be reported?*
A. Scaled scores ranging from 100-999. Minimum passing score is 400.

Q. *When is the test given?*
A. By appointment, Monday through Saturday, throughout the year.

Q. *Where is the test given?*
A. Sylvan Technology Centers in the United States, Canada, and Puerto Rico.

# CHAPTER 6

## *Examination Development*

### Examination Committee

The Joint Generalist Examination Committee, which prepares the Medical Technologist and Medical Laboratory Technician examinations, is composed of medical technologists, medical laboratory technicians, and pathologists. The committee represents diverse geographical areas and diverse types of practice. The responsibility of item writing, evaluation, and selection rests with the examination committee members. Question writing requires an understanding of the examination population and mastery of the subject as well as mastery of written communication skills. Question review by the entire committee ensures that the item adheres to appropriate technical and/or scientific principles. The committee is also responsible for maintaining the currency of the content of the examinations and is supported by the Board of Registry staff, which provides expertise in psychometrics and examination production.

### Criterion-Referenced Testing

The Board of Registry's process of examination construction and analysis is based on the concept of criterion-referenced testing. Generally, a criterion-referenced examination is designed to ascertain an individual's knowledge with respect to a set of previously defined competencies summarizing the knowledge and skill represented on the examination. Each examination question is designed to test some aspect of the competencies that have been developed as criteria against which examinees are measured. Thus, every question on an examination becomes a "criterion" against which the examinee is measured. If an examinee answers an item correctly, he or she has met the criterion; if an examinee answers incorrectly, he or she has not met the criterion. Since it is unlikely that one question would be the absolute measure of a competency, the Board of Registry examinations are carefully planned so that several items measure each competency.

In criterion-referenced testing, the domain of practice of the Medical Technologist or Medical Laboratory Technician is delineated in the competency statements and content guidelines (see

Chapter 7, "Examination Content Guidelines"). These content guidelines are the basis for writing examination questions.

## Purpose of the Examination

The Board of Registry certification examinations measure an examinee's level of skill and knowledge (competency) at a particular point in time. Because of its ties to a competency statement, each examination question contributes to the pass/fail decision. Since questions must accurately distinguish between qualified and unqualified candidates, each question is carefully written, reviewed, and evaluated. A very comprehensive process is used to ensure that each question measures that which it is intended to measure.

## Components of Competency

Examination items are written from competency statements. The Board of Registry competency statements were developed based on selected components of competence.

The three components are (1) knowledge, (2) technical skill, and (3) cognitive skill. The components expand into competency statements in which knowledge is represented in the content areas and technical skill is represented by task definitions (see Chapter 7).

### Knowledge

This is the first dimension of competency and a criterion against which examinees are measured. Knowledge is the content base upon which the field of practice in Medical Technology is built. Content areas of Medical Technology typically cover Blood Banking, Body Fluids (including Urinalysis), Chemistry, Hematology, Immunology, and Microbiology.

### Technical Skill

The second component of competency and a criterion against which the examinee is measured may be defined as the ability to complete an assigned activity or apply knowledge to a procedure. The implication is that laboratory tasks can be defined and that one's ability to perform them can be measured on a test. While these are not the only tasks completed by laboratory staff, they are the areas that are considered essential to test on the examinations.

### Cognitive Skill

The third component of competence is the ability to deal with data at various cognitive skill levels. Cognitive skill refers to the cognitive or mental processes required to answer the question. Questions are classified into three cognitive skill levels, based on the structure of the question. The three cognitive skill levels used by the Board of Registry are defined as follows:

*Recall (level 1):* The ability to recognize previously learned (memorized) knowledge ranging from specific facts to complete theories.

*Interpretive skills (level 2):* The ability to use recalled knowledge to understand or apply verbal, numeric, or visual data.

*Problem solving (level 3)*: The ability to use recalled knowledge and the interpretation/ application of distinct criteria to resolve a problem or situation and/or make an appropriate decision.

The cognitive skill level of a question is influenced by the construction of the stem in concert with the responses. Thus, concepts such as coagulation provide the content for the development of questions on all three cognitive skill levels. The sample questions in the figure below demonstrate this point. All items on a Board of Registry examination were written to test one of the competency statements listed in Chapter 7.

---

**Cognitive Skill:** *Recall (level 1)*

The prothrombin time test requires that the patient's citrated plasma be combined with:

  a. platelet lipids
  b. thromboplastin
  c. Ca++ and platelet lipids
*d. Ca++ and thromboplastin


**Cognitive Skill:** *Interpretation (level 2)*

A patient develops unexpected bleeding following three transfusions. The following test results were obtained:

Prolonged PT and APTT
Decreased fibrinogen
Increased fibrin split products
Decreased platelets

What is the most probable cause of these results?

  a. familial afibrinogenemia
  b. primary fibrinolysis
*c. DIC
  d. liver disease


**Cognitive Skill:** *Problem Solving (level 3)*

A patient develops severe unexpected bleeding following four transfusions. The following test results were obtained:

Prolonged PT and APTT
Decreased fibrinogen
Increased fibrin split products
Decreased platelets

Given these results, which of the following blood products should be recommended to the physician for this patient?

  a. platelets
  b. factor VIII
*c. cryoprecipitate
  d. fresh frozen plasma

*Correct answer*

---

## Question Development

The Board of Registry examinations consist of multiple-choice questions. A multiple-choice question may be defined as a measuring device that contains a STEM and four RESPONSES, one of which is the *best* answer. The form is flexible so that an item may ask a specific question, describe a situation, report laboratory results, etc.

The stem of a multiple-choice question:

1. Asks a question.
2. Gives an incomplete statement.
3. States an issue.
4. Describes a situation.

The content of the stem focuses on a central theme or problem, using clear and precise language, without excessive length that can confuse or distract examinees. The stem may describe clinical data and laboratory results that require interpretation or problem solving. The question or issue presented in the stem is relevant to the knowledge and task delineated in a competency statement.

The responses present the "best" answer and the "distractors." Each multiple-choice question has four independent responses. The best answer is the one agreed upon by the experts; however, the other three distractors may seem plausible to the examinee who has partial, incomplete, or inappropriate knowledge. The distractors may therefore be considered logical misconceptions of the best answer. The responses are written to be parallel in content, length, and category of information.

As you review the questions included in this book, it may be useful to note the construction of the question, carefully reviewing both the stem and responses as you practice selecting the best answer.

## Color Plates and Other Visual Materials

Some of the questions on the examination will refer to visual materials such as graphs, charts, or color photographs. On the computerized test, visual material will appear on the screen with the question. Subject areas that may have color photographs include Hematology, Urinalysis, and Microbiology (including Bacteriology, Parasitology, and Mycology). Although color photographs are not provided in this book, there are examples on the computer disk.

An example of a question that contains visual material appears in Figure 1.

## Preparation of Examinations

The Board of Registry maintains databases containing more than 10,000 examination questions. This computerized database system has extensive identification and sorting capabilities. There are 100 multiple-choice questions in each computerized Medical Laboratory Technician or Medical Technologist examination.

Board of Registry examinations are carefully constructed according to the specific predetermined criteria summarized in the competency statements and content outlines. Each examination is constructed according to a multidimensional examination blueprint. The blueprint delineates the number of questions that will be used to measure each content area. The examination is balanced with regard to knowledge, technical skills, and cognitive skills. The computer algorithm implements

**Figure 1**

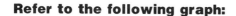

**Refer to the following graph:**

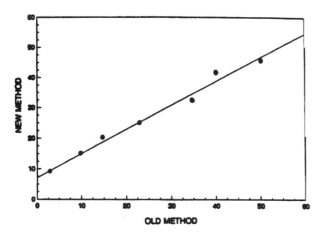

A new methodology for amylase has been developed and compared with the existing method as illustrated in the graph shown above. The new method can be described as:

  a. poor correlation with constant bias
*b. good correlation with constant bias
  c. poor correlation with no bias
  d. good correlation with no bias

*Correct answer*

these criteria for each examination. While different questions may be presented to individuals, the overall content distribution will match the test plan indicated in the content guidelines.

# CHAPTER 7

## *Examination Content Guidelines*

The content of each examination is determined based on the competency statements and content outlines developed and published by the Board of Registry. These competency statements and content outlines are provided to show you the topics that will be covered on the examinations.

## Taxonomy Levels for Medical Laboratory Technician and Medical Technologist Examination Questions

**Taxonomy 1**
> *Recall:* Ability to recall or recognize previously learned (memorized) knowledge ranging from specific facts to complete theories.

**Taxonomy 2**
> *Interpretive Skills:* Ability to utilize recalled knowledge to interpret or apply verbal, numeric, or visual data.

**Taxonomy 3**
> *Problem Solving:* Ability to utilize recalled knowledge and the interpretation/application of distinct criteria to resolve a problem or situation and/or make an appropriate decision.

## Medical Laboratory Technician Competency Statements

In regard to laboratory operations and the performance of laboratory tests involving Microbiology, Hematology, Chemistry, Urinalysis and Body Fluids, Immunology, and Blood Bank at career entry the Medical Laboratory Technician:

**Applies**
- principles of basic laboratory procedures in order to perform tests
- principles of special procedures related to testing
- knowledge to identify sources of error in laboratory testing

- knowledge of fundamental biological characteristics as they pertain to laboratory testing
- principles of theory and practice related to laboratory operations (safety)
- knowledge of standard operating procedures

## Selects
- procedural course of action appropriate for the type of sample and test requested
- methods/reagents/media/blood products according to established procedures
- instruments to perform test appropriate to test methodology according to established procedures
- appropriate controls for test performed
- routine laboratory procedures to verify test results according to established protocol
- special laboratory procedures to verify test results

## Prepares
- reagents/media/blood products according to established procedures
- instruments to perform tests
- controls appropriate for testing procedures

## Calculates
- results from test data obtained from laboratory procedures

## Correlates Laboratory Data
- and clinical data to assess test results
- and quality control data to assess test results
- with other laboratory data to assess test results
- with physiologic processes to assess/validate test results

## Evaluates Laboratory Data
- and clinical data to specify additional tests
- to verify test results
- to check for possible source of errors
- to determine possible inconsistent results
- to recognize health and disease states
- to assess validity/accuracy of procedures for a given test
- to determine appropriate instrument adjustments
- to recognize common procedural/technical problems
- to take corrective action according to predetermined criteria
- to recognize and report the need for additional testing
- to make identifications

## Medical Laboratory Technician Content Outline
*All percentages are approximate ranges to be included on the examination.*

### VI. BLOOD BANK (20% OF TOTAL EXAM)

1. **Red Blood Cells (55% of subtest; 11% of total exam)**
   A. Immunologic genetic theory and principles
   B. Specimen and component selection, collection, preparation, transport, and storage

C. Laboratory examinations
    1. Basic tests
    2. Special tests

## 2. Other Components (15% of subtest; 3% of total exam)
A. Immunologic genetic theory and principles
B. Specimen and component selection, collection, preparation, transport, and storage
C. Laboratory examinations

## 3. Hemotherapy (25% of subtest; 5% of total exam)
A. Donors
B. Therapeutic phlebotomy
C. Adverse reactions
D. Transfusion practice

## 4. Laboratory Operations (5% of subtest; 1% of total exam)
A. Quality assurance
B. Safety
C. Instruments
D. Laboratory mathematics


# II. URINALYSIS AND BODY FLUIDS (10% OF TOTAL EXAM)

## 1. Urine (75% of subtest; 7.5% of total exam)
A. Anatomy and physiology
B. Specimen selection, collection, transport, storage, and processing
C. Laboratory examinations
    1. Physical
    2. Chemical
    3. Microscopic

## 2. Other Body Fluids (20% of subtest; 2% of total exam)
A. Anatomy and physiology
B. Specimen selection, collection, transport, storage, and processing
C. Laboratory examinations
    1. Basic tests
    2. Special tests
    3. Principles of microscopy
D. Related conditions and disorders affecting CSF, feces, and other body fluids

## 3. Laboratory Operations (5% of subtest; 0.5% of total exam)
A. Quality assurance
B. Safety
C. Instruments
D. Laboratory mathematics

## III. CHEMISTRY (20% OF TOTAL EXAM)

1. **Carbohydrates, Lipids and Lipoproteins, Heme Derivatives (20% of subtest; 4% of total exam)**
   A. Biochemical theory and physiology
   B. Specimen selection, collection, transport, storage, and processing
   C. Laboratory examinations
      1. Basic tests
      2. Special tests
   D. Biochemical manifestation of disease

2. **Protein and Enzymes (23% of subtest; 5% of total exam)**
   A. Biochemical theory and physiology
   B. Specimen selection, collection, transport, storage, and processing
   C. Laboratory examinations
      1. Basic tests
      2. Special tests
   D. Biochemical manifestation of disease

3. **Acid-Base Electrolytes (23% of subtest; 5% of total exam)**
   A. Biochemical theory and physiology
   B. Specimen selection, collection, transport, storage, and processing
   C. Laboratory examinations
      1. Basic tests
      2. Special tests
   D. Biochemical manifestation of disease

4. **Special Chemistry & Instrumentation (29% of subtest; 5% of total exam)**
   A. Special chemistry (endocrinology, TDM, and others)
      1. Biochemical theory and physiology
      2. Specimen selection, collection, transport, storage, and processing
      3. Laboratory examinations
      4. Biochemical manifestation of disease
   B. Instrumentation
      1. Principles of operation
      2. Essential components

5. **Laboratory Operations (5% of subtest; 1% of total exam)**
   A. Quality assurance
   B. Safety
   C. Instruments
   D. Laboratory mathematics

## IV. HEMATOLOGY (20% OF TOTAL EXAM)

1. **Erythrocytes (33% of subtest; 7% of total exam)**

A. Anatomy and physiology of hematopoiesis
B. Specimen selection, collection, transport, storage, and processing
C. Laboratory examinations
   1. Basic tests
   2. Special tests
D. Hematopoietic diseases

2. **Leukocytes (33% of subtest; 7% of total exam)**
   A. Anatomy and physiology of hematopoiesis
   B. Specimen selection, collection, transport, storage, and processing
   C. Laboratory examinations
      1. Basic tests
      2. Special tests
   D. Hematopoietic diseases

3. **Thrombocytes & Hemostasis (29% of subtest; 5% of total exam)**
   A. Anatomy and physiology of hematopoiesis
   B. Specimen selection, collection, transport, storage, and processing
   C. Laboratory examinations
      1. Basic tests
      2. Special tests
   D. Hematopoietic disorders/Hemostatic diseases

4. **Laboratory Operations (5% of subtest; 1% of total exam)**
   A. Quality assurance
   B. Safety
   C. Instruments
   D. Laboratory mathematics


## V. IMMUNOLOGY (10% OF TOTAL EXAM)

1. **Immune System (45% of subtest; 4.5% of total exam)**
   A. Anatomy and physiology
      1. Humoral
      2. Cellular
      3. Complement
   B. Immunologic manifestation of disease

2. **Laboratory Examination (50% of subtest; 5% of total exam)**
   A. Specimen selection, collection, transport, storage, and processing
   B. Basic tests

3. **Laboratory Operations (5% of subtest; 0.5% of total exam)**
   A. Quality assurance
   B. Safety
   C. Instruments
   D. Laboratory mathematics

## VI. MICROBIOLOGY (20% OF TOTAL EXAM)

1. **Bacteria (70% of subtest; 14% of total exam)**
   A. Morphology, cultural and growth characteristics
   B. Specimen and/or media selection, collection, transport, storage, and processing
   C. Laboratory examinations
      1. Basic tests
      2. Special tests
   D. Infectious diseases

2. **Other Organisms (25% of subtest; 5% of total exam)**
   A. Fungi
      1. Morphology, cultural and growth characteristics
      2. Specimen and/or media selection, collection, transport, storage, and processing
      3. Laboratory examinations
      4. Infectious diseases
   B. Mycobacteria
      1. Morphology, cultural and growth characteristics
      2. Specimen and/or media selection, collection, transport, storage, and processing
      3. Laboratory examinations
      4. Infectious diseases
   C. Parasites
      1. Morphology, cultural and growth characteristics
      2. Specimen and/or media selection, collection, transport, storage, and processing
      3. Laboratory examinations
      4. Infectious diseases
   D. Viruses, rickettsiae, and other microorganisms
      1. Morphology, cultural and growth characteristics
      2. Specimen and/or media selection, collection, transport, storage, and processing
      3. Laboratory examinations
      4. Infectious disease

3. **Laboratory Operations (5% of subtest; 1% of total exam)**
   A. Quality assurance
   B. Safety
   C. Instruments
   D. Laboratory mathematics

## Examination Reporting

After the examination has been administered and scored, a report is sent to the examinee. The examinee Performance Report provides the scaled score on the total examination and pass/fail status for all candidates.

In addition, failing candidates receive scaled scores for each subtest (see content outline for subtests). This information may help the examinee identify areas of strengths and weaknesses in order to develop a study plan for future examinations.

# Medical Technologist Competency Statements

In regard to laboratory operations and the performance of laboratory tests involving Microbiology, Hematology, Chemistry, Urinalysis and Body Fluids, Immunology, and Blood Bank at career entry the Medical Technologist:

## Applies
- principles of basic laboratory procedures in order to perform tests
- principles of special procedures related to testing
- knowledge to identify sources of error in laboratory testing
- knowledge of fundamental biological characteristics as they pertain to laboratory testing
- principles of theory and practice related to laboratory operations (management/safety/ education/research and development)
- knowledge of standard operating procedures

## Selects
- procedural course of action appropriate for the type of sample and test requested
- methods/reagents/media/blood products according to established procedures
- instruments to perform test appropriate to test methodology according to established procedures
- appropriate controls for test performed
- routine laboratory procedures to verify test results according to established protocol
- special laboratory procedures to verify test results
- instruments for new laboratory procedures

## Prepares
- reagents/media/blood products according to established procedures
- instruments to perform tests
- controls appropriate for testing procedures

## Calculates
- results from test data obtained from laboratory procedures

## Correlates Laboratory Data
- and clinical data to assess test results
- and quality control data to assess test results
- with other laboratory data to assess test results
- with physiologic processes to assess/validate test results and procedures

## Evaluates
- laboratory and clinical data to specify additional tests
- laboratory data to recognize common procedural/technical problems
- laboratory data to verify test results
- laboratory data to check for possible source of errors
- laboratory data to determine possible inconsistent results
- laboratory data to recognize health and disease states
- laboratory data to assess validity/accuracy of procedures for a given test

- laboratory data to determine appropriate instrument adjustments
- laboratory data to take corrective action according to predetermined criteria
- laboratory data to recognize and report the need for additional testing
- laboratory data to determine alternate methods for a given test
- various methods to establish new testing procedures
- laboratory and clinical data to ensure personnel safety
- laboratory operational procedures
- test results obtained by alternate methodologies
- laboratory data to establish reference range criteria for existing or new tests
- laboratory data to make identifications/recommendations

## Medical Technologist Content Outline

*All percentages are approximate ranges to be included on the examination.*

### I. BLOOD BANK (20% OF TOTAL EXAM)

1. **Red Blood Cells (55% of subtest; 11% of total exam)**
   A. Immunologic genetic theory and principles
   B. Specimen and component selection, collection, preparation, transport, and storage
   C. Laboratory examinations
      1. Basic tests
      2. Special tests

2. **Other Components (15% of subtest; 3% of total exam)**
   A. Immunologic genetic theory and principles
   B. Specimen and component selection, collection, preparation, transport, and storage
   C. Laboratory examinations

3. **Hemotherapy (25% subtest; 5% of total exam)**
   A. Donors
   B. Therapeutic phlebotomy
   C. Adverse reactions
   D. Transfusion practice

4. **Laboratory Operations (5% subtest; 1% of total exam)**
   A. Quality assurance
   B. Safety
   C. Management
   D. Research and development
   E. Instruments
   F. Education
   G. Laboratory mathematics

## II. URINALYSIS AND BODY FLUIDS (10% OF TOTAL EXAM)

1. **Urine (75% of subtest; 7.5% of total exam)**
   A. Anatomy and physiology
   B. Specimen selection, collection, transport, storage, and processing
   C. Laboratory examination
      1. Physical
      2. Chemical
      3. Microscopic

2. **Other Body Fluids (20% of subtest; 2% of total exam)**
   A. Anatomy and physiology
   B. Specimen selection, collection, transport, storage, and processing
   C. Laboratory examinations
      1. Basic tests
      2. Special tests
      3. Principles of microscopy
   D. Related conditions and disorders affecting CSF, feces, and other body fluids

3. **Laboratory Operations (5% of subtest; 0.5% of total exam)**
   A. Quality assurance
   B. Safety
   C. Management
   D. Research and development
   E. Instruments
   F. Education
   G. Laboratory mathematics

## III. CHEMISTRY (20% OF TOTAL EXAM)

1. **Carbohydrates, Lipids and Lipoproteins, Heme Derivatives (20% of subtest; 4% of total exam)**
   A. Biochemical theory and physiology
   B. Specimen selection, collection, transport, storage, and processing
   C. Laboratory examinations
      1. Basic tests
      2. Special tests
   D. Biochemical manifestation of disease

2. **Protein and Enzymes (23% of subtest; 5% of total exam)**
   A. Biochemical theory and physiology
   B. Specimen selection, collection, transport, storage, and processing
   C. Laboratory examinations
      1. Basic tests
      2. Special tests
   D. Biochemical manifestation of disease

3. **Acid-Base Electrolytes (23% ofsubtest; 5% of total exam)**
   A. Biochemical theory and physiology
   B. Specimen selection, collection, transport, storage, and processing
   C. Laboratory examinations
      1. Basic tests
      2. Special tests
   D. Biochemical manifestation of disease

4. **Special Chemistry & Instrumentation (29% of subtest; 5% of total exam)**
   A. Special chemistry (endocrinology, TDM, and others)
      1. Biochemical theory and physiology
      2. Specimen selection, collection, transport, storage, and processing
      3. Laboratory examinations
      4. Biochemical manifestation of disease
   B. Instrumentation
      1. Principles of operation
      2. Essential components

5. **Laboratory Operations (5% of subtest; 1% of total exam)**
   A. Quality assurance
   B. Safety
   C. Management
   D. Research and development
   E. Instruments
   F. Education
   G. Laboratory mathematics

## IV. HEMATOLOGY (20% OF TOTAL EXAM)

1. **Erythrocytes (33% of subtest; 7% of total exam)**
   A. Anatomy and physiology of hematopoiesis
   B. Specimen selection, collection, transport, storage, and processing
   C. Laboratory examinations
      1. Basic tests
      2. Special tests
   D. Hematopoietic diseases

2. **Leukocytes (33% of subtest; 7% of total exam)**
   A. Anatomy and physiology of hematopoiesis
   B. Specimen selection, collection, transport, storage, and processing
   C. Laboratory examinations
      1. Basic tests
      2. Special tests
   D. Hematopoietic diseases

**3. Thrombocytes & Hemostasis (29% of subtest; 5% of total exam)**
   A. Anatomy and physiology of hematopoiesis
   B. Specimen selection, collection, transport, storage, and processing
   C. Laboratory examinations
      1. Basic tests
      2. Special tests
   D. Hematopoietic disorders/Hemostatic disorders

**4. Laboratory Operations (5% of subtest; 1% of total exam)**
   A. Quality assurance
   B. Safety
   C. Management
   D. Research and development
   E. Instruments
   F. Education
   G. Laboratory mathematics

## V. IMMUNOLOGY (10% OF TOTAL EXAM)

**1. Immune System (45% of subtest; 4.5% of total exam)**
   A. Anatomy and physiology
      1. Humoral
      2. Cellular
      3. Complement
   B. Immunologic manifestation of disease

**2. Laboratory Examination (50% of subtest; 5% of total exam)**
   A. Specimen selection, collection, transport, storage, and processing
   B. Basic tests

**3. Laboratory Operations (5% of subtest; 0.5% of total exam)**
   A. Quality assurance
   B. Safety
   C. Management
   D. Research and development
   E. Instruments
   F. Education
   G. Laboratory mathematics

## VI. MICROBIOLOGY (20% OF TOTAL EXAM)

**1. Bacteria (55% of subtest; 11% of total exam)**
   A. Morphology, cultural and growth characteristics
   B. Specimen and/or media selection, collection, transport, storage, and processing

C. Laboratory examinations
    1. Basic tests
    2. Special tests
D. Infectious diseases

**2. Other Organisms (40% of subtest; 8% of total exam)**
A. Fungi
    1. Morphology, cultural and growth characteristics
    2. Specimen and/or media selection, collection, transport, storage, and processing
    3. Laboratory examinations
    4. Infectious diseases
B. Mycobacteria
    1. Morphology, cultural and growth characteristics
    2. Specimen and/or media selection, collection, transport, storage, and processing
    3. Laboratory examinations
    4. Infectious diseases
C. Parasites
    1. Morphology, cultural and growth characteristics
    2. Specimen and/or media selection, collection, transport, storage, and processing
    3. Laboratory examinations
    4. Infectious diseases
D. Viruses, rickettsiae, and other microorganisms
    1. Morphology, cultural and growth characteristics
    2. Specimen and/or media selection, collection, transport, storage, and processing
    3. Laboratory examinations
    4. Infectious diseases

**3. Laboratory Operations (5% of subtest; 1% of total exam)**
A. Quality assurance
B. Safety (general)
C. Management
D. Research and development
E. Instruments
F. Education
G. Laboratory mathematics

## Examination Reporting

After the examination has been administered and scored, a report is sent to the examinee. The examinee Performance Report provides the scaled score on the total examination and pass/fail status for all candidates.

In addition, failing candidates receive scaled scores for each subtest (see content outline for subtests). This information may help the examinee identify areas of strengths and weaknesses in order to develop a study plan for future examinations.

*All Board of Registry examinations use conventional units for results and reference ranges.*

# CHAPTER 8

*Examination Scoring*

## Setting the Absolute Standard

In 1980, the Board of Registry adopted a policy of criterion-referenced testing, which measures an examinee's performance compared to an absolute standard or criterion. Absolute standards are established by the examination committee through a systematic evaluation of the content and skill represented in each question.

For the Board of Registry examinations, the absolute standard is the pass point. The pass point is represented as a scaled score of 400. Any individual who meets or exceeds the level of performance represented by the pass point passes the examination. Those who do not meet this standard fail the examination.

All examinations are equated to the absolute standard. This ensures that all candidates meet the same standard regardless of the difficulty of the questions seen by each candidate.

## Question Development and Analysis

The Board of Registry uses standard procedures for psychometric analysis to ensure that each examinee receives a fair examination.

Examination questions are evaluated through item analysis statistics. Item statistics are used to identify unacceptable items. To ensure the continued quality of the examination, questions are reviewed periodically, and those found to be unsatisfactory are excluded from the examination item pool.

Item statistical analysis includes traditional item analysis and item response theory (IRT) analysis. The Rasch model is used for the IRT analysis. Both approaches to analysis include an assessment of item difficulty. Difficulty is assessed by the percentage of examinees selecting each response. The correct response or best answer should draw the highest proportion of the population, while the distractors may draw a smaller percentage of the population. This provides an index of how easy or difficult the question was for a particular population. The IRT analysis then translates the percentage into an absolute log-odds unit of difficulty, so that the relative difficulty of items can be monitored across tests.

For traditional item analysis, discrimination provides an indication of how well the question differentiates between those examinees who did well on the total examination and those who did not. The computation compares or correlates the performance of candidates who selected the best answer to the question with the performance of those candidates who did well on the total examination. A positive correlation is anticipated for the correct response (best answer), and negative correlations are anticipated for the distractors. This is based on the assumption that those who did well on the question should do well on the test.

IRT analysis provides a fit statistic that is an assessment of how well the item fits the expectations of the Rasch model. The basic expectation is that examinees who are more able will answer any item correctly more frequently than examinees who are less able. The second expectation is that easier items will be answered correctly by more examinees than harder items. When these two relatively simple expectations are *not* met, the "fit statistic" flags the item for review.

## Score Reporting

Examinee Performance Reports are generated and distributed to the examinees within 10 days following the examination date. (Test results are not released by telephone to anyone.) The purpose of the report is to provide examinees with information about their performance on the examination.

The following explanation refers to the sample Examinee Performance Reports shown on page 35 and page 36. The first paragraph provides an explanation of how to interpret the profile. Key information is presented under "YOUR PERFORMANCE SUMMARY." A scaled minimum pass score (MPS) of 400 is the standard against which all examinees are measured. Individuals who achieve or exceed the pass point pass the examination; others fail. The decision to pass or fail is based on the candidate ability measure for the total test. Pass or fail status is noted under STATUS.

A performance report for a candidate who passed is shown on page 35. A report for a candidate who failed is shown on page 36. Subtest scaled scores for Blood Banking (BBNK), Chemistry (CHEM), Hematology (HEMA), Immunology (IMMU), Microbiology (MICR), and Urinalysis (UA) are included. This provides the failing candidate with information concerning strengths and weaknesses, which may be useful for future study.

Sample of Examination Performance Report—Pass

# BOARD OF REGISTRY

Joel M. Shilling, M.D.
Chair

P. O. Box 12277, Chicago, IL 60612-0277

(312) 738-1336     (312) 738-5808 FAX

```
EXAMINEE PERFORMANCE REPORT
MEDICAL LABORATORY TECHNICIAN EXAMINATION


999-99-9999    MLT(ASCP) 99999
JONES, JULIE L
600 W MAIN STREET
SOMEPLACE, USA


THIS REPORT PROVIDES INFORMATION CONCERNING YOUR EXAMINATION
PERFORMANCE.  A SCALED MINIMUM PASS SCORE (MPS) OF 400 ON THE TOTAL
TEST WAS REQUIRED TO PASS.

YOUR PERFORMANCE SUMMARY FOR THE TOTAL MLT EXAMINATION TAKEN ON
02/08/1993:

      MPS              YOUR SCORE              STATUS
      400                 485                   PASS
```

Representatives from:
American Society of Clinical Pathologists - Technicians/Technologists/Pathologists
American Academy of Microbiology • American Association of Blood Banks • American Society of Cytopathology • American Society of Hematology
Clinical Laboratory Management Association • National Registry in Clinical Chemistry • National Society for Histotechnology

Sample of Examination Performance Report—Fail

# BOARD OF REGISTRY

P. O. Box 12277, Chicago, IL 60612-0277

Joel M. Shilling, M.D.
Chair

(312) 738-1336    (312) 738-5808 FAX

```
EXAMINEE PERFORMANCE REPORT
MEDICAL LABORATORY TECHNICIAN EXAMINATION

999-99-999    MLT(ASCP)  99999
JONES, JULIE L
600 W MAIN STREET
SOMEPLACE, USA

THIS REPORT PROVIDES INFORMATION CONCERNING YOUR EXAMINATION
PERFORMANCE. A SCALED MINIMUM PASS SCORE (MPS) OF 400 ON THE TOTAL
TEST WAS REQUIRED TO PASS.

YOUR PERFORMANCE SUMMARY FOR THE TOTAL MLT EXAMINATION TAKEN ON
02/08/1993:
```

| MPS | YOUR SCORE | STATUS |
|-----|-----------|--------|
| 400 | 326 | FAIL |

SUBTEST PERFORMANCE SUMMARY

| SUBTESTS | PERCENT OF TOTAL TEST | SCALED SCORES |
|----------|----------------------|---------------|
| BLOOD BANKING | [20%] | 401 |
| CHEMISTRY | [20%] | 242 |
| HEMATOLOGY | [20%] | 281 |
| IMMUNOLOGY | [10%] | 495 |
| MICROBIOLOGY | [20%] | 356 |
| URINALYSIS | [10%] | 240 |

Representatives from:
American Society of Clinical Pathologists - Technicians/Technologists/Pathologists
American Academy of Microbiology • American Association of Blood Banks • American Society of Cytopathology • American Society of Hematology
Clinical Laboratory Management Association • National Registry in Clinical Chemistry • National Society for Histotechnology

# CHAPTER 9

## Blood Bank

The following items have been identified as appropriate for both entry level medical technologists and medical laboratory technicians.

1. Isoimmunization to platelet antigen ($Pl^{A1}$) and the placental transfer of maternal antibodies would be expected to cause newborn:

   a. erythroblastosis
   b. leukocytosis
   c. leukopenia
   d. thrombocytopenia

2. Following plasmapheresis, how long must a person wait before being eligible to donate a unit of Whole Blood?

   a. 8 weeks
   b. 2 weeks
   c. 48 hours
   d. 24 hours

3. Each unit of Whole Blood will yield approximately how many units of cryoprecipitated AHF?

   a. 40
   b. 80
   c. 130
   d. 250

4. Addition of which of the following will enhance the shelf-life of whole blood?

   a. heparin
   b. adenine
   c. hydroxyethyl starch
   d. lactated Ringer's solution


5. Pretransfusion compatibility testing must include:

   a. antibody screening by antiglobulin test
   b. autocontrol
   c. minor crossmatch
   d. D$^u$ test on recipient


6. Severe intravascular hemolysis is most likely caused by antibodies of which blood group system?

   a. ABO
   b. Rh
   c. Kell
   d. Duffy


7. Under extreme emergency conditions when there is no time to determine ABO group for transfusion, the technologist should:

   a. refuse to release any blood until the patient's sample has been typed
   b. release O, Rh-negative whole blood
   c. release O, Rh-negative red blood cells
   d. release O, Rh-positive red blood cells


8. An obstetrical patient has had three previous pregnancies. Her first baby was healthy, the second was jaundiced at birth and required an exchange transfusion, while the third was stillborn. Which of the following is the most likely cause?

   a. ABO incompatibility
   b. immune deficiency disease
   c. congenital spherocytic anemia
   d. Rh incompatibility


9. With regard to inheritance, most blood group systems are:

   a. sex-linked dominant
   b. sex-linked recessive
   c. autosomal recessive
   d. autosomal codominant

10. The optimum storage temperature for Cryoprecipitated AHF is:

    a. 22°C
    b. 4°C
    c. –12°C
    d. –20°C


11. The optimum storage temperature for Platelets is:

    a. 22°C
    b. 4°C
    c. –12°C
    d. –20°C


12. The optimum storage temperature for Red Blood Cells, Frozen is:

    a. 4°C
    b. –12°C
    c. –20°C
    d. –80°C


13. The optimum storage temperature for Whole Blood is:

    a. 4°C
    b. –12°C
    c. –20°C
    d. –80°C


14. Quality control tests must be performed daily on:

    a. reagent red blood cells
    b. oral thermometers
    c. banked whole blood
    d. centrifuge timers


15. Criteria determining Rh immune globulin eligibility include:

    a. mother is Rh-positive
    b. infant is Rh-negative
    c. mother has not been previously immunized to the D antigen
    d. infant has a positive direct antiglobulin test

16. Which of the following constitutes permanent rejection status of a donor?

    a. a tattoo 5 months previously
    b. recent close contact with a patient with viral hepatitis
    c. two units of blood transfused 4 months previously
    d. confirmed positive test for HBsAg 10 years previously


17. The major crossmatch will detect a(n):

    a. group A patient mistyped as group O
    b. irregular antibody in the donor unit
    c. Rh-negative donor unit mislabeled as Rh-positive
    d. recipient antibody directed against antigens on the donor red cells


18. Cells of the $A_3$ subgroup will:

    a. react with *Dolichos biflorus*
    b. not be agglutinated by anti-A
    c. give a mixed field reaction with anti-A,B
    d. not be agglutinated by anti-H


19. Mixed-field reactions with anti-A and anti-A,B and negative reactions with anti-B and anti-$A_1$ lectin (*Dolichos biflorus*) are observed. Without further testing, the most likely conclusion is that the patient is group:

    a. $A_1$
    b. $A_2$
    c. $A_3$
    d. $A_{el}$


20. Anti-Fy$^a$ is:

    a. usually a cold-reactive agglutinin
    b. more reactive when tested with enzyme-treated red blood cells
    c. capable of causing hemolytic transfusion reactions
    d. often an autoagglutinin


21. A patient received two units of Red Blood Cells and had a delayed hemolytic transfusion reaction. Pretransfusion records indicate a negative antibody screen. Repeat testing of the pretransfusion specimen detected an antibody at the antiglobulin phase. What is the most likely explanation for the original results?

    a. red cells were overwashed
    b. centrifugation time was prolonged
    c. patient's serum was omitted from the original testing
    d. antiglobulin reagent was neutralized

22. Which one of the following is an indicator of polyagglutination?

    a. RBCs typing as D$^u$ positive
    b. presence of red cell autoantibody
    c. decreased serum bilirubin
    d. agglutination with normal adult ABO-compatible sera


23. Anti-Sd$^a$ is strongly suspected if:

    a. the patient has been previously transfused
    b. the agglutinates are mixed-field and refractile
    c. the patient is group A or B
    d. only a small number of panel cells are reactive


24. Mixed-field agglutination at the anti–human globulin phase of a crossmatch may be attributed to:

    a. recently transfused cells
    b. intrauterine exchange transfusion
    c. an antibody such as anti-Sd$^a$
    d. fetomaternal hemorrhage


25. In suspected cases of hemolytic disease of the newborn, what significant information can be obtained from the baby's blood smear?

    a. estimation of WBC, RBC, and platelet counts
    b. marked increase in immature neutrophils (shift to the left)
    c. a differential to estimate the absolute number of lymphocytes present
    d. determination of the presence of spherocytes and elevated numbers of nucleated red blood cells


26. As a preventive measure against graft-versus-host disease, red blood cells prepared for infants who have received intrauterine transfusions should be:

    a. saline-washed
    b. irradiated
    c. frozen and deglycerolized
    d. group and Rh compatible with the mother


27. Which of the following is the preferred specimen for the initial compatibility testing in exchange transfusion therapy?

    a. maternal serum
    b. eluate prepared from infant's red blood cells
    c. paternal serum
    d. infant's postexchange serum

28. When the main objective of an exchange transfusion is to remove the infant's antibody-sensitized red blood cells and to control hyperbilirubinemia, the blood product of choice is ABO compatible:

a. Fresh Whole Blood
b. Red Blood Cells washed
c. Fresh Frozen Plasma
d. Heparinized Red Blood Cells

29. Which one of the following histories represents an acceptable donor?

| | Hct | BP | Temp | Pulse | Age | Sex |
|---|---|---|---|---|---|---|
| a. | 39 | 110/70 | 99.8 | 75 | 40 | F |
| b. | 37 | 135/85 | 98.6 | 80 | 35 | M |
| c. | 41 | 90/50 | 99.4 | 65 | 65 | M |
| d. | 45 | 115/80 | 98.6 | 102 | 17 | M |

30. According to AABB standards, 75% of all Platelet, Pheresis units tested shall contain how many platelets per μL?

a. $5.5 \times 10^{10}$
b. $6.5 \times 10^{10}$
c. $3.0 \times 10^{11}$
d. $5.0 \times 10^{11}$

31. Following the second spin in the preparation of Platelets, the platelets should be:

a. allowed to sit undisturbed for 1 hour
b. agitated immediately
c. pooled immediately
d. transfused within 48 hours

32. Which of the following is proper procedure for preparation of Platelets from Whole Blood?

a. light spin followed by a hard spin
b. light spin followed by two hard spins
c. two light spins
d. hard spin followed by a light spin

33. The purpose of a low-dose irradiation of blood components is to:

a. prevent posttransfusion purpura
b. prevent graft-versus-host (GVH) disease
c. sterilize components
d. prevent noncardiogenic pulmonary edema

34. Platelets prepared in a polyolefin type container, stored at 22°C-24°C in 50 mL of plasma, and gently agitated can be used for up to:

    a. 24 hours
    b. 48 hours
    c. 3 days
    d. 5 days

35. The enzyme responsible for conferring H activity on the red cell membrane is alpha-:

    a. galactosyl transferase
    b. N-acetylgalactosaminyl transferase
    c. L-fucosyl transferase
    d. glucosyl transferase

36. Refer to the following data:

| Forward Group | | | Reverse Group | | |
|---|---|---|---|---|---|
| Anti-A | Anti-B | Anti-A$_1$ Lectin | A$_1$ cells | A$_2$ Cells | B Cells |
| 4+ | neg | 4+ | neg | 2+ | 4+ |

The ABO discrepancy seen above is most likely due to:

    a. anti-A$_1$
    b. rouleaux
    c. anti-H
    d. unexpected IgG antibody present

Questions 37-39 refer to the following blood panel:

| Cell | D | C | E | c | e | M | N | S | s | Le^a | Le^b | P_1 | K | k | Fy^a | Fy^b | Jk^a | Jk^b | Xg^a | | IS | 37 C | AHG |
|------|---|---|---|---|---|---|---|---|---|------|------|-----|---|---|------|------|------|------|------|---|----|------|-----|
| 1 | 0 | + | 0 | + | + | + | 0 | 0 | + | 0 | + | 0 | 0 | + | 0 | + | 0 | + | + | | 0 | 0 | 1+ |
| 2 | + | + | 0 | 0 | + | 0 | + | 0 | + | + | 0 | + | 0 | + | + | 0 | + | + | + | | 0 | 0 | 0 |
| 3 | + | + | 0 | 0 | + | + | + | + | + | 0 | + | + | 0 | + | 0 | + | 0 | + | + | | 0 | 0 | 0 |
| 4 | + | 0 | + | + | 0 | + | + | + | 0 | 0 | + | 0 | + | + | 0 | + | + | 0 | + | | 0 | 0 | 1+ |
| 5 | 0 | 0 | + | + | + | 0 | + | 0 | + | + | 0 | + | 0 | + | + | 0 | 0 | + | + | | 0 | 0 | 1+ |
| 6 | 0 | 0 | 0 | + | + | + | 0 | 0 | + | 0 | 0 | + | 0 | + | 0 | 0 | + | 0 | + | | 0 | 0 | 1+ |
| 7 | 0 | 0 | 0 | + | + | + | + | 0 | + | + | 0 | + | + | 0 | 0 | + | + | + | 0 | | 0 | 0 | 1+ |
| 8 | 0 | 0 | 0 | + | + | + | 0 | 0 | + | 0 | + | 0 | 0 | + | + | 0 | + | + | + | | 0 | 0 | 1+ |
| 9 | 0 | 0 | 0 | + | + | + | + | + | 0 | 0 | 0 | 0 | 0 | + | + | + | + | 0 | + | | 0 | 0 | 1+ |
| 10 | 0 | 0 | 0 | + | + | + | 0 | + | + | 0 | + | 0 | 0 | + | + | 0 | + | 0 | + | | 0 | 0 | 1+ |
| Patient | | | | | | | | | | | | | | | | | | | | | 0 | 0 | 0 |

37. A 25-year-old Caucasian woman, gravida 3, para 2, required two units of Whole Blood. The antibody screen was positive and the results of the antibody panel are shown above. Which of the following antibodies may be the cause of the positive antibody screen?

    a. anti-M and anti-K
    b. anti-c and anti-E
    c. anti-s and anti-c
    d. anti-Fy^b and anti-c


38. A 25-year-old Caucasian woman, gravida 3, para 2, required two units of Whole Blood. The antibody screen was positive and the results of the antibody panel are shown above. What is the most probable genotype of this patient?

    a. *rr*
    b. *r'r'*
    c. *R_0r*
    d. *R_1R_1*


39. A 25-year-old Caucasian woman, gravida 3, para 2, required two units of Whole Blood. The antibody screen was positive and the results of the antibody panel are shown above. Which common antibody has NOT been ruled out by the panel?

    a. anti-S
    b. anti-Le^a
    c. anti-Jk^a
    d. anti-K

40. A patient's serum reacted weakly positive (1+$^w$) with 16 of 16 group O panel cells at the AHG test phase. The autocontrol was negative. Tests with ficin-treated panel cells demonstrated no reactivity at the AHG phase. Which antibody is most likely responsible for these results?

a. anti-Ch
b. anti-k
c. anti-e
d. anti-Js$^a$

41. Use of EDTA plasma prevents activation of the classical complement pathway by:

a. causing rapid decay of complement components
b. chelating Mg$^{++}$ ions, which prevents the assembly of C6
c. chelating Ca$^{++}$ ions, which prevents assembly of C1
d. preventing chemotaxis

42. A Kleihauer-Betke stain of a postpartum blood film revealed 0.3% fetal cells. What is the estimated volume (mL) of the fetomaternal hemorrhage expressed as whole blood?

a. 5
b. 15
c. 25
d. 35

43. The most effective component to treat a patient with fibrinogen deficiency is:

a. Fresh Frozen Plasma
b. Platelets
c. Fresh Whole Blood
d. Cryoprecipitated AHF

44. An assay of plasma from a bag of cryoprecipitated AHF yields a concentration of 9 international units (IU) of Factor VIII per mL of cryoprecipitated AHF. If the volume is 9 mL, what is the Factor VIII content of the bag in IU?

a. 9
b. 18
c. 27
d. 81

45. The approximate percentage of the original plasma content of Factor VIII recovered in cryoprecipitated AHF is:

   a. 10%-20%
   b. 20%-40%
   c. 40%-80%
   d. 80%-100%

46. A newborn demonstrates petechiae, ecchymosis, and mucosal bleeding. The preferred blood component for this infant would be:

   a. Red Blood Cells
   b. Fresh Frozen Plasma
   c. Platelets
   d. Cryoprecipitated AHF

47. A 65-year-old woman experienced shaking, chills, and a fever of 103°F approximately 40 minutes following the transfusion of a second unit of Red Blood Cells. The most likely explanation for the patient's symptoms is:

   a. transfusion of bacterially contaminated blood
   b. congestive heart failure due to fluid overload
   c. anaphylactic transfusion reaction
   d. severe febrile transfusion reaction

48. An acid elution stain was made using a 1-hour postdelivery maternal blood sample. Two thousand cells were counted and thirty of these cells appeared to contain fetal hemoglobin. It is the policy of the medical center to add one vial of Rh immune globulin to the calculated dose when the estimated volume of the hemorrhage exceeds 20 mL of whole blood. Calculate the number of vials of Rh immune globulin that would be indicated under these circumstances.

   a. 2
   b. 3
   c. 4
   d. 5

49. The Liley method of predicting the severity of hemolytic disease of the newborn is based on the amniotic fluid:

   a. bilirubin concentration by standard methods
   b. change in optical density measured at 450 nm
   c. Rh determination
   d. ratio of lecithin to sphingomyelin

50. A unit of Fresh Frozen Plasma was inadvertently thawed and then immediately refrigerated at 4°C on Monday morning. On Tuesday evening this unit may still be transfused as a replacement for:

    a. all coagulation factors
    b. Factor V
    c. Factor VIII
    d. Factor IX

51. According to AABB standards, which of the following donors may be accepted as a blood donor?

    a. hip replacement 5 months previous
    b. spontaneous abortion at 2 months of pregnancy, 3 months ago
    c. resides with a known hepatitis patient
    d. received a blood transfusion 22 weeks previously

52. Which of the following is the correct storage temperature for the component listed?

    a. Cryoprecipitated AHF, 4°C
    b. Fresh Frozen Plasma (FFP), –20°C
    c. Red Blood Cells frozen, –40°C
    d. Platelets, 37°C

53. Refer to the following data:

| Antisera | Reactions |
|----------|-----------|
| Anti-C | + |
| Anti-D | + |
| Anti-E | + |
| Anti-c | + |
| Anti-e | + |

Which of the following is a possible genotype for an individual whose red cells give the reactions shown above?

    a. $R_1R_1$
    b. $R_1r'$
    c. $R_0r''$
    d. $R_1R_2$

54. Which of the following blood components contains the most Factor VIII concentration relative to volume?

    a. Single-Donor Plasma
    b. Cryoprecipitated AHF
    c. Fresh Frozen Plasma
    d. Platelets


55. Which of the following blood components must be prepared within 8 hours after phlebotomy?

    a. Red Blood Cells
    b. Fresh Frozen Plasma
    c. Red Blood Cells frozen
    d. Cryoprecipitated AHF


56. Although ABO compatibility is preferred, ABO incompatible product may be administered when transfusing:

    a. Single-Donor Plasma
    b. Cryoprecipitated AHF
    c. Fresh Frozen Plasma
    d. Granulocytes


57. Which of the following blood components is the best source of Factor IX?

    a. Platelets
    b. Prothrombin complex
    c. Cryoprecipitated AHF
    d. Single-Donor Plasma


58. Coughing, cyanosis, and difficult breathing are symptoms of which of the following transfusion reactions?

    a. febrile
    b. allergic
    c. circulatory overload
    d. hemolytic


59. Hypotension, nausea, flushing, fever, and chills are symptoms of which of the following transfusion reactions?

    a. allergic
    b. circulatory overload
    c. hemolytic
    d. anaphylactic

60. Hives and itching are symptoms of which of the following transfusion reactions?

    a. febrile
    b. allergic
    c. circulatory overload
    d. anaphylactic

61. Hemoglobinuria, hypotension, and generalized bleeding are symptoms of which of the following transfusion reactions?

    a. allergic
    b. circulatory overload
    c. hemolytic
    d. anaphylactic

62. Fever and chills are symptoms of which of the following transfusion reactions?

    a. citrate toxicity
    b. circulatory overload
    c. allergic
    d. febrile

63. Cold agglutinin syndrome is best associated with which of the following blood groups?

    a. Duffy
    b. P
    c. I/i
    d. Rh

64. The following results were obtained:

| | Anti-A | Anti-B | Anti-D | Rh Control | DAT | Ab Screen |
|---|---|---|---|---|---|---|
| Infant | 4+ | 0 | 2+ | 0 | 0 | NT |
| Mother | 0 | 0 | +$^w$(mf) | 0 | 0 | 0 |

NT = not tested

Which of the following is the most probable explanation for these results?

    a. hemolytic disease of the newborn due to antibody against a high-frequency antigen
    b. large fetomaternal hemorrhage
    c. hemolytic disease of the newborn due to anti-D
    d. mother's cells are polyagglutinable

65. Antibodies involved in warm autoimmune hemolytic anemia are often associated with which blood group system?

   a. Rh
   b. I
   c. P
   d. Duffy

66. The following results were obtained:

| | Anti-A | Anti-B | Anti-D | Rh Control | DAT | Ab Screen |
|---|---|---|---|---|---|---|
| Infant | 0 | 0 | 0 | NT | 4+ | NT |
| Mother | 4+ | 0 | 0 | 0 | NT | Anti-D |

NT = not tested

Which of the following is the most probable explanation for these results?

   a. ABO hemolytic disease of the newborn
   b. Rh hemolytic disease of the newborn, infant has received intrauterine transfusions
   c. Rh hemolytic disease of the newborn, infant has a false-negative Rh typing
   d. large fetomaternal hemorrhage

67. The use of Red Blood Cells, Deglycerolized would be most beneficial when transfusing a patient:

   a. with sickle cell anemia
   b. who is at high risk for hepatitis B infection
   c. who is sensitized to platelet antigens
   d. with warm autoantibody

68. A method currently in routine use for freezing Red Blood Cells is:

   a. low concentration of glycerol (5% w/v)
   b. low concentration of glycerol (10% w/v)
   c. high concentration of glycerol (40% w/v)
   d. high concentration of glycerol (70% w/v)

69. Rejuvenation of a unit of Red Blood Cells is a method used to:

   a. remove antibody attached to RBCs
   b. inactivate viruses and bacteria
   c. restore 2,3-DPG and ATP to normal levels
   d. filter blood clots and other debris

70. A unit of Red Blood Cells is issued at 9:00 AM. At 9:10 AM the unit is returned to the Blood Bank. The container has NOT been entered, but the unit has NOT been refrigerated during this time span. The best course of action for the technologist is to:

    a. culture the unit for bacterial contamination
    b. discard the unit if not used within 24 hours
    c. store the unit at room temperature
    d. record the return and place the unit back into inventory

71. Cryoprecipitated AHF, if maintained in the frozen state at −18°C or below, has a shelf life of:

    a. 42 days
    b. 6 months
    c. 12 months
    d. 36 months

72. The quality assurance program for Red Blood Cells, Deglycerolized should include regularly scheduled monitoring to determine:

    a. sterility
    b. hematocrit
    c. potassium concentration
    d. acceptable glycerol removal

73. Which of the following is a characteristic of polyagglutinable red cells?

    a. can be classified by reactivity with *Ulex europaeus*
    b. are agglutinated by most adult sera
    c. are always an acquired condition
    d. autocontrol is always positive

74. Which of the following situations could result in an ABO discrepancy that is caused by problems with the patient's red cells?

    a. an unexpected antibody
    b. rouleaux
    c. agammaglobulinemia
    d. Tn activation

75. Which of the following is characteristic of Tn polyagglutinable red cells?

    a. If group O, they may appear to have acquired a group A antigen.
    b. They show strong reactions with anti-$A_1$ lectin.
    c. They react with *Arachis hypogaea* lectin.
    d. The polyagglutination is a transient condition.

76. Mixed field agglutination encountered in ABO grouping would most likely be due to:

    a. Bombay phenotype ($O_h$)
    b. T activation
    c. $A_3$ red cells
    d. positive indirect antiglobulin test

77. The use of leukocyte-depleted Red Blood Cells and Platelet Concentrates is indicated for which of the following patient groups?

    a. CMV-seropositive postpartum mothers
    b. victims of acute trauma with massive bleeding
    c. patients with history of febrile transfusion reactions
    d. burn victims with anemia and low serum protein

78. Blood selected for exchange transfusion must:

    a. lack red blood cell antigens corresponding to maternal antibodies
    b. be less than 3 days old
    c. be irradiated to prevent graft-vs-host disease
    d. be ABO compatible with the father

79. ABO-hemolytic disease of the newborn:

    a. usually requires an exchange transfusion
    b. most often occurs in firstborn children
    c. frequently results in stillbirth
    d. is usually seen only in the newborns of group O mothers

80. While performing routine postpartum testing for an Rh immune globulin (RhIg) candidate, a weakly positive antibody screening test was found. Anti-D was identified. This antibody is most likely the result of:

    a. massive fetomaternal hemorrhage occurring at the time of this delivery
    b. antenatal administration of RhIg at 28 weeks' gestation
    c. contamination of the blood sample with Wharton's jelly
    d. mother having a positive direct Coombs' test

81. A blood component used in the treatment of hemophilia A is:

    a. Factor VIII concentrate
    b. Fresh Frozen Plasma
    c. Platelets
    d. Whole Blood

82. A 24-year-old man with hemophilia is involved in an auto accident and is actively bleeding. Factor VIII assay results are 8%. The blood product of choice is:

    a. Single-Donor Plasma
    b. Fresh Frozen Plasma
    c. Whole Blood
    d. Cryoprecipitated AHF

83. An adult male patient who is actively bleeding has the following test results:

| ABO | AB |
|---|---|
| Rh | Negative |
| Antibody screening | Negative |

Six units of Red Blood Cells are ordered stat. The Blood Bank has the following Red Blood Cell units available:

| A, Rh-positive | 12 |
|---|---|
| B, Rh-positive | 2 |
| AB, Rh-positive | 4 |
| A, Rh-negative | 4 |
| B, Rh-negative: | 2 |

Which of the following should be crossmatched for this patient while more blood is being ordered?

    a. 6 A, Rh-positive
    b. 4 A, Rh-negative and 2 A, Rh-positive
    c. 4 AB, Rh-positive and 2 A, Rh-negative
    d. 4 A, Rh-negative and 1 O, Rh-negative and 1 B, Rh-negative

84. Which of the following blood components is most appropriate to transfuse to an 8-year-old male hemophiliac who is about to undergo minor surgery?

    a. Cryoprecipitated AHF
    b. Red Blood Cells
    c. Platelets
    d. heat-treated Factor VIII concentrate

85. According to AABB standards, platelets prepared from whole blood shall have at least:

    a. $5.5 \times 10^{10}$ platelets per unit in at least 75% of the units tested
    b. $6.5 \times 10^{10}$ platelets per unit in 75% of the units tested
    c. $7.5 \times 10^{10}$ platelets per unit in 100% of the units tested
    d. $8.5 \times 10^{10}$ platelets per unit in 95% of the units tested

86. Based upon Kleihauer-Betke test results, which of the following formulas is used to determine the volume of fetomaternal hemorrhage in mL of Whole Blood?

    a. % of fetal cells x 30
    b. % of fetal cells x 50
    c. % of maternal cells x 50
    d. % of maternal cells x 30

87. According to AABB standards, what is the minimum pH required for platelets?

    a. 4
    b. 5
    c. 6
    d. 7

88. During the preparation of platelet concentrates from Whole Blood, the blood should be:

    a. chilled to 6°C
    b. kept at room temperature
    c. warmed to 37°C
    d. heated to 57°C

89. A temperature rise of 1°C or more occurring in association with a transfusion is usually indicative of which of the following transfusion reactions?

    a. febrile
    b. circulatory overload
    c. hemolytic
    d. anaphylactic

90. Which of the following transfusion reactions is characterized by high fever, shock, hemoglobinuria, DIC, and renal failure?

    a. bacterial contamination
    b. circulatory overload
    c. hemolytic
    d. anaphylactic

91. Which of the following transfusion reactions occurs after infusion of only a few milliliters of blood and gives no history of fever?

    a. febrile
    b. circulatory overload
    c. anaphylactic
    d. hemolytic

92. During initial investigation of a suspected hemolytic transfusion reaction, it was observed that the posttransfusion serum was yellow in color and the direct antiglobulin test was negative. What is the next step in this investigation?

    a. Repeat compatibility testing on suspected unit(s).
    b. Perform plasma hemoglobin and haptoglobin determinations.
    c. Use enhancement media to repeat the antibody screen.
    d. No further serologic testing is necessary.

93. A granulocyte transfusion is indicated if the patient has:

    a. leukemia
    b. an absolute granulocyte count of 350/μL or less
    c. a viral infection
    d. a leukocyte count of 1,000/μL

94. Transfusion of which of the following is needed to help correct hypofibrinogenemia due to DIC?

    a. Whole Blood
    b. Fresh Frozen Plasma
    c. Cryoprecipitated AHF
    d. Platelets

95. According to AABB standards, Fresh Frozen Plasma must be infused within what period of time following thawing?

    a. 24 hours
    b. 36 hours
    c. 48 hours
    d. 72 hours

96. In a quality assurance program, at least 75% of the bags of Cryoprecipitated AHF must contain a minimum of how many international units of Factor VIII?

    a. 60
    b. 70
    c. 80
    d. 90

97. In the liquid state, plasma must be stored at:

    a. 56°C
    b. 37°C
    c. 22°C
    d. 1°C-6°C

98. Cryoprecipitated AHF must be transfused within what period of time following thawing and pooling?

    a. 4 hours
    b. 8 hours
    c. 12 hours
    d. 24 hours


99. In the autoadsorption procedure for the removal of cold autoagglutinins from serum, pre-treatment of the patient's red cells with which one of the following reagents is helpful?

    a. ficin
    b. phosphate-buffered saline at pH 9.0
    c. low ionic strength saline (LISS)
    d. albumin


100. In an emergency situation, Rh-negative red cells are transfused into an Rh-positive person of the genotype CDe/CDe. The first antibody MOST likely to develop is:

    a. anti-c
    b. anti-d
    c. anti-e
    d. anti-E


101. A 10% red cell suspension in saline is used in a compatibility test. Which of the following would most likely occur?

    a. a false-positive result due to antigen excess
    b. a false-positive result due to the prozone phenomenon
    c. a false-negative result due to the prozone phenomenon
    d. a false-negative result due to antigen excess


102. The most serious transfusion reactions are due to incompatibility in which of the following blood group systems?

    a. ABO
    b. Rh
    c. MN
    d. Duffy

103. A 29-year-old male is hemorrhaging severely. He is AB, Rh-negative. Six units of blood are required stat. Of the following types available in the Blood Bank, which would be most preferable for crossmatch?

a. AB, Rh-positive
b. A, Rh-negative
c. A, Rh-positive
d. O, Rh-negative

104. The following results were obtained on a patient's blood group and type during routine ABO and Rh testing:

| Cell Testing | Serum Testing |
| --- | --- |
| Anti-A = neg | $A_1$ cells = 4+ |
| Anti-B = 4+ | B cells = 2+ |
| Anti-D = neg | |
| Autocontrol = neg | |

Select the course of action to resolve this problem:

a. Draw a new blood sample from the patient and repeat all test procedures.
b. Test the patient's serum with $A_2$ cells and the patient's red cells with anti-$A_1$ lectin.
c. Repeat the ABO antigen grouping using three-time washed saline-suspended cells.
d. Perform antibody screening procedure at immediate spin using group O cells.

105. An antibody that causes in vitro hemolysis and reacts with the red cells of three of ten crossmatched donor units is most likely:

a. anti-Le$^a$
b. anti-s
c. anti-k
d. anti-E

106. In a delayed transfusion reaction, the causative antibody is generally too weak to be detected in routine compatibility testing and antibody screening tests but becomes detectable at what point after transfusion?

a. 3 to 6 hours
b. 1 to 5 days
c. 60 to 90 days
d. after 120 days

107. The most frequent transfusion-associated disease complication of blood transfusions is:

    a. cytomegalovirus (CMV)
    b. syphilis
    c. hepatitis
    d. AIDS

108. A 22-year-old man is admitted to the emergency room in shock following massive hemorrhage from knife wounds to his chest and abdomen. An emergency transfusion is required. Which of the following is the product of choice?

    a. O, Rh-positive Red Blood Cells
    b. O, Rh-negative Red Blood Cells
    c. O, Rh-positive Whole Blood
    d. O, Rh-negative Whole Blood

109. The following compatibility results were obtained:

| | 22°C | 37°C | AHG |
|---|---|---|---|
| Donor | 0 | 0 | 0 |
| Screening cells | 0 | 0 | 0 |
| Autocontrol | 0 | 0 | 3+ |

The most probable explanation for these findings is that the:

    a. patient has an antibody directed against an antigen present on donor RBCs
    b. donor has an antibody directed against an antigen present on patient RBCs
    c. patient has a positive direct antiglobulin test
    d. donor has a positive direct antiglobulin test

110. An antibody identification study is performed with the five-cell panel shown below:

| | | ANTIGENS | | | | | |
|---|---|---|---|---|---|---|---|
| | | 1 | 2 | 3 | 4 | 5 | TEST RESULTS |
| | I | + | 0 | 0 | + | + | + |
| PANEL CELLS | II | 0 | 0 | + | 0 | + | 0 |
| | III | 0 | + | + | + | 0 | 0 |
| | IV | 0 | + | + | 0 | + | + |
| | V | + | + | + | 0 | 0 | + |
| | AUTO | | | | | | 0 |

An antibody against which of the following antigens could NOT be excluded?

a. 1
b. 2
c. 3
d. 4

111. A patient received two units of Red Blood Cells and had a delayed transfusion reaction. Antibody screening records indicate that no agglutination was detected during testing except after the addition of IgG-sensitized cells. Repeat testing of the pretransfusion specimen detected an antibody at the antiglobulin phase. What is a possible explanation?

a. red cells were overwashed
b. centrifugation time was prolonged
c. patient's serum was omitted from the original testing
d. antiglobulin reagent was neutralized

112. A patient is group $A_2B$, Rh-positive and has an antiglobulin-reacting anti-$A_1$ in his serum. He is bleeding profusely in the operating room and group $A_2B$ Red Blood Cells are NOT available. Which of the following types of blood should be given as a first choice?

a. B, Rh-positive
b. B, Rh-negative
c. $A_1B$, Rh-positive
d. O, Rh-negative

113. Which of the following might cause a false-negative indirect antiglobulin test (IAT)?

a. overreading
b. IgG-coated screening cells
c. saline wash stored in a glass container
d. too heavy a cell suspension

114. How many units of Red Blood Cells are required to raise the hematocrit of a 70-kg non-bleeding man from 24% to 30%?

a. 1
b. 2
c. 3
d. 4

115. After receiving a unit of Whole Blood, a patient immediately developed flushing, nervousness, fever spike of 102°F, shaking, chills, and back pain. The plasma hemoglobin was elevated and there was hemoglobinuria. Laboratory investigation of this adverse reaction would most likely show:

    a. an error in ABO grouping
    b. an error in Rh typing
    c. presence of anti-Jk$^a$ antibody in patient's serum
    d. presence of gram-negative bacteria in blood bag

116. A patient whose saline and albumin crossmatches were compatible had a severe hemolytic reaction. Of the following antibodies, the one most likely present is anti-:

    a. Le$^b$
    b. K
    c. M
    d. P

117. In the direct (DAT) and indirect (IAT) antiglobulin techniques, false-negative reactions may result if the:

    a. patient's blood specimen was contaminated with bacteria
    b. patient's blood specimen was collected into tubes containing silicon gel
    c. saline used for washing the serum/cell mixture has been stored in glass or metal containers
    d. addition of AHG is delayed for 40 minutes or more after washing the serum/cell mixture

118. Which of the following antigens gives enhanced reactions with its corresponding antibody following treatment of the red cells with proteolytic enzymes?

    a. Fy$^a$
    b. E
    c. S
    d. M

119. A request is received to crossmatch five units of Red Blood Cells on a man who is group AB, Rh-positive. The blood inventory shows the following:

| | |
|---|---|
| A, Rh-positive | 23 units |
| A, Rh-negative | 6 units |
| B, Rh-positive | 4 units |
| AB, Rh-positive | 2 units |
| O, Rh-positive | 30 units |
| O, Rh-negative | 4 units |

Assuming all the blood crossmatched is compatible, the desirable sequence of blood units that can be issued for transfusion would be:

a.  5 units of group O, Rh-positive
b.  5 units of group A, Rh-positive
c.  2 units of group AB, Rh-positive; 3 units of group A, Rh-positive
d.  2 units of group AB, Rh-positive; 3 units of group B, Rh-positive

120. The results of a Kleihauer-Betke stain indicate a fetomaternal hemorrhage of 35 mL of Whole Blood. How many vials of Rh immune globulin would be required?

a.  1
b.  2
c.  3
d.  4

121. Which of the following would be the component of choice for treatment of von Willebrand's disease?

a.  Platelets
b.  Factor IX concentrate
c.  Cryoprecipitated AHF
d.  Fresh Frozen Plasma

122. Which of the following blood components is the best source of fibrinogen for transfusion to a patient with hypofibrinogenemia?

a.  Fresh Frozen Plasma
b.  Whole Blood
c.  Platelets
d.  Cryoprecipitated AHF

123. Which of the following is consistent with standard blood bank procedure governing the infusion of Fresh Frozen Plasma?

a.  Only blood group-specific plasma may be administered.
b.  Group O may be administered to recipients of all blood groups.
c.  Group AB may be administered to AB recipients only.
d.  Group A may be administered to both A and O recipients.

124. Which of the following is an immediate nonimmunologic adverse effect of a transfusion?

a.  hemolytic reaction
b.  febrile nonhemolytic reaction
c.  congestive heart failure
d.  urticaria

125. A 40-year-old man with autoimmune hemolytic anemia due to anti-E has a hemoglobin level of 10.8 gm/dL. This patient will most likely be treated with:

a. Whole Blood
b. Red Blood Cells
c. Fresh Frozen Plasma
d. no transfusion

126. Below are the results of the history obtained from a prospective female blood donor:

| | |
|---|---|
| Age | 18 |
| Temperature | 99.0 |
| Pulse | 80 beats/min |
| Hct | 36% |
| Hgb | 12.5 g/dL |
| History | Tetanus toxoid immunization 1 week ago |

How many of the above results will exclude this donor from giving blood for a routine transfusion?

a. none
b. one
c. two
d. three

127. A group A, Rh-positive infant of a group O, Rh-positive mother has a weakly positive direct antiglobulin test and a moderately elevated bilirubin at birth. The most likely cause is:

a. ABO incompatibility
b. Rh incompatibility
c. blood group incompatibility due to an antibody to a low-frequency antigen
d. neonatal jaundice NOT associated with blood group incompatibility

128. Prior to blood donation, the intended venipuncture site must be cleaned with a scrub solution containing:

a. hypochlorite
b. isopropyl alcohol
c. 10% acetone
d. PVP iodine complex

129. When removed from the refrigerator, a unit of donor blood was observed to have an accumulation of cream-colored material at the top of the plasma. The most probable cause of the accumulation is:

    a.  ingestion of a fatty meal shortly before blood donation
    b.  fungal contamination of the anticoagulant solution
    c.  bacterial contamination during collection of the blood
    d.  failure to mix the blood with anticoagulant during collection


130. A blood specimen from a pregnant woman is found to be group B, Rh-negative and the serum contains anti-D with a titer of 512. What would be the most appropriate type of blood to have available for a possible exchange transfusion for her infant?

    a.  O, Rh-negative
    b.  O, Rh-positive
    c.  B, Rh-negative
    d.  B, Rh-positive


131. A patient who is group AB, Rh-negative needs two units of Fresh Frozen Plasma. Which of the following units of plasma would be MOST acceptable for transfusion?

    a.  group O, Rh-negative
    b.  group A, Rh-negative
    c.  group B, Rh-positive
    d.  group AB, Rh-positive


132. Washed Red Blood Cells would be the product of choice for a patient with:

    a.  multiple red cell alloantibodies
    b.  an increased risk of hepatitis infection
    c.  warm autoimmune hemolytic anemia
    d.  anti-IgA antibodies


133. When evaluating a suspected transfusion reaction, which of the following is the ideal sample collection time for a bilirubin determination?

    a.  6 hours posttransfusion
    b.  12 hours posttransfusion
    c.  24 hours posttransfusion
    d.  48 hours posttransfusion

134. The test for weak D is performed by incubating a patient's red cells with:

   a. several different dilutions of anti-D serum
   b. anti-D serum followed by washing and antiglobulin serum
   c. anti-D$^u$ serum
   d. antiglobulin serum

135. Refer to the following data:

|        | Rh Genotype |
|--------|-------------|
| Mother | cde/cde     |
| Father | CDe/cde     |

   These parents would most likely have a child with the genotype:

   a. $R_1R_1$
   b. $R_0r$
   c. $r'r$
   d. $rr$

136. A 35-year-old man with von Willebrand's disease has an acute nosebleed and a hemoglobin level of 9.9 gm/dL. From the following list, select the blood component that is the MOST appropriate choice for transfusion to this patient.

   a. Platelets
   b. Fresh Frozen Plasma
   c. Cryoprecipitated AHF
   d. Red Blood Cells

137. A patient's red cells are typed as follows:

| Anti-D | 4+ |
|--------|----|
| Anti-C | 0  |
| Anti-E | 0  |

   Which of the following genotypes would correspond to these results?

   a. $R_0R_0$
   b. $R_1r$
   c. $R_1R_2$
   d. $R_2r$

138. Whole Blood for exchange transfusion of a newborn with hemolytic disease due to ABO incompatibility should be:

    a. group O with no hemolytic anti-A or anti-B
    b. same ABO group as the mother
    c. same ABO group as the baby
    d. group AB with no detectable antibodies


139. Four units of blood are needed for elective surgery. The patient's serum contains anti-C, anti-e, anti-Fy$^a$, and anti-Jk$^b$. Which of the following would be the best source of donor blood?

    a. autologous donations
    b. test 100 group O, Rh-negative donors
    c. test 100 group-compatible donors
    d. rare donor file


140. Refer to the following diagram:

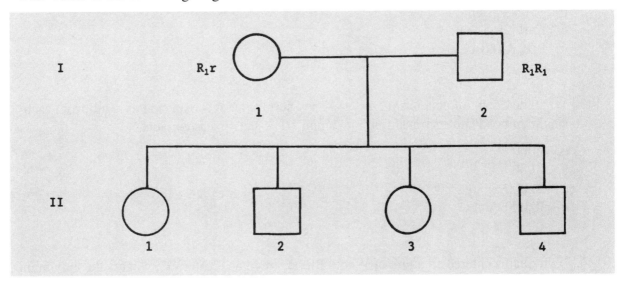

    Given the most probable genotypes of the parents, which of the following statements best describes the most probable Rh genotypes of the four children?

    a. two are $R_1r$, two are $R_1R_1$
    b. three are $R_1r$, one is $rr$
    c. one ir $R_0r$, one is $R_1r$, two are $R_1R_1$
    d. one is $R_0r'$, one is $R_1R_1$, two are $R_1r$


141. Which unit should be selected for exchange transfusion if the newborn is group A, Rh-positive and the mother is group A, Rh-positive with anti-c?

    a. A, CDe/CDe
    b. A, cDE/cDE
    c. O, cde/cde
    d. A, cde/cde

142. Polyspecific reagents used in the direct antiglobulin test should have specificity for:

   a. IgG and IgA
   b. IgG and C3d
   c. IgM and IgA
   d. IgM and C3d


143. In the direct antiglobulin test, the antiglobulin reagent is used to:

   a. mediate hemolysis of indicator Red Blood Cells by providing complement
   b. precipitate antierythrocyte antibodies
   c. measure antibodies in a test serum by fixing complement
   d. detect preexisting antibodies on erythrocytes


144. Human blood groups were discovered around 1900 by:

   a. Jules Bordet
   b. Louis Pasteur
   c. Karl Landsteiner
   d. P. L. Mollison


145. What increment of platelets/μL, per m² body surface area, is expected to result from each single unit of Platelets transfused into a non-HLA-sensitized recipient?

   a. 3,000
   b. 10,000
   c. 20,000
   d. 30,000


146. If the seal is entered on a unit of Whole Blood stored at 1°C to 6°C, what is the maximum allowable storage period, in hours?

   a. 6
   b. 24
   c. 48
   d. 72


147. A Whole Blood unit from a donor that contains a clinically significant red cell alloantibody should be:

   a. discarded
   b. adsorbed with antigen-positive red cells before issue
   c. processed into components containing minimal plasma
   d. labeled with the antibody specificity

148. Which of the following Rh antigens has the highest frequency in Caucasians?

   a. D
   b. E
   c. c
   d. e


149. Which of the following blood group systems is most commonly associated with delayed hemolytic transfusion reactions?

   a. Lewis
   b. Kidd
   c. MNS
   d. I


150. Which of the following immunoglobulins is present in the highest concentration in normal human serum?

   a. IgM
   b. IgG
   c. IgA
   d. IgE


151. A mother is group A, with anti-D in her serum. What is the preferred blood product if an intrauterine transfusion is indicated?

   a. O, Rh-negative Red Blood Cells
   b. O, Rh-negative Red Blood Cells, irradiated
   c. A, Rh-negative Red Blood Cells
   d. A, Rh-negative Red Blood Cells, irradiated


152. The most appropriate laboratory test for early detection of acute hemolysis is:

   a. a visual inspection for free plasma hemoglobin
   b. plasma haptoglobin concentration
   c. examination for hematuria
   d. serum bilirubin concentration


153. Even in the absence of prior transfusion or pregnancy, individuals with the Bombay phenotype ($O_h$) will always have naturally occurring:

   a. anti-Rh
   b. anti-$K_o$
   c. anti-U
   d. anti-H

154. HLA antibodies are:

    a. naturally occurring
    b. induced by multiple transfusions
    c. directed against granulocyte antigens only
    d. frequently cause hemolytic transfusion reactions


155. Genes of the major histocompatibility complex (MHC):

    a. code for HLA-A, HLA-B, and HLA-C antigens only
    b. are linked to genes in the ABO system
    c. are the primary genetic sex determinants
    d. contribute to the coordination of cellular and humoral immunity


156. During storage, the concentration of 2,3-diphosphoglycerate (2,3-DPG) decreases in a unit of:

    a. Platelets
    b. Fresh Frozen Plasma
    c. Red Blood Cells
    d. Cryoprecipitated AHF


157. Which of the following antigens is MOST likely to be involved in hemolytic disease of the newborn?

    a. $Le^a$
    b. $P_1$
    c. M
    d. Kell


158. Fresh Frozen Plasma:

    a. contains all labile coagulative factors except Cryoprecipitated AHF
    b. has a higher risk of transmitting hepatitis than does Whole Blood
    c. should be transfused within 24 hours of thawing
    d. need not be ABO-compatible


159. Cryoprecipitated AHF:

    a. is indicated for fibrinogen deficiencies
    b. should be stored at 4°C prior to administration
    c. will not transmit hepatitis B virus
    d. is indicated for the treatment of hemophilia B

160. An important determinant of platelet viability following storage is:

   a. plasma potassium concentration
   b. plasma pH
   c. prothrombin time
   d. activated partial thromboplastin time


161. According to AABB standards, Platelets must be:

   a. gently agitated if stored at room temperature
   b. separated within 12 hours of Whole Blood collection
   c. suspended in sufficient plasma to maintain a pH of 5.0 or lower
   d. prepared only from Whole Blood units that have been stored at 4°C for 6 hours


162. Platelet transfusions are of most value in treating:

   a. hemolytic transfusion reaction
   b. posttransfusion purpura
   c. functional platelet abnormalities
   d. immune thrombocytopenic purpura


163. An unexplained fall in hemoglobin and mild jaundice in a patient transfused with Red Blood Cells 1 week ago would most likely indicate:

   a. paroxysmal nocturnal hemoglobinuria
   b. posttransfusion hepatitis infection
   c. presence of HLA antibodies
   d. delayed hemolytic transfusion reaction


164. Fresh Frozen Plasma from a group A, Rh-positive donor may be safely transfused to a patient who is group:

   a. A, Rh-negative
   b. B, Rh-negative
   c. AB, Rh-positive
   d. AB, Rh-negative


165. The drug cephalosporin can cause a positive direct antiglobulin test by which of the following mechanisms?

   a. immune-complex formation
   b. complement fixation
   c. autoantibody production
   d. membrane modification

166. Which of the following would most likely be responsible for an incompatible major cross-match?

    a.  recipient's red cells possess a low-frequency antigen
    b.  anti-K (Kell) antibody in donor serum
    c.  recipient's red cells are polyagglutinable
    d.  donor red cells have a positive direct antiglobulin test

167. Rh immune globulin administration would NOT be indicated in an Rh-negative woman who has a(n):

    a.  first trimester abortion
    b.  husband who is Rh-positive
    c.  anti-D titer of 1:4096
    d.  positive direct Coombs' test

168. A fetomaternal hemorrhage of 35 mL of fetal Rh-positive packed RBCs has been detected in an Rh-negative woman. How many vials of Rh immune globulin should be given?

    a.  0
    b.  1
    c.  2
    d.  3

169. What information is essential on the label of recipient blood samples drawn for compatibility testing?

    a.  biohazard sticker for AIDS patients
    b.  patient's room number
    c.  patient's hospital identification number
    d.  patient's date of birth

170. Which of the following red cell antigens are found on glycophorin-A?

    a.  M, N
    b.  $Le^a$, $Le^b$
    c.  S, s
    d.  P, $P_1$, $P^k$

171. Current testing on all donor blood must include:

    a.  complete Rh phenotyping
    b.  indirect antiglobulin test
    c.  direct antiglobulin test
    d.  serological test for syphilis

172. Irradiation of a unit of Red Blood Cells is done to prevent the replication of donor:

    a. granulocytes
    b. lymphocytes
    c. red cells
    d. Platelets


173. AHG (Coombs) control cells:

    a. can be used as a positive control for anti-C3 reagents
    b. can be used only for the indirect Coombs' test
    c. are coated only with IgG antibody
    d. must be used to confirm all positive Coombs' reactions


174. During the issue of an autologous unit of Whole Blood, the supernatant plasma is observed to be dark red in color. What would be the best course of action?

    a. The unit may be issued only for autologous use.
    b. Remove the plasma and issue the unit as red blood cells.
    c. Issue the unit only as washed red blood cells.
    d. Quarantine the unit until further testing determines disposition.


175. An Rh-positive patient's serum is known to contain anti-LW. Red Blood Cells selected for crossmatch should be from which of the following genotypes?

    a. $R_1R_1$
    b. $R_2R_2$
    c. $R_0R_0$
    d. $rr$


176. A first-time blood donor is noticed to experience rapid breathing and involuntary twitching of his fingers shortly after starting phlebotomy. The phlebotomist should:

    a. raise his feet above his head
    b. administer oxygen
    c. have him rebreathe air from a paper bag
    d. have him inhale from an ammonia capsule


177. The most important step in the safe administration of blood is to:

    a. perform compatibility testing accurately
    b. get an accurate patient history
    c. exclude disqualified donors
    d. accurately identify the donor unit and intended recipient

178. What is the most probable racial origin of this donor with the following typing results?

Le(a–b–); Fy(a–b–); Js(a+b+)

   a. Black
   b. Oriental
   c. American Indian
   d. Caucasian


179. The Kell (K1) antigen is:

   a. absent from the red cells of neonates
   b. strongly immunogenic
   c. destroyed by enzymes
   d. has a frequency of 50% in the random population


180. The antibody in the Lutheran system that is best detected at lower temperatures is:

   a. anti-Lu$^a$
   b. anti-Lu$^b$
   c. anti-Lu$^3$
   d. anti-Lu


181. Which of the following HTLA antibodies is considered to be most clinically significant?

   a. anti-Yt$^a$
   b. anti-Ch
   c. anti-Yk
   d. anti-Cs


182. A donor is tested with Rh antisera, with the following results:

| | |
|---|---|
| Anti-D | + |
| Anti-C | + |
| Anti-E | 0 |
| Anti-c | + |
| Anti-e | + |
| Rh control | 0 |

What is his most probable Rh genotype?

   a. $R_1R_1$
   b. $R_1r$
   c. $R_0r$
   d. $R_2r$

183. While performing an antibody screen, a test reaction is observed that is suspected to be rouleaux. A saline replacement test is done and the reaction remains. What is the best interpretation?

    a. The original reaction was rouleaux and may be ignored.
    b. The replacement test is invalid and should be repeated.
    c. The original reaction was due to true agglutination.
    d. The antibody screen is negative.

184. Which of the following is a characteristic of anti-i?

    a. often associated with hemolytic disease of the newborn
    b. frequently a cold agglutinin
    c. reacts best at 37°C
    d. is usually IgG

185. The test currently used to detect donors who are infected with the AIDS virus is:

    a. anti-HBc
    b. anti-HIV 1,2
    c. HBsAg
    d. ALT

186. What is/are the minimum pretransfusion testing requirement(s) for autologous donations collected and transfused by the same facility?

    a. ABO and Rh typing only
    b. ABO/Rh type, antibody screen
    c. ABO/Rh type, antibody screen, crossmatch
    d. no pretransfusion testing is required for autologous donations

187. For plateletpheresis donors, the pretransfusion platelet count must be at least:

    a. $150 \times 10^3/\mu L$
    b. $200 \times 10^3/\mu L$
    c. $250 \times 10^3/\mu L$
    d. $300 \times 10^3/\mu L$

188. A patient admitted to the trauma unit requires emergency release of Fresh Frozen Plasma (FFP). His blood donor card states that he is group AB, Rh-positive. Which of the following blood groups of FFP should be issued?

    a. A
    b. B
    c. AB
    d. O

189. Refer to the following data:

| Hemoglobin | 7.4 g/dL |
|---|---|
| Reticulocyte count | 22% |

| Direct Antiglobulin Test | Antibody Screen—IAT |
|---|---|
| Polyspecific = 3+ | SC I = 3+ |
| IgG = 3+ | SC II = 3+ |
| C3 = 0 | Auto = 3+ |

Which clinical condition is consistent with the lab results shown above?

a. cold hemagglutinin disease
b. warm autoimmune hemolytic anemia
c. penicillin-induced hemolytic anemia
d. delayed hemolytic transfusion reaction

190. The mechanism that best explains hemolytic anemia due to penicillin is:

a. drug adsorption
b. membrane modification
c. immune complex formation
d. autoantibody production

191. Laboratory studies of maternal and cord blood yield the following results:

| Maternal Blood | Cord Blood |
|---|---|
| O, Rh-negative | B, Rh-positive |
| Anti-E in serum | DAT = 2+ |
| Anti-E in eluate | |

If exchange transfusion is necessary, the best choice of blood is:

a. B, Rh-negative, E positive
b. B, Rh-positive, E positive
c. O, Rh-negative, E negative
d. O, Rh-positive, E negative

192. The blood sample of choice for the pretransfusion testing of neonates with HDN is:

a. maternal serum
b. maternal eluate
c. cord blood serum
d. cord blood eluate

193. What is the most likely cause of the following ABO discrepancy?

| Patient's cells vs | Patient's serum vs |
|---|---|
| Anti-A = 0 | $A_1$ cells = 0 |
| Anti-B = 0 | B cells = 0 |

   a. recent transfusion with group O blood
   b. antigen depression due to leukemia
   c. false-negative cell typing due to rouleaux
   d. hypogammaglobulinemia due to advanced patient age

194. A patient is typed as group O, Rh-positive and crossmatched with 6 units of blood. At the indirect antiglobulin (IAT) phase of testing, both antibody screening cells and two cross-matched units are incompatible. What is the most likely cause of the incompatibility?

   a. recipient alloantibody
   b. recipient autoantibody
   c. donors have positive DATs
   d. rouleaux

195. Consider the following ABO typing results:

| Patient's cells vs | Patient's serum vs |
|---|---|
| Anti-A = 4+ | $A_1$ cells = 1+ |
| Anti-B = 0 | B cells = 4+ |

Additional testing was performed using patient serum:

| | IS | RT |
|---|---|---|
| Screening cell I | 1+ | 2+ |
| Screening cell II | 1+ | 2+ |
| Autocontrol | 1+ | 2+ |

What should be done next?

   a. antibody identification
   b. neutralization
   c. cold autoadsorption
   d. elution

196. For which of the following transfusion candidates would CMV-seronegative blood be MOST likely indicated?

    a. renal dialysis patients
    b. pregnant women
    c. transplant candidates
    d. CMV-seropositive patients


197. Posttransfusion purpura is caused by:

    a. anti-A
    b. white cell antibodies
    c. anti-P1$^{A1}$
    d. platelet washout


198. Posttransfusion anaphylactic reactions occur most often in patients with:

    a. leukocyte antibodies
    b. erythrocyte antibodies
    c. IgA deficiency
    d. Factor VIII deficiency


199. The antibodies of the Kidd blood group system:

    a. react best by the indirect antiglobulin test
    b. are predominantly IgM
    c. often cause allergic transfusion reactions
    d. do not generally react with antigen-positive, enzyme-treated RBCs


200. Which of the following prospective donors would be accepted for donation?

    a. 32-year-old woman who received a transfusion in a complicated delivery 5 months ago
    b. 19-year-old sailor who has been stateside for 1 year and stopped taking his antimalarial medication 1 year ago
    c. 22-year-old college student who has a temperature of 99.2°F and states that he feels well but is nervous about donating
    d. 45-year-old woman who has just recovered from a bladder infection and is still taking antibiotics


201. Transfusion of plateletpheresis products from HLA-compatible donors is the preferred treatment for:

    a. recently diagnosed cases of TTP with severe thrombocytopenia
    b. acute leukemia in relapse with neutropenia, thrombocytopenia and sepsis
    c. immune thrombocytopenic purpura
    d. severely thrombocytopenic patients, known to be refractory to random donor platelets

202. Why are donors deferred for 6 months following receipt of blood products?

    a. to permit adequate screening for transfusion-acquired viral infections
    b. donation may cause recurrence of the condition that required transfusion
    c. to allow clearance of all transfused cells in the donor
    d. to allow donor recovery from the condition that required transfusion

203. A 37-year-old female with systemic lupus erythematosus (SLE) is admitted with anemia. Blood samples are received with a crossmatch request for 4 units of Red Blood Cells. The patient is group B, Rh-negative. The following results were obtained in pretransfusion testing:

| | IS | 37°C | IAT |
|---|---|---|---|
| Screening cell I | 0 | 0 | 3+ |
| Screening cell II | 0 | 0 | 3+ |
| Autocontrol | 0 | 0 | 3+ |

The most probable cause of these results is:

    a. rouleaux
    b. a warm autoantibody
    c. a cold autoantibody
    d. multiple alloantibodies

204. A 42-year-old female is undergoing surgery tomorrow and her physician requests that 4 units of Red Blood Cells be crossmatched. The following results were obtained:

| | IS | 37°C | IAT |
|---|---|---|---|
| Screening cell I | 0 | 0 | 0 |
| Screening cell II | 0 | 0 | 0 |
| Autocontrol | 0 | 0 | 0 |
| Crossmatch | | | |
|   Donor 1 | 4+ | 1+ | +/- |
|   Donors 2, 3, 4 | 0 | 0 | 0 |

What is the most likely cause of the incompatibility of donor 1?

    a. single alloantibody
    b. multiple alloantibodies
    c. Rh incompatibilities
    d. donor 1 has a positive DAT

205. Examine the following results of ABO typing tests and state the most probable cause of the discrepancy.

| Patient's cells vs | Patient's serum vs |
|---|---|
| Anti-A = 0 | $A_1$ cells = 2+ |
| Anti-B = 0 | B cells = 4+ |
| Anti-A,B = +/− | O cells = 0 |

    a. acquired B antigen
    b. the patient is a newborn
    c. chimerism
    d. weak subgroup of A with anti-$A_1$

206. A 14-year-old male trauma victim is in need of three units of Red Blood Cells. The following results were obtained during pretransfusion testing:

| | IS | 37°C | IAT |
|---|---|---|---|
| Screening cell I | 0 | 0 | 0 |
| Screening cell II | 0 | 0 | 0 |
| Autocontrol | 0 | 0 | 0 |
| Crossmatch | | | |
|     Donor 1 | 0 | 0 | 0 |
|     Donor 2 | 0 | 0 | ± |
|     Donor 3 | 0 | 0 | 0 |

What is the FIRST step in resolving this problem?

    a. perform an enzyme panel on the patient's serum
    b. choose more donors to crossmatch
    c. repeat the crossmatch
    d. perform a DAT on donor 2

207. The Western Blot is a confirmatory test for the presence of:

    a. CMV antibody
    b. anti-HIV-1
    c. HBsAg
    d. serum protein abnormalities

208. A commonly used screening method for anti-HIV-1 detection is:

    a. latex agglutination
    b. radioimmunoassay (RIA)
    c. thin-layer chromatography (TLC)
    d. enzyme-linked immunosorbent assay (ELISA)

209. Which of the following red cell typings would most commonly be found in the black donor population?

a. Lu(a–b–)
b. Jk(a–b–)
c. Fy(a–b–)
d. K–k–

210. An individual's Red Blood Cells give the following reactions with Rh antisera:

| Antisera | Reaction |
|----------|----------|
| Anti-D | 4+ |
| Anti-C | 3+ |
| Anti-E | 0 |
| Anti-c | 3+ |
| Anti-e | 3+ |
| Rh-control | 0 |

The most probable genotype of this individual is:

a. CDe/cDE
b. cDE/cde
c. cDe/cde
d. CDe/cde

211. A patient is typed with the following results:

| Patient's cells with | Patient's serum with |
|----------------------|----------------------|
| Anti-A = 0 | $A_1$ red cells = 2+ |
| Anti-B = 0 | B red cells = 4+ |
| Anti-A,B = 2+ | Antibody screening = negative |

The most probable reason for these findings is that the patient is group:

a. O—confusion due to faulty group O antiserum
b. O—with an anti-$A_1$ antibody
c. $A_x$—with an anti-$A_1$ antibody
d. $A_1$—with an anti-A antibody

212. The primary indication for granulocyte transfusion is:

a. prophylactic treatment for infection
b. additional supportive therapy in those patients who are responsive to antibiotic therapy
c. clinical situations where bone marrow recovery is not anticipated
d. severe neutropenia with an infection nonresponsive to antibiotic therapy

213. A patient in the immediate post–bone marrow transplant period has a hematocrit of 21%. The red cell product of choice for this patient would be:

a. packed
b. saline washed
c. microaggregated filtered
d. irradiated

214. A sample gives the following results:

| Cells with | Serum with |
|---|---|
| Anti-A = 3+ | $A_1$ cells = 4+ |
| Anti-B = 4+ | B cells = negative |

Which lectin should be used first to resolve this discrepancy?

a. *Ulex europaeus*
b. *Arachis hypogaea*
c. *Dolichos biflorus*
d. *Vicia graminea*

215. A man suffering from gastrointestinal bleeding has received 20 units of Red Blood Cells in the past 24 hours and is still oozing postoperatively. The following results were obtained:

| | |
|---|---|
| PT | 20 seconds (control, 12 seconds) |
| APTT | 43 seconds (control, 31 seconds) |
| Platelet count | 160 x $10^3$/μL |
| Hgb | 10 g/dL |
| Factor VIII | 85% |

What blood product should be administered?

a. Fresh Frozen Plasma
b. Red Blood Cells
c. Factor VIII concentrate
d. Platelets

216. Anti-I usually results in a positive direct antiglobulin test (DAT) because of:

a. anti-I agglutinating the cells
b. C3d bound to the red cells
c. T-activation
d. C3c remaining on the red cells after cleavage of C3b

217. B lymphocytes are associated with:

 a. graft rejection
 b. macrophage stimulation
 c. delayed hypersensitivity reaction
 d. synthesis of antibody

218. Plastic bag overwraps are recommended when thawing units of FFP in 37°C water baths because they prevent:

 a. the FFP bag from cracking when it contacts the warm water
 b. water from slowly traveling across the bag membrane (dialysis)
 c. the entry ports from becoming contaminated with water
 d. the label from peeling off as the water circulates in the bath

219. A unit of Red Blood Cells expiring in 35 days is split into five small aliquots using a sterile pediatric quad set and a sterile connecting device. Each aliquot must be labeled as expiring in:

 a. 6 hours
 b. 12 hours
 c. 5 days
 d. 35 days

220. Refer to the following information:

| Postpartum | D | Rh Control | $D^u$ | $D^u$ Control | Rosette Fetal Screen |
|---|---|---|---|---|---|
| Mother | neg | neg | +micro | neg | 20 rosettes/5 fields |
| Newborn | 4+ | neg | NT | NT | NT |

NT = not tested

What is the best interpretation for the laboratory data given above?

 a. mother is Rh-positive
 b. mother is $D^u$ variant
 c. mother has had a fetal-maternal hemorrhage
 d. mother has a positive DAT

221. A woman who was requested to be a directed donor had a mastectomy with radiotherapy for breast carcinoma 5 years ago. Currently, she is well and has a hemoglobin of 14 g/dL and a hematocrit of 41%. The blood bank should:

 a. accept the unit of blood for directed donation
 b. accept the unit of blood for general use
 c. accept the donor for only washed RBCs
 d. defer the donor permanently

222. A cause for permanent deferral of blood donation is:

    a. diabetes
    b. residence in an endemic malaria region
    c. history of jaundice of uncertain cause
    d. history of therapeutic rabies vaccine


223. The following reactions were obtained:

| Cells tested with | Serum tested with |
|---|---|
| Anti-A = 4+ | A₁ cells = 2+ |
| Anti-B = 3+ | B cells = 4+ |
| Anti-A,B = 4+ | |

Then the technologist washed the patient's cells with saline, and added two drops of saline to the reverse grouping. Upon repeat testing, the following results were obtained:

| Cells tested with | Serum tested with |
|---|---|
| Anti-A = 4+ | A₁ cells = 0 |
| Anti-B = 0 | B cells = 4+ |
| Anti-A,B = 4+ | |

The results are consistent with:

    a. acquired immunodeficiency disease
    b. Bruton's agammaglobulinemia
    c. multiple myeloma
    d. acquired "B" antigen


224. Upon inspection, a unit of Platelets is noted to have visible clots, but otherwise appears normal. The technologist should:

    a. issue without concern
    b. filter to remove the clots
    c. centrifuge to express off the clots
    d. quarantine for Gram stain and culture


225. Which plateletpheresis product should be irradiated?

    a. autologous unit collected prior to surgery
    b. random stock unit going to a patient with DIC
    c. a directed donation given by a mother for her son
    d. a directed donation given by an unrelated family friend

226. The following test results are noted for a unit of blood labeled group A, Rh-negative:

Cells plus

| | |
|---|---|
| Anti-A | 4+ |
| Anti-B | 0 |
| Anti-D | 3+ |
| Rh control | 0 |

What should be done next?

a. transfuse as a group A, Rh-negative
b. transfuse as a group A, Rh-positive
c. notify the collecting facility
d. discard the unit

227. A technologist typed 10 units for c antigen. All 10 units test c-negative after a 37°C incubation. The technologist should:

a. record the units as c-negative
b. wash the antigen typings and add AHG
c. recheck the antisera with positive and negative controls
d. titrate the antisera to check its avidity

228. Leukocyte-reduced Red Blood Cells are ordered for a newly diagnosed bone marrow candidate. What is the best way to prepare this product?

a. crossmatch only CMV seronegative units
b. irradiate the unit with 1500 rads
c. wash the unit with saline prior to infusion
d. transfuse through a 3 Log leukocyte-removing filter

229. When Platelets are stored on a rotator set on an open bench top, the ambient air temperature must be recorded:

a. once a day
b. twice a day
c. every 4 hours
d. every hour

230. Which of the following tests is most commonly used to demonstrate antibodies that have become attached to a patient's red cells in vivo?

a. direct antiglobulin
b. complement fixation
c. indirect antiglobulin
d. immunofluorescence

231. Some blood group antibodies characteristically hemolyze appropriate red cells in the presence of:

   a. complement
   b. anticoagulants
   c. preservatives
   d. penicillin

232. The minimum hemoglobin concentration in g/dL in a fingerstick from a male blood donor is:

   a. 12.0
   b. 12.5
   c. 13.5
   d. 15.0

233. The purpose of testing with anti-A,B is to detect:

   a. anti-A$_1$
   b. anti-A$_2$
   c. subgroups of A
   d. subgroups of B

234. A mother is Rh-negative and the father Rh-positive. Their baby is Rh-negative. It may be concluded that:

   a. the father is homozygous Rh-positive
   b. the mother is heterozygous Rh-negative
   c. the father is heterozygous Rh-positive
   d. at least one of the three Rh typings must be erroneous

235. In performing an antibody screening test and/or compatibility test, the use of a patient's specimen collected in an EDTA tube will:

   a. prevent the detection of all clinically significant antibodies
   b. require the use of LISS
   c. require an extended incubation time period
   d. prevent the detection of complement-dependent antibodies

236. Which of the following represents an acceptably identified patient for sample collection and transfusion?

   a. A handwritten band with patient's name and hospital identification number is affixed to the patient's leg.
   b. The addressographed hospital band is taped to the patient's bed.
   c. An unbanded patient responds positively when his name is called.
   d. The chart transported with the patient contains his armband not yet attached.

237. Rh-immune globulin is requested for an Rh-negative mother who has the following results:

| | D | D Control | $D^u$ | $D^u$ Control |
|---|---|---|---|---|
| Mother's postpartum sample | 0 | 0 | $1+^{mf}$ | 0 |

mf = mixed field

What is the most likely explanation?

a. Mother is a genetic weak D.
b. Mother had a fetomaternal hemorrhage of D+ cells.
c. Mother's red cells are coated weakly with IgG.
d. Anti-D reagent is contaminated with an atypical antibody.


238. Samples from the same patient were received on 2 consecutive days. Test results are summarized below:

| | Day 1 | Day 2 |
|---|---|---|
| Anti-A | 4+ | 0 |
| Anti-B | 0 | 4+ |
| Anti-D | 3+ | 3+ |
| Rh control | 0 | 0 |
| $A_1$ cells | 0 | 4+ |
| B cells | 4+ | 0 |
| Antibody screen | Negative | Negative |

How should the request for crossmatch be handled?

a. crossmatch A, Rh-positive units with sample from day 1
b. crossmatch B, Rh-positive units with sample from day 2
c. crossmatch AB, Rh-positive units with both samples
d. collect a new sample and repeat the tests


239. The following results are seen on a maternal postpartum sample:

| | Rh | Rh Control | $D^u$ | $D^u$ Control |
|---|---|---|---|---|
| Mother's cells | 0 | 0 | + (mixed field) | 0 |

The most appropriate course of action is to:

a. report as Rh-negative
b. report as $D^u$-positive
c. perform an elution
d. investigate for a fetomaternal hemorrhage

240. The following test results were obtained on a patient sample. The anti-D used was a chemically modified reagent.

Anti-A         4+
Anti-B         Negative
Anti-D         4+
A$_1$ cells    Negative
B cells        4+

The best interpretation is that:

a. the sample is Rh-positive
b. the sample is Rh-negative
c. the Rh result is invalid
d. a high-protein Rh control must be run

241. Review the following schematic diagram:

Patient Serum + Reagent Group "O" Cells
Incubate → Read for Agglutination
Wash → Add AHG → Agglutination Observed

The next step would be to:

a. add "check cells" as a confirmatory measure
b. identify the cause of the agglutination
c. perform an elution technique
d. perform a direct antiglobulin test

242. The most common cause of posttransfusion hepatitis can be detected in donors by testing for:

a. anti-HCV
b. HB$_s$Ag
c. anti-HAV IgM
d. anti-HB$_e$

243. A unit of packed cells is split into two aliquots under closed sterile conditions at 8 AM. The expiration time for each aliquot is now:

a. 4 PM on the same day
b. 8 PM on the same day
c. 8 AM the next morning
d. the original date of the unsplit unit

244. A group B, Rh-negative patient has a positive DAT. Which of the following situations would occur?

  a. all major crossmatches would be incompatible
  b. the D$^u$ test and control would be positive
  c. the antibody screening test would be positive
  d. the forward and reverse ABO groupings would not agree


245. Which blood component is most effective in treating a patient with von Willebrand's disease?

  a. Platelets
  b. Stored Plasma
  c. Cryoprecipitated AHF
  d. Whole Blood


246. A group B, Rh-negative patient in shock from acute blood loss would benefit most from a transfusion of:

  a. group O, Rh-positive Red Blood Cells
  b. group B, Rh-negative FFP
  c. group B, Rh-positive Red Blood Cells
  d. group B, Rh-negative Whole Blood


247. To qualify as a donor for autologous transfusion, a patient's hemoglobin should be at least:

  a. 8 g/dL
  b. 11 g/dL
  c. 13 g/dL
  d. 15 g/dL


248. After checking the inventory, it was noted that there were no units on the shelf marked "May Issue as Uncrossmatched: For Emergency Only." Which of the following should the technician now place on this shelf?

  a. one unit of each of the ABO blood groups
  b. units of group O, Rh-positive Whole Blood
  c. units of group O, Rh-negative Red Blood Cells
  d. any units expiring at midnight

*The remaining questions (\*) have been identified as more appropriate for the entry level medical technologist.*

*249. Hydroxyethyl starch (HES) is a rouleaux-promoting agent used to:

    a. increase the harvest of granulocytes in leukapheresis
    b. treat patients following hemolytic transfusion reaction
    c. resolve ABO typing discrepancies
    d. stabilize the pH of stored Platelets

Questions 250-251 refer to the following panel:

| Cell | D | C | E | c | e | M | N | S | s | $Le^a$ | $Le^b$ | $P_1$ | K | k | $Fy^a$ | $Fy^b$ | $Jk^a$ | $Jk^b$ | IS | 37 C | AHG |
|---|---|---|---|---|---|---|---|---|---|---|---|---|---|---|---|---|---|---|---|---|---|
| 1 | 0 | + | 0 | + | + | + | 0 | 0 | + | 0 | + | 0 | 0 | + | 0 | + | 0 | + | 0 | 0 | 0 |
| 2 | + | + | 0 | 0 | + | 0 | + | 0 | + | + | 0 | + | 0 | + | + | 0 | 0 | + | 0 | 0 | 2+ |
| 3 | + | + | 0 | 0 | + | + | + | + | + | 0 | + | + | + | 0 | + | + | + | + | 0 | 0 | 3+ |
| 4 | + | + | + | + | 0 | 0 | + | + | 0 | 0 | + | + | 0 | + | 0 | + | 0 | + | 0 | 1+ | 4+ |
| 5 | 0 | 0 | + | + | + | 0 | + | 0 | + | 0 | + | + | 0 | + | + | + | + | + | 0 | 1+ | 4+ |
| 6 | 0 | 0 | 0 | + | + | + | 0 | 0 | + | 0 | 0 | + | 0 | + | 0 | 0 | + | 0 | 0 | 0 | 0 |
| 7 | 0 | 0 | 0 | + | + | 0 | + | 0 | + | 0 | + | + | + | + | 0 | + | 0 | + | 0 | 0 | 2+ |
| 8 | 0 | 0 | 0 | + | + | + | 0 | + | 0 | + | 0 | + | 0 | + | 0 | + | + | 0 | 0 | 0 | 0 |
| 9 | 0 | 0 | 0 | + | + | + | 0 | + | 0 | 0 | + | + | + | + | + | 0 | + | + | 0 | 0 | 3+ |
| 10 | + | + | + | 0 | + | + | 0 | + | 0 | + | 0 | 0 | 0 | + | + | 0 | + | 0 | 0 | 1+ | 4+ |
| Autocontrol | | | | | | | | | | | | | | | | | | | 0 | 0 | 0 |

*250. Based on the results of the above panel, the most likely antibodies are:

    a. anti-M and anti-K
    b. anti-E, anti-$Fy^a$, and anti-K
    c. anti-$Fy^a$ and anti-M
    d. anti-E and anti-$Le^b$

*251. Based on the results of the above panel, which technique would be most helpful in determining antibody specificity?

    a. proteolytic enzyme treatment
    b. urine neutralization
    c. autoadsorption
    d. saliva inhibition

*252. Which of the following medications is most likely to cause production of autoantibodies?

    a. penicillin
    b. cephalothin
    c. methyldopa
    d. tetracycline

*253. Which of the following is the best source of HLA-compatible leukocytes or Platelets?

    a. mother
    b. father
    c. siblings
    d. cousins

*254. Leukocyte-poor Red Blood Cells would most likely be indicated for patients with a history of:

    a. febrile transfusion reaction
    b. iron deficiency anemia
    c. hemophilia A
    d. von Willebrand's disease

*255. A patient has become refractory to platelet transfusion. Which of the following are probable causes?

    a. transfusion of Rh-incompatible Platelets
    b. decreased pH of the Platelets
    c. development of an alloantibody with anti-D specificity
    d. development of antibodies to HLA

*256. Which of the following would most likely indicate that a patient's red cells are a subgroup of A?

    a. positive autocontrol
    b. heavy rouleaux in the serum
    c. positive antibody screening test
    d. discrepancy between cell and serum ABO grouping

*257. Transfusion of Ch+ (Chido-positive) red cells to a patient with anti-Ch has been reported to cause:

    a. no clinically significant red cell destruction
    b. clinically significant immune red cell destruction
    c. decreased $^{51}$Cr red cell survivals
    d. febrile transfusion reactions

*258. What happens to an antibody in an in vitro neutralization study when a soluble antigen preparation is added?

    a. inhibition
    b. dilution
    c. complement fixation
    d. hemolysis


*259. Proteolytic enzyme treatment of red cells usually destroys which antigen?

    a. Jk$^a$
    b. E
    c. Fy$^a$
    d. k


*260. Results of a serum sample tested against a panel of reagent red cells gives presumptive evidence of an alloantibody directed against a high incidence antigen. Further investigation to confirm the specificity should include which of the following?

    a. serum testing against red cells from random donors
    b. serum testing against red cells known to lack high incidence antigens
    c. serum testing against enzyme-treated autologous red cells
    d. testing of an eluate prepared from the patient's red cells


*261. A test panel composed of HBsAg, anti-HAV-IgM, and anti-HBc is designed to:

    a. indicate immunity to hepatitis
    b. estimate the degree of infectivity
    c. aid in the diagnosis of past hepatitis infection
    d. aid in the diagnosis of acute viral hepatitis


*262. One of the most useful techniques in the identification and classification of high-titer, low-avidity (HTLA) antibodies is:

    a. reagent red cell panels
    b. adsorption and elution
    c. titration and inhibition
    d. cold autoadsorption


*263. Which of the following measures should be employed if a donor experiences perioral paresthesia during an apheresis procedure?

    a. increase flow rate
    b. reduce flow rate
    c. elevate donor's feet
    d. have donor breathe into a paper bag

*264. What percent of group O donors would be compatible with a serum sample that contained anti-X and anti-Y if X antigen is present on red cells of 5 of 20 donors and Y antigen is present on red cells of 1 of 10 donors?

a. 2.5
b. 6.8
c. 25.0
d. 68.0

*265. The following results were obtained when testing a sample from a 20-year-old, first-time blood donor. What is the most likely cause of this ABO discrepancy?

| Forward Group | Reverse Group |
|---|---|
| Anti-A = 0 | $A_1$ cells = 0 |
| Anti-B = 0 | B cells = 3+ |

a. loss of antigen due to disease
b. acquired B
c. phenotype $O_h$ "Bombay"
d. weak subgroup of A

*266. A patient is group O, Rh-negative with anti-D and anti-K in her serum. What percentage of the general Caucasian donor population would be compatible with this patient?

a. 0.5
b. 2.0
c. 3.0
d. 6.0

*267. Anti-D and anti-C are identified in the serum of a transfused pregnant woman, gravida 1, para 1. Nine months ago she received Rh immune globulin (RhIg) after delivery. Tests of the patient, her husband, and the child revealed the following:

| | Anti-D | Anti-C | Anti-E | Anti-c | Anti-e |
|---|---|---|---|---|---|
| Patient | neg | neg | neg | + | + |
| Father | + | neg | neg | + | + |
| Child | + | neg | neg | + | + |

The most likely explanation for the presence of anti-C is that this antibody is:

a. actually anti-$C^w$
b. from the RhIg dose
c. actually anti-G
d. naturally occurring

*268. Which of the following phenotypes will react with anti-f?

    a.  *rr*
    b.  $R_1R_1$
    c.  $R_2R_2$
    d.  $R_1R_2$

*269. A woman types as Rh-positive. She has an anti-c titer of 32 at AHG. Her baby has a negative DAT and is not affected by hemolytic disease of the newborn. What is the father's most likely Rh phenotype?

    a.  *rr*
    b.  *r"r*
    c.  $R_1r$
    d.  $R_2r$

*270. Which red cell genotype has the least amount of LW antigen?

    a.  CDe/CDe
    b.  Cde/cDE
    c.  cDE/cde
    d.  cde/cde

*271. Plasma exchange is recommended in the treatment of patients with macroglobulinemia in order to remove:

    a.  antigen
    b.  excess IgM
    c.  excess IgG
    d.  abnormal Platelets

*272. Glycophorin B is associated with the antigenic activity of:

    a.  MN
    b.  Ss
    c.  $Wr^aWr^b$
    d.  $Lu^a/Lu^b$

*273. In a prenatal workup, the following results were obtained:

| Forward Group | Reverse Group |
|---|---|
| Anti-A = 4+ | $A_1$ cells = neg |
| Anti-B = 2+ | B cells = 3+ |
| Anti-D = 4+ | |
| Rh control = neg | |
| | |
| DAT: neg | |
| Antibody screen: neg | |

ABO discrepancy was thought to be due to an antibody directed against acriflavine. Which test would resolve this discrepancy?

a. $A_1$ lectin
b. wash patient's RBCs and repeat testing
c. anti-A,B and extend incubation of the reverse group
d. repeat reverse group using $A_2$ cells


*274. Refer to the following data:

| Forward Group | Reverse Group |
|---|---|
| Anti-A = 4+ | $A_1$ cells = neg |
| Anti-B = neg | $A_2$ cells = 2+ |
| Anti-$A_1$ lectin = 4+ | B cells = 4+ |

Which of the following antibody screen results would you expect with the ABO discrepancy seen above?

a. negative
b. positive with all screen cells at the 37°C phase
c. positive with all screen cells at the RT phase; autocontrol is negative
d. positive with all screen cells and the autocontrol cells at the RT phase


*275. To confirm the specificity of anti-$Le^b$, an inhibition study using Lewis substance was performed with the following results:

| | Le(b+) cells |
|---|---|
| Patient serum + Lewis substance | + |
| Patient serum + Saline control | 0 |

What conclusion can be made from these results?

a. Anti-$Le^b$ is confirmed.
b. Anti-$Le^b$ is not confirmed.
c. A second antibody is suspected due to the positive control.
d. Anti-$Le^b$ cannot be confirmed due to the positive control.

*276. Serologic results on an untransfused patient were:

| | |
|---|---|
| Antibody screening | Negative |
| Direct antiglobulin test | 3+ |
| Ether eluate | Negative |

Which drug would most likely be involved?

a. methyldopa
b. aspirin
c. insulin
d. cephalothin

*277. A weakly reactive anti-D is detected in a postpartum serum specimen from an Rh-negative woman. During her prenatal period, all antibody screening tests were negative. These findings indicate:

a. that she is a candidate for Rh immune globulin
b. that she is NOT a candidate for Rh immune globulin
c. a need for further investigation to determine candidacy for Rh immune globulin
d. the presence of Rh-positive cells in her circulation

*278. In the process of identifying an antibody, the technologist observed 2+ reactions with three of the ten cells in a panel after the immediate spin phase. These reactions disappeared following incubation at 37°C and after the anti–human globulin test phase. The antibody most likely is:

a. anti-$P_1$
b. anti-Le$^a$
c. anti-C
d. anti-Fy$^a$

*279. The phenomenon of an Rh-positive person whose serum contains anti-D is best explained by antigen:

a. deletion
b. mosaicism
c. suppression
d. inhibition

*280. Mixed field agglutination is a characteristic observation for which of the following antibodies?

a. anti-K
b. anti-Sd$^a$
c. anti-Js$^a$
d. anti-e

*281. Hemolysis of the red cell occurs when which components of complement are attached?

a. C1
b. C3
c. C4-C2
d. C8-C9


*282. The observed phenotypic frequencies at the Jk locus in a particular population are:

| Phenotype | Number of Persons |
|---|---|
| Jk(a+b–) | 122 |
| Jk(a+b+) | 194 |
| Jk(a–b+) | 84 |

What is the gene frequency of the $Jk^a$ in this population?

a. 0.31
b. 0.45
c. 0.55
d. 0.60


*283. How many Caucasians in a population of 100,000 will have the following combination of phenotypes?

| System | Phenotype | Phenotype Frequency (%) |
|---|---|---|
| ABO | O | 45 |
| Gm | Fb | 48 |
| PGM1 | 2-1 | 37 |
| EsD | 2-1 | 18 |

a. 1
b. 14
c. 144
d. 1438


*284. In a random population, 16% of the people are Rh-negative (*rr*).What percentage of the Rh-positive population would be heterozygous for the D antigen?

a. 36
b. 48
c. 57
d. 66

*285. A patient presented with the following laboratory data:

Decreased levels of Factor VIII antigen
Decreased levels of Factor VIII clotting activity
Prolonged template bleeding time
Impaired aggregation of Platelets in response to ristocetin

What is the treatment of choice for this disease?

a. Platelets
b. lyophilized Factor VIII concentrate
c. Factor IX complex
d. Cryoprecipitated AHF


*286. Which of the following is the first step in hemoglobin clearance from the plasma following an intravascular hemolytic transfusion reaction?

a. reduction in plasma haptoglobin concentration
b. increase in plasma hemoglobin
c. urinary excretion of hemosiderin
d. urinary excretion of hemoglobin


*287. A patient diagnosed as having mild hemophilia A (8% Factor VIII:C) was transfused with Factor VIII concentrates in preparation for abdominal surgery. It was calculated that he would require 1200 units of Factor VIII to raise his plasma concentration to 50%. Following infusion his Factor VIII concentration rose to 65%, and remained at 50% for approximately 30 hours without further infusion. What would be the most likely explanation for this observation?

a. patient really had von Willebrand's disease
b. Factor VIII concentrates had twice the specified Factor VIII concentration
c. patient had an inhibitor to the Factor VIII complex
d. patient had idiopathic thrombocytopenic purpura


*288. Which of the following would be the best source of Platelets for transfusion in the case of alloimmune neonatal thrombocytopenia?

a. father
b. mother
c. pooled platelet-rich plasma
d. polycythemic donor


*289. Which of the following patient groups is at risk for developing graft-versus-host disease?

a. full-term infants
b. patients with history of febrile transfusion reactions
c. patients with a positive direct antiglobulin test
d. recipients of blood donated by immediate family members

*290. Inhibition testing can be used to confirm antibody specificity for which of the following antibodies?

   a. anti-Lu$^a$
   b. anti-M
   c. anti-Le$^a$
   d. anti-Fy$^a$


*291. Anti-N is identified in a patient's serum. If random crossmatches are performed on 10 donor units, how many would be expected to be compatible?

   a. 0
   b. 3
   c. 7
   d. 10


*292. Resistance to malaria is best associated with which of the following blood groups?

   a. Rh
   b. I/i
   c. P
   d. Duffy


*293. Paroxysmal cold hemoglobinuria (PCH) is best associated with which of the following blood groups?

   a. Kell
   b. Duffy
   c. P
   d. I/i


*294. The linked HLA genes on each chromosome constitute a(n):

   a. allele
   b. trait
   c. phenotype
   d. haplotype


*295. The mating of an Xg(a+) man and an Xg(a–) woman will produce ONLY:

   a. Xg(a–) sons and Xg(a–) daughters
   b. Xg(a+) sons and Xg(a+) daughters
   c. Xg(a–) sons and Xg(a+) daughters
   d. Xg(a+) sons and Xg(a–) daughters

*296. When the red cells of an individual fail to react with anti-U, they usually fail to react with:

    a. anti-M
    b. anti-Le$^b$
    c. anti-S
    d. anti-P$_1$

*297. The HLA complex shows strong associations with which blood groups?

    a. MN
    b. Bg
    c. Duffy
    d. Rodgers

*298. Which of the following is a characteristic of anti-i?

    a. is often associated with warm autoimmune hemolytic anemia
    b. can often be found in the serum of patients with infectious mononucleosis
    c. can often be detected at lower temperatures in the serum of normal individuals
    d. is found only in the serum of group O individuals

*299. In which of the following situations would the phthalate ester separation technique be most useful?

    a. positive DAT due to methyldopa
    b. recently transfused patient with multiple alloantibodies
    c. incompatibility due to cold autoantibodies
    d. febrile transfusion reaction caused by leukocyte antibodies

*300. DR antigens in the HLA system are:

    a. significant in organ transplantation
    b. not detectable in the lymphocytotoxicity test
    c. expressed on Platelets
    d. expressed on granulocytes

*301. In paternity testing, a "direct exclusion" is established when a genetic marker is:

    a. absent in the child, but present in the mother and alleged father
    b. absent in the child, present in the mother, and absent in the alleged father
    c. present in the child, absent in the mother, and present in the alleged father
    d. present in the child, but absent in the mother and alleged father

*302. Granulocytes for transfusion should:

    a. be administered through a microaggregate filter
    b. be ABO and Rh compatible with the recipient's serum
    c. be infused within 72 hours of collection
    d. never be transfused to patients with a history of febrile transfusion reactions


*303. A patient has life-threatening anemia due to warm autoantibodies. The patient's serum was reactive 2+ in the antiglobulin phase of testing with all cells on a routine panel. A technique that would be beneficial in preparing the patient's serum for compatibility testing is:

    a. autoadsorption using the patient's ZZAP-treated red cells
    b. autoadsorption using the patient's LISS-treated red cells
    c. adsorption using enzyme-treated red cells from a normal donor
    d. adsorption using methyldopa-treated red cells


*304. HLA typing is important in screening for:

    a. ABO incompatibility
    b. a kidney donor
    c. Rh incompatibility
    d. a blood donor


*305. In a hematologically stable adult with a 1.8 m$^2$ body surface area, one unit of Platelets should increase the platelet count by:

    a. 500-1000/μL
    b. 1500-3000/μL
    c. 5000-10,000/μL
    d. 15,000-20,000/μL


*306. Congestive heart failure, severe headache, and/or peripheral edema occurring soon after transfusion is indicative of which type of transfusion reaction?

    a. hemolytic
    b. febrile
    c. anaphylactic
    d. circulatory overload


*307. A 33-year-old woman is found to have a positive antibody screening test during a prenatal evaluation. Which of the following techniques would be most useful in determining if the antibody involved could cause hemolytic disease of the newborn?

    a. treating the serum with dithiothreitol (DTT)
    b. one-stage papain procedure
    c. two-stage papain procedure
    d. adsorption-elution technique

*308. A specimen of cord blood is submitted to the transfusion service for routine testing. The following results are obtained:

| | |
|---|---|
| Anti-A | 4+ |
| Anti-B | 0 |
| Anti-A,B | 4+ |
| Anti-D | 3+ |
| Rh control | 0 |
| Direct antiglobulin test | 2+ |

It is known that the father is group B, with the genotype of cde/cde. Of the following four antibodies, which one is the most likely cause of the positive direct antiglobulin test?

a. anti-A
b. anti-D
c. anti-c
d. anti-C


*309. In chronic granulomatous disease (CGD), granulocyte function is impaired. An association exists between this clinical condition and a depression of which of the following antigens?

a. Rh
b. P
c. Kell
d. Duffy


*310. One week after birth, an infant with a positive DAT and a bilirubin level of 18.5 mg/dL is in need of an exchange transfusion. Since the mother could not be located at the time, the next course of action would be to:

a. crossmatch blood using the baby's serum
b. crossmatch blood using an eluate from the baby's red cells
c. locate the father as a potential donor
d. use group O, Rh-positive blood for the exchange


*311. A person's saliva incubated with the following antibodies and tested with the appropriate $A_2$, O, and B indicator cells, gives the following test results:

| Antibody Specificity | Test Results |
|---|---|
| Anti-A | Reactive |
| Anti-B | Inhibited |
| Anti-H | Inhibited |

The person's red cell ABO phenotype is:

a. A
b. AB
c. B
d. O

*312. A blood specimen was found to be A, Rh-positive with a negative antibody screen. Six units of group A, Rh-positive Red Blood Cells were crossmatched and one unit was incompatible in the antiglobulin phase. The same result was obtained when the test was repeated. Which should be done FIRST?

a. repeat the ABO grouping on the incompatible unit using a more sensitive technique
b. test a panel of red cells that possesses low-frequency antigens
c. perform a direct antiglobulin test on the donor unit
d. obtain a new specimen and repeat the crossmatch

*313. The red cells of a nonsecretor (se/se) will most likely type as:

a. *Le(a–b–)*
b. *Le(a+b+)*
c. *Le(a+b–)*
d. *Le(a–b+)*

*314. The serum of a group O Cde/Cde donor contains anti-D. In order to prepare specific anti-D reagent from this donor's serum, which of the following cells would be suitable for the adsorption?

a. group O, cde/cde cells
b. group O, Cde/cde cells
c. group A₂B, CDe/cde cells
d. group A₁B, cde/cde cells

*315. The patient has a positive antibody screen. Prior to transfusion granulocytes MUST be:

a. washed to remove the plasma
b. retyped for Rh antigen only
c. crossmatched with the recipient's serum
d. filtered to remove RBCs and lymphocytes

*316. Which of the following is the proper storage requirement for Granulocytes?

a. 1°C to 6°C
b. 10°C to 18°C
c. room temperature with constant agitation
d. room temperature without agitation

*317. Once collected, Granulocytes MUST be administered within:

a. 6 hours
b. 24 hours
c. 7 days
d. 35 days

*318. Therapeutic plasmapheresis is performed to:

a. harvest granulocytes
b. harvest Platelets
c. treat patients with polycythemia
d. treat patients with plasma abnormalities

*319. A reason a patient's crossmatch may be incompatible while the antibody screen is negative is:

a. the patient has an antibody against a high frequency antigen
b. the incompatible donor unit has a positive direct antiglobulin test
c. cold agglutinins are interfering in the crossmatch
d. the patient's serum contains warm autoantibody

*320. A unit of very rare red cells has been deglycerolized for 10 hours. The patient's condition has stabilized and transfusion of these cells is no longer necessary. Which of the following is the most appropriate course of action?

a. Urge the attending physician to transfuse the patient due to the value of the rare cells.
b. Discard the unit.
c. Extend the expiration time and date an additional 24 hours.
d. Document the value of the rare cells and refreeze before 20 hours have elapsed.

*321. A mother has the red cell phenotype DCe with anti-c (titer of 32 at AHG) in her serum. The father has the phenotype DCce, and the baby is Rh-negative and not affected with hemolytic disease of the newborn. What is the baby's most probable Rh genotype?

a. dCe
b. dCce
c. DCe
d. DCce

*322. To confirm the specificity of a serum antibody identified as anti-$P_1$, a neutralization study was performed and the following results were obtained:

|  | $P_1$ + RBCs |
|---|---|
| Serum + $P_1$ substance | Negative |
| Serum + saline | Negative |

What conclusion can be made from these results?

a. Anti-P$_1$ is confirmed.
b. Anti-P$_1$ is ruled out.
c. A second antibody is suspected due to the results of the negative control.
d. Anti-P$_1$ cannot be confirmed due to the results of the negative control.


*323. To prepare anti-Kell as a reagent from a serum containing anti-I and anti-Kell, the serum should be absorbed with:

a. Kell-positive, I-positive cells at 22°C
b. Kell-positive, I-negative cells at 4°C
c. Kell-negative, I-positive cells at 4°C
d. Kell-negative, I-positive cells at 37°C


*324. In a case of cold autoimmune hemolytic anemia, the patient's serum would most likely react 4+ at immediate spin with:

a. group A cells, B cells, and O cells, but not his own cells
b. cord cells but not his own or other adult cells
c. all cells of a group O cell panel and his own cells
d. only penicillin-treated panel cells, not his own cells


*325. Which direct antiglobulin test result on a recently transfused patient is most associated with an anamnestic antibody response?

| | Polyspecific | IgG | C3 | Control |
|---|---|---|---|---|
| a. | +$^{mf}$ | +$^{mf}$ | 0 | 0 |
| b. | 1+ | 0 | 1+ | 0 |
| c. | 2+ | 2+ | 0 | 0 |
| d. | 4+ | 4+ | 4+ | 0 |


*326. For a patient who has suffered an acute hemolytic transfusion reaction, the primary treatment goal should be to:

a. prevent alloimmunization
b. diminish chills and fever
c. prevent hemoglobinemia
d. reverse hypotension and minimize renal damage

*327. A family has been typed for HLA because one of the children needs a bone marrow transplant. Typing results are listed below:

Father    A1,3;B8,35
Mother    A2,23;B12,18
Child 1   A1,2:B8,12
Child 2   A1,23;B8,18
Child 3   A3,23;B18,?

What expected antigen is missing in child 3?

a.  A1
b.  A2
c.  B12
d.  B35


*328. In a paternity case, the child has a genetic marker that is absent in the mother and cannot be demonstrated in the alleged father. What type of paternity exclusion is this known as?

a.  indirect (second order)
b.  direct (first order)
c.  prior probability
d.  Hardy-Weinberg


*329. A 10-year-old girl was hospitalized because her urine had a distinct red color. The patient had recently recovered from an upper respiratory infection and appeared very pale and lethargic. Tests were performed with the following results:

Hemoglobulin            5 g/dL
Reticulocyte count      15%
DAT                     Weak reactivity with polyspecific and anti-C3d only
Antibody screen         Negative
Methemalbumin           Present
Ham's test              Negative
Sucrose hemolysis test  Negative
Donath-Landsteiner test Positive; P-cells showed no hemolysis

The patient probably has:

a.  paroxysmal cold hemoglobinuria (PCH)
b.  paroxysmal nocturnal hemoglobinuria (PNH)
c.  warm autoimmune hemolytic anemia
d.  hereditary erythroblastic multinuclearity with a positive acidified serum test (HEMPAS)

*330. What is the approximate probability of finding compatible blood among random Rh-positive units for a patient who has anti-c and anti-K? (Consider that 20% of Rh-positive donors are C-negative and 90% are K-negative.)

a. 1%
b. 10%
c. 18%
d. 45%

*331. A neonate is to be transfused for the first time with group O Red Blood Cells. Which of the following is appropriate when compatibility testing is performed?

a. screen and crossmatch with mother's serum
b. screen and crossmatch with baby's serum
c. crossmatch is NOT necessary if initial screening of mother's or baby's serum was negative
d. screening or crossmatching is NOT necessary; issue group and Rh compatible blood

*332. A patient who has been typed as Rh-negative has a negative antibody screen. However, crossmatching reveals an antibody that reacts 4+ in the AHG phase with 1 of 10 Rh-negative donors. What is the most likely cause of this incompatibility?

a. The patient has an antibody to a low-frequency antigen.
b. The donor has been mistyped for ABO.
c. The donor is actually Rh-positive.
d. The donor Red Blood Cells are polyagglutinable.

*333. Which of the following is the correct interpretation of this saliva neutralization testing?

| Indicator Cells | A | B | O |
| --- | --- | --- | --- |
| Saliva plus anti-A | + | 0 | 0 |
| Saliva plus anti-B | 0 | + | 0 |
| Saliva plus anti-H | 0 | 0 | 0 |

a. group A secretor
b. group B secretor
c. group AB secretor
d. group O secretor

*334. Mixed leukocyte culture (MLC) is a biological assay for detecting which of the following?

a. HLA-A antigens
b. HLA-B antigens
c. HLA-D antigens
d. immunoglobulins

*335. A poor increment in the platelet count 1 hour following platelet transfusion is most commonly caused by:

    a. splenomegaly
    b. alloimmunization to HLA antigens
    c. disseminated intravascular coagulation
    d. defective Platelets


*336. Washed Red Blood Cells are indicated in which of the following situations?

    a. an IgA-deficient patient with a history of transfusion-associated anaphylaxis
    b. a pregnant woman with a history of hemolytic disease of the newborn
    c. a patient with a positive DAT and red cell autoantibody
    d. a newborn with a hematocrit of less than 30%


*337. Anti-$A_1$ lectin (*Dolichos biflorus*) will react with which of the following red cells?

    a. T-activated
    b. Tn-activated
    c. $O_h$
    d. $A_x$


*338. Examination of immune parameters during the course of HIV infection reveals:

    a. a progressive decrease in T-helper cell numbers as clinical disease worsens
    b. qualitative defects in B-cell function
    c. a progressive increase in T-helper cell numbers as clinical disease worsens
    d. normal B-cell function


*339. Refer to the cell panel on the next page:


Based on the results, which of the following antibodies is MOST likely present?

    a. anti-C
    b. anti-E
    c. anti-D
    d. anti-Kell


*340. One of the most effective methods for the elution of warm autoantibodies from RBCs utilizes:

    a. 10% sucrose
    b. LISS
    c. an organic solvent
    d. distilled water

| Cell | D | C | E | c | e | M | N | S | s | Leᵃ | Leᵇ | P₁ | K | k | Fyᵃ | Fyᵇ | Jkᵃ | Jkᵇ | IS | 37 C | AHG | Enzyme AHG |
|---|---|---|---|---|---|---|---|---|---|---|---|---|---|---|---|---|---|---|---|---|---|---|
| 1 | 0 | + | 0 | + | + | + | 0 | 0 | + | 0 | + | 0 | 0 | + | 0 | + | 0 | + | 0 | 0 | 2+ | 3+ |
| 2 | + | + | 0 | 0 | + | + | + | + | + | 0 | + | + | 0 | + | + | 0 | 0 | + | 0 | 0 | 3+ | 4+ |
| 3 | + | + | 0 | + | + | + | 0 | + | + | + | 0 | + | + | 0 | + | + | + | 0 | 0 | 0 | 2+ | 3+ |
| 4 | + | + | 0 | 0 | + | + | 0 | + | 0 | 0 | + | + | 0 | + | 0 | + | + | + | 0 | 0 | 3+ | 4+ |
| 5 | 0 | 0 | 0 | + | + | + | 0 | + | + | 0 | + | 0 | 0 | + | + | + | + | + | 0 | 0 | 2+ | 0 |
| 6 | 0 | 0 | 0 | + | + | 0 | + | + | 0 | 0 | + | + | + | + | + | + | + | 0 | 0 | 0 | 2+ | 0 |
| 7 | + | 0 | 0 | + | + | 0 | + | + | + | 0 | + | + | 0 | + | 0 | 0 | + | + | 0 | 0 | 0 | 0 |
| 8 | + | 0 | + | + | 0 | 0 | + | 0 | + | + | 0 | + | 0 | + | 0 | + | 0 | + | 0 | 0 | 0 | 0 |
| 9 | + | 0 | + | + | + | + | + | 0 | + | 0 | + | + | 0 | + | + | + | + | + | 0 | 0 | 2+ | 0 |
| 10 | 0 | 0 | 0 | + | + | + | + | + | 0 | 0 | + | 0 | 0 | + | + | 0 | + | 0 | 0 | 0 | 2+ | 0 |
| Autocontrol | | | | | | | | | | | | | | | | | | | 0 | 0 | 0 | 0 |

*341. A patient's Red Blood Cells gave the following reactions:

| Anti-D | Anti-C | Anti-E | Anti-c | Anti-e | Anti-f |
|---|---|---|---|---|---|
| + | + | + | + | + | 0 |

The most probable genotype of this patient is:

a. $R_1R_2$
b. $R_2r''$
c. $R_2r$
d. $R_2R_2$

*342. Which of the following would be most useful for removing an autoantibody for red cell phenotyping?

a. bromelin
b. chloroquine
c. LISS
d. phthalate esters

*343. An individual has been sensitized to the Cellano (k) antigen and has produced anti-k. What is her most probable Kell genotype?

a. $KK$
b. $Kk$
c. $kk$
d. $K_0K_0$

*344. Which of the following HTLA antibodies is neutralizable by pooled human plasma?

a. anti-Ytᵃ
b. anti-Ch
c. anti-Yk
d. anti-Cs

*345. For serial plasmapheresis donors, the total serum protein must be at least:

a. 4.5 g/dL
b. 5.0 g/dL
c. 5.5 g/dL
d. 6.0 g/dL

*346. A 42-year-old male of average body mass has a history of chronic anemia requiring transfusion support. Two units of Red Blood Cells are transfused. If the pretransfusion hemoglobin was 7.0 g/dL, the expected posttransfusion hemoglobin concentration should be:

a. 8.0 g/dL
b. 9.0 g/dL
c. 10.0 g/dL
d. 11.0 g/dL

*347. A 56-year-old female with cold hemagglutinin disease has a positive direct antiglobulin test (DAT). When the DAT is repeated using monospecific antiglobulin sera, which of the following is most likely to be detected?

a. IgM
b. IgG
c. C3d
d. C4d

*348. Which of the following best reflects the discrepancy seen when a person's red cells demonstrate the acquired-B phenotype?

| | Forward Grouping | Reverse Grouping |
|---|---|---|
| a. | B | O |
| b. | AB | A |
| c. | O | B |
| d. | B | AB |

*349. Consider the following ABO typing results:

| Patient's cells vs | Patient's serum vs |
|---|---|
| Anti-A = 4+ | $A_1$ cells = 1+ |
| Anti-B = 0 | B cells = 4+ |

Additional testing was performed using patient serum:

|  | IS | RT |
|---|---|---|
| Screening cell I | 1+ | 2+ |
| Screening cell II | 1+ | 2+ |
| Autocontrol | 1+ | 2+ |

What is the MOST LIKELY cause of this discrepancy?

a. $A_2$ with anti-$A_1$
b. cold alloantibody
c. cold autoantibody
d. acquired-A phenomenon


*350. A blood donor has the genotype *hh*, *AB*. What is his red blood cell phenotype?

a. A
b. B
c. O
d. AB


*351. A patient has had massive trauma involving replacement of one blood volume with Red Blood Cells and crystalloid. She is currently experiencing oozing from mucous membranes and surgical incisions. Laboratory values are as follows:

| PT | Normal |
|---|---|
| APTT | Normal |
| Bleeding time | Prolonged |
| Platelet count | $20 \times 10^3/\mu L$ |
| Hemoglobin | 11.4 g/dL |

What is the blood component of choice for this patient?

a. Platelets
b. Cryoprecipitated AHF
c. Fresh Frozen Plasma
d. Prothrombin Complex

*352. A 26-year-old female is admitted with anemia of undetermined origin. Blood samples are received with a crossmatch request for six units of Red Blood Cells. The patient is group A, Rh-negative and has no history of transfusion or pregnancy. The following results were obtained in pretransfusion testing:

|                   | IS | 37°C | IAT |
|-------------------|----|------|-----|
| Screening cell I  | 0  | 0    | 3+  |
| Screening cell II | 0  | 0    | 3+  |
| Autocontrol       | 0  | 0    | 3+  |
| All 6 donors      | 0  | 0    | 3+  |

The best way to find compatible blood is to:

a. do an antibody identification panel
b. use the saline replacement technique
c. use the prewarm technique
d. perform a warm autoadsorption

*353. A paternity investigation produces the following red cell phenotyping results:

|                | ABO | Rh   |
|----------------|-----|------|
| Alleged father | B   | DcE  |
| Mother         | O   | DCe  |
| Child          | O   | DCce |

What conclusions can be made?

a. There is no exclusion of paternity.
b. Paternity may be excluded on the basis of ABO typing.
c. Paternity may be excluded on the basis of Rh typing.
d. Paternity may be excluded on the basis of both ABO and Rh typing.

*354. A patient was given two units of blood in an emergency. The blood was type specific, but not crossmatched. Further study revealed an anti-K in the pretransfusion sample. One unit was K-positive. Serum obtained immediately posttransfusion failed to react with K-positive cells. This is due to the antibody being:

a. cleared by the spleen
b. inactivated in the liver
c. destroyed by the action of complement
d. adsorbed by the donor cells

*355. The objective, "The student will be able to prepare correctly a creatinine working standard from a stock solution," is an example of which behavioral domain?

a. psychomotor
b. affective
c. intellectual
d. cognitive

*356. The first step in the development of long-term objectives for a continuing education program must include:

a. total cost of the program
b. total number of hours in the program
c. a list of topics to be covered
d. a statement of competencies to be achieved

*357. Which of the following phenotyped individuals would be the most appropriate saliva donor to neutralize an auto anti-H in the serum of a group A, Le(a–b+) patient?

a. Group A, Le(a–b–)
b. Group A, Le(a+b–)
c. Group O, Le(a+b–)
d. Group O, Le(a–b+)

*358. A child with an *E coli* infection develops a positive antibody screen. Reactivity is seen at immediate spin and 37°C with 1 of 10 random donor units and is unchanged by enzymes. The antibody is:

a. anti-K
b. anti-M
c. anti-$P_1$
d. anti-Fy$^a$

*359. The following laboratory data are obtained on a patient with a history of recent anemia and hemoglobinuria:

| Antibody screen | Negative at all phases |
| DAT | Negative |

Acid Hemolysin Test

|  | Tube 1 | Tube 2 | Tube 3 |
| --- | --- | --- | --- |
| Serum | Normal | Normal | Inactivated normal |
| Acid | No | Yes | Yes |
| Cells | Patient | Patient | Patient |
| Result | Negative | Hemolysis | Negative |

What interpretation can be made from these results?

a. They confirm the patient has complement-sensitive PNH red cells.
b. They confirm the presence of a cold autoantibody.
c. They are inconclusive because the normal serum may lack complement.
d. They are inconclusive because of a suspect acid solution.

*360. What is the most appropriate interpretation for the laboratory data given below?

|  | D | D Control | Dᵘ | Dᵘ Control | Rosette Fetal Screen |
|---|---|---|---|---|---|
| Mother | neg | neg | neg | neg | 1 rosette per 5 fields |
| Newborn | neg | neg | neg | neg | Not tested |

a. mother is not a candidate for RhIg
b. mother needs one vial of RhIg
c. mother needs two vials of RhIg
d. the fetal-maternal hemorrhage needs to be quantitated

*361. A serologic centrifuge is recalibrated for ABO testing after major repairs. Given the data below, the centrifuge time for this machine should be:

|  | 15 sec | 20 sec | 25 sec | 30 sec |
|---|---|---|---|---|
| Is button delineated? | Yes | Yes | Yes | Yes |
| Is supernatant clear? | No | Yes | Yes | Yes |
| Button easy to resuspend? | Yes | Yes | Yes | No |
| Strength of reaction? | +m | 1+ | 1+ | 1+ |

a. 15 seconds
b. 20 seconds
c. 25 seconds
d. 30 seconds

*362. Which of the following procedures would be most helpful to confirm a weak ABO subgroup?

a. adsorption-elution
b. neutralization-inhibition
c. elution-diffusion
d. immunodiffusion-precipitation

*363. Given the following data on a mother and her newborn, who would be the best source of Platelets if the newborn requires an urgent transfusion?

|  | Mother | Newborn |
|---|---|---|
| ABO/Rh | A, Rh-negative | O, Rh-positive |
| Known antibody | Anti-Pl^A1 | Not tested |
| DAT | Negative | Negative |
| Platelet count | 412 x 10³/μL | 6.0 x 10³/μL |

a. father
b. mother
c. random donor
d. autologous donor

| Cell | D | C | E | c | e | M | N | S | s | Le^a | Le^b | P_1 | K | k | Fy^a | Fy^b | Jk^a | Jk^b | Serum Alb IS | 37 C | AHG | prewarm AHG |
|---|---|---|---|---|---|---|---|---|---|---|---|---|---|---|---|---|---|---|---|---|---|---|
| 1 | 0 | + | 0 | + | + | + | 0 | 0 | + | 0 | + | 0 | 0 | + | 0 | + | 0 | + | 0 | 0 | 1+ | 0 |
| 2 | + | + | 0 | 0 | + | 0 | + | 0 | + | + | 0 | + | 0 | + | + | 0 | 0 | + | 0 | 1+ | 2+ | 0 |
| 3 | + | + | 0 | 0 | + | + | + | + | + | 0 | + | + | + | 0 | + | + | + | + | 0 | 0 | 1+ | 0 |
| 4 | + | + | + | + | 0 | 0 | + | + | 0 | 0 | + | + | 0 | + | 0 | + | 0 | + | 0 | 0 | 1+ | 0 |
| 5 | 0 | 0 | + | + | + | 0 | + | 0 | + | 0 | + | + | 0 | + | + | + | + | + | 0 | 0 | 1+ | 0 |
| 6 | 0 | 0 | 0 | + | + | + | 0 | 0 | + | 0 | 0 | + | 0 | + | 0 | 0 | + | 0 | 0 | 0 | 0 | 0 |
| 7 | 0 | 0 | 0 | + | + | 0 | + | 0 | + | 0 | + | + | + | + | 0 | + | 0 | + | 0 | 0 | 1+ | 0 |
| 8 | 0 | 0 | 0 | + | + | + | 0 | + | 0 | + | 0 | + | 0 | + | 0 | + | + | 0 | 0 | 1+ | 2+ | 0 |
| 9 | 0 | 0 | 0 | + | + | + | 0 | + | 0 | 0 | + | + | + | + | + | 0 | + | + | 0 | 0 | 1+ | 0 |
| 10 | + | + | + | 0 | + | + | 0 | + | 0 | + | 0 | 0 | 0 | + | + | 0 | + | 0 | 0 | 1+ | 2+ | 0 |
| Autocontrol | | | | | | | | | | | | | | | | | | | 0 | 0 | 0 | 0 |

*364. A pregnant woman has a positive antibody screen and the panel results are given above. What is the association of the antibody(ies) with hemolytic disease of the newborn (HDN)?

a. causes severe HDN
b. causes mild HDN
c. is not associated with HDN
d. HDN cannot be determined


*365. Anti-E is identified in a panel at the antiglobulin phase. When check cells are added to the negative tubes, no agglutination is seen. The most appropriate course of action would be to:

a. quality control the AHG reagent and check cells, then repeat the panel
b. open a new vial of check cells for subsequent testing that day
c. open a new vial of AHG for subsequent testing that day
d. record the check cell reactions and report the antibody panel result


*366. A multiply transfused patient developed a headache, nausea, fever and chills during his last transfusion. What component is most appropriate to prevent this reaction in the future?

a. Red Blood Cells
b. Irradiated Red Blood Cells
c. Leukocyte-Reduced Red Blood Cells
d. CMV-seronegative Red Blood Cells

*367. Given the following objective:

"After listening to the audiotape, the student will be able to describe the interaction between T and B lymphocytes in the immune system to the satisfaction of the instructor."

Which of the following test questions reflects the intent of this objective?

a. How are T and B lymphocytes separated in vitro?
b. How many T lymphocytes does a normal person have in peripheral blood?
c. What are the morphological characteristics of B lymphocytes?
d. How are antibodies produced after a viral infection?

*368. A patient received four units of blood 2 years ago and now has multiple antibodies. He has not been transfused since that time. It would be most helpful to the patient to:

a. phenotype his cells to determine which additional alloantibodies may be produced
b. recommend the use of directed donors, who are more likely to be compatible
c. use proteolytic enzymes to destroy the "in vitro" activity of some of the antibodies
d. freeze the patient's serum to use for antigen typing of compatible units

*369. A trauma patient who has just received 10 units of blood may develop:

a. anemia
b. polycythemia
c. leukocytosis
d. thrombocytopenia

*370. The process of separation of antibody from its antigen is known as:

a. diffusion
b. absorption
c. lyophilization
d. elution

*371. What is the most appropriate diluent for preparing a solution of 8% bovine albumin for a red cell control?

a. deionized water
b. distilled water
c. normal saline
d. Alsever's solution

*372. A patient's serum reacts with two of the three antibody screening cells at the AHG phase. Eight of the ten units crossmatched were incompatible at the AHG phase. All reactions are markedly enhanced by enzymes. These results are most consistent with:

a. anti-M
b. anti-E
c. anti-c
d. anti-Fy$^a$

*373. Ten units of group A Platelets were transfused to a group AB patient. The pretransfusion platelet count was 12 x 10$^3$/μL and the posttransfusion count was 18 x 10$^3$/μL. From this information, the laboratorian would most likely conclude that the patient:

a. needs group AB Platelets to be effective
b. clinical data do not suggest a need for Platelets
c. has developed antibodies to the transfused Platelets
d. should receive irradiated Platelets

*374. On Monday, a patient's Kell antigen typing result was positive. Two days later, the patient's Kell typing was negative. The patient was transfused with two units of Fresh Frozen Plasma on Tuesday. The technician might conclude that the:

a. transfusion of FFP affected the Kell typing
b. wrong patient was drawn
c. results are normal
d. anti-Kell reagent was omitted on Monday

*375. What is the most appropriate control for a positive direct antiglobulin test?

a. check cells and antihuman globulin
b. patient cells and antihuman globulin
c. check cells and saline
d. patient cells and saline

*376. A father donating Platelets for his son is connected to a continuous flow machine, which uses the principle of centrifugation to separate platelets from whole blood. As the platelets are harvested, all other remaining elements are returned to the donor. This method of platelet collection is known as:

a. apheresis
b. autologous
c. homologous
d. fractionation

*377. A high protein major crossmatch at the antiglobulin phase was negative. When one drop of check cells was added, no agglutination was seen. The MOST likely explanation is that the:

a. albumin in the high protein tube neutralized the AHG reagent
b. centrifuge speed was set too high
c. residual patient serum inactivated the AHG reagent
d. laboratorian did not add enough check cells


*378. How would the hematocrit of a patient with chronic anemia be affected by the transfusion of a unit of Whole Blood containing 475 mL of blood vs two units of Red Blood Cells each with a total volume of 250 mL?

a. Patient's hematocrit would be equally affected by the Whole Blood or the Red Blood Cells.
b. Red Blood Cells would provide twice the increment in hematocrit as the Whole Blood.
c. Whole Blood would provide twice the increment in hematocrit as the Red Blood Cells.
d. Whole Blood would provide a change in hematocrit slightly less than the Red Blood Cells.


*379. Five days after transfusion, a patient becomes mildly jaundiced and experiences a drop in hemoglobin and hematocrit with no apparent hemorrhage. Below are the results of the transfusion reaction workup:

| | Anti-A | Anti-B | Anti-A, B | Anti-D | $A_1$ cells | B cells | Ab Screen | DAT |
|---|---|---|---|---|---|---|---|---|
| Patient pretransfusion | neg | 4+ | neg | 3+ | 4+ | neg | neg | neg |
| Patient posttransfusion | neg | 4+ | neg | 3+ | 4+ | neg | +/-w | 1+w |
| Donor 1 | neg | neg | neg | 3+ | 4+ | 4+ | neg | |
| Donor 2 | neg | 4+ | neg | 3+ | 4+ | neg | neg | |

In order to reach a conclusion, the technologist should first:

a. retype the pre- and posttransfusion patient and donor 1 samples
b. request an EDTA tube be drawn from the patient and repeat the DAT
c. repeat the pretransfusion antibody screen on the patient's sample
d. identify the antibody in the serum and eluate from the posttransfusion sample

# *Blood Bank* **Answer Key**

| | | | | |
|---|---|---|---|---|
| 1. d | 42. b | 83. b | 124. c | 165. d |
| 2. c | 43. d | 84. d | 125. d | 166. d |
| 3. b | 44. d | 85. a | 126. b | 167. c |
| 4. b | 45. c | 86. b | 127. a | 168. d |
| 5. a | 46. c | 87. c | 128. d | 169. c |
| 6. a | 47. d | 88. b | 129. a | 170. a |
| 7. c | 48. c | 89. a | 130. a | 171. d |
| 8. d | 49. b | 90. a | 131. d | 172. b |
| 9. d | 50. d | 91. c | 132. d | 173. c |
| 10. d | 51. b | 92. d | 133. a | 174. d |
| 11. a | 52. b | 93. b | 134. b | 175. d |
| 12. d | 53. d | 94. c | 135. d | 176. c |
| 13. a | 54. b | 95. a | 136. c | 177. d |
| 14. a | 55. b | 96. c | 137. a | 178. a |
| 15. c | 56. b | 97. d | 138. a | 179. b |
| 16. d | 57. b | 98. a | 139. a | 180. a |
| 17. d | 58. c | 99. a | 140. a | 181. a |
| 18. c | 59. c | 100. a | 141. a | 182. b |
| 19. c | 60. b | 101. d | 142. b | 183. c |
| 20. c | 61. c | 102. a | 143. d | 184. b |
| 21. c | 62. d | 103. b | 144. c | 185. b |
| 22. d | 63. c | 104. d | 145. b | 186. a |
| 23. b | 64. b | 105. a | 146. b | 187. a |
| 24. c | 65. a | 106. b | 147. c | 188. c |
| 25. d | 66. c | 107. c | 148. d | 189. b |
| 26. b | 67. c | 108. b | 149. b | 190. a |
| 27. a | 68. c | 109. c | 150. b | 191. d |
| 28. a | 69. c | 110. a | 151. b | 192. a |
| 29. c | 70. d | 111. c | 152. a | 193. d |
| 30. c | 71. c | 112. a | 153. d | 194. a |
| 31. a | 72. d | 113. d | 154. b | 195. c |
| 32. a | 73. b | 114. b | 155. d | 196. c |
| 33. b | 74. d | 115. a | 156. c | 197. c |
| 34. d | 75. a | 116. b | 157. d | 198. c |
| 35. c | 76. c | 117. d | 158. c | 199. a |
| 36. c | 77. c | 118. b | 159. a | 200. c |
| 37. b | 78. a | 119. c | 160. b | 201. d |
| 38. d | 79. d | 120. b | 161. a | 202. a |
| 39. d | 80. b | 121. c | 162. c | 203. b |
| 40. a | 81. a | 122. d | 163. d | 204. a |
| 41. c | 82. d | 123. d | 164. a | 205. d |

| | | | | |
|---|---|---|---|---|
| 206. d | 241. b | 276. d | 311. c | 346. b |
| 207. b | 242. a | 277. c | 312. c | 347. c |
| 208. d | 243. d | 278. b | 313. c | 348. b |
| 209. c | 244. b | 279. b | 314. d | 349. c |
| 210. d | 245. c | 280. b | 315. c | 350. c |
| 211. c | 246. d | 281. d | 316. d | 351. a |
| 212. d | 247. b | 282. c | 317. b | 352. d |
| 213. d | 248. c | 283. d | 318. d | 353. c |
| 214. c | 249. a | 284. b | 319. b | 354. d |
| 215. a | 250. b | 285. d | 320. d | 355. a |
| 216. b | 251. a | 286. a | 321. a | 356. d |
| 217. d | 252. c | 287. a | 322. d | 357. d |
| 218. c | 253. c | 288. b | 323. c | 358. a |
| 219. d | 254. a | 289. d | 324. c | 359. a |
| 220. c | 255. d | 290. c | 325. a | 360. a |
| 221. d | 256. d | 291. b | 326. d | 361. b |
| 222. c | 257. a | 292. d | 327. d | 362. a |
| 223. c | 258. a | 293. c | 328. b | 363. b |
| 224. d | 259. c | 294. d | 329. a | 364. c |
| 225. c | 260. b | 295. c | 330. c | 365. a |
| 226. c | 261. d | 296. c | 331. c | 366. c |
| 227. c | 262. c | 297. b | 332. a | 367. d |
| 228. d | 263. b | 298. b | 333. d | 368. a |
| 229. c | 264. d | 299. b | 334. c | 369. d |
| 230. a | 265. d | 300. a | 335. b | 370. d |
| 231. a | 266. d | 301. d | 336. a | 371. c |
| 232. b | 267. c | 302. b | 337. b | 372. c |
| 233. c | 268. a | 303. a | 338. a | 373. c |
| 234. c | 269. a | 304. b | 339. a | 374. b |
| 235. d | 270. d | 305. c | 340. c | 375. d |
| 236. a | 271. b | 306. d | 341. a | 376. a |
| 237. b | 272. b | 307. a | 342. b | 377. c |
| 238. d | 273. b | 308. c | 343. a | 378. b |
| 239. d | 274. c | 309. c | 344. b | 379. d |
| 240. a | 275. b | 310. b | 345. d | |

# CHAPTER 10

# *Chemistry*

*The following items have been identified as appropriate for both entry level medical technologists and medical laboratory technicians.*

1. The urinary excretion product measured as an indicator of epinephrine production is:

   a. dopamine
   b. dihydroxyphenylalanine (DOPA)
   c. homovanillic acid
   d. vanillylmandelic acid

2. Which two conditions can "physiologically" elevate serum alkaline phosphatase?

   a. rickets, hyperparathyroidism
   b. obstructive jaundice, biliary cirrhosis
   c. growth, third trimester of pregnancy
   d. viral hepatitis, infectious mononucleosis

3. The $T_3$ resin uptake test is a measure of:

   a. circulating $T_3$
   b. bound $T_3$
   c. binding capacity of thyroxine-binding globulin
   d. total thyroxine-binding globulin

4. During an evaluation of adrenal function, a patient had plasma cortisol determinations in the morning after awakening and in the evening. Laboratory results indicated that the morning value was higher than the evening concentration. This is indicative of:

    a. a normal finding
    b. Cushing's syndrome
    c. Addison's disease
    d. hypopituitarism

5. In the liver, bilirubin is converted to:

    a. urobilinogen
    b. urobilin
    c. bilirubin-albumin complex
    d. bilirubin diglucuronide

6. The following results were obtained in a creatinine clearance evaluation:

| | |
|---|---|
| Urine concentration | 84 mg/dL |
| Urine volume | 1440 mL/24 hr |
| Serum concentration | 1.4 mg/dL |
| Body surface area | 1.60 m$^2$ (average = 1.73 m$^2$) |

The creatinine clearance in mL/min is:

    a. 6
    b. 22
    c. 60
    d. 65

7. The electrophoretic pattern of a plasma sample compared with a serum sample shows a:

    a. broad prealbumin peak
    b. sharp fibrinogen peak
    c. diffuse pattern because of the presence of anticoagulants
    d. decreased globulin fraction

8. The biuret reaction for the analysis of serum protein depends on the number of:

    a. free amino groups
    b. free carboxyl groups
    c. peptide bonds
    d. tyrosine residues

9. Total iron-binding capacity measures the serum iron transporting capacity of:

   a. hemoglobin
   b. ceruloplasmin
   c. transferrin
   d. ferritin

10. In the Jendrassik-Grof method for the determination of serum bilirubin concentration, quantitation is obtained by measuring the green color of:

    a. azobilirubin
    b. bilirubin glucuronide
    c. urobilin
    d. urobilinogen

11. Absorbance (A) of a solution may be converted to percent transmittance (%T) using the formula:

    a. $1 + \log \%T$
    b. $2 + \log \%T$
    c. $1 - \log \%T$
    d. $2 - \log \%T$

12. Aspartate aminotransferase (AST) and alanine aminotransferase (ALT) are both elevated in which of the following diseases?

    a. muscular dystrophy
    b. viral hepatitis
    c. pulmonary emboli
    d. infectious mononucleosis

13. Calcium concentration in the serum is regulated by:

    a. insulin
    b. parathyroid hormone
    c. thyroxine
    d. vitamin C

14. Which of the following steroids is an adrenal cortical hormone?

    a. angiotensinogen
    b. corticosterone
    c. progesterone
    d. pregnanetriol

15. Blood $PCO_2$ may be measured by:

    a. direct colorimetric measurement of dissolved $CO_2$
    b. calculations of blood pH and total $CO_2$ concentration
    c. measurement of $CO_2$-saturated hemoglobin
    d. measurement of $CO_2$ consumed at the cathode


16. In the potentiometric measurement of hydrogen ion concentration, reference electrodes that may be used include:

    a. silver-silver chloride
    b. quinhydrone
    c. hydroxide
    d. hydrogen


17. In a spectrophotometer, light of a specific wavelength can be isolated from white light with a(n):

    a. double beam
    b. diffraction grating
    c. aperture
    d. slit


18. The osmolality of a urine or serum specimen is measured by a change in the:

    a. freezing point
    b. sedimentation point
    c. midpoint
    d. osmotic pressure


19. Which of the following serum constituents is unstable if a blood specimen is left standing at room temperature for 8 hours before processing?

    a. cholesterol
    b. triglyceride
    c. creatinine
    d. glucose


20. A urine screening test for porphobilinogen is positive. The MOST likely disease state is:

    a. lead poisoning
    b. porphyria cutanea tarda
    c. acute porphyria attack
    d. erythrocytic protoporphyria

21. In electrophoretic analysis, buffers:

    a. stabilize electrolytes
    b. maintain basic pH
    c. act as a carrier for ions
    d. produce an effect on protein configuration


22. A condition in which erythrocyte protoporphyrin is increased is:

    a. acute intermittent porphyria
    b. iron deficiency anemia
    c. porphyria cutanea tarda
    d. acute porphyric attack


23. The stimulant that causes localized sweating for the sweat test is:

    a. polyvinyl alcohol
    b. lithium sulfate
    c. potassium sulfate
    d. pilocarpine nitrate


24. In the sweat test, the sweating stimulant is introduced to the skin by application of:

    a. filter paper moistened with pilocarpine nitrate
    b. an electric current
    c. copper electrodes
    d. filter paper moistened in deionized water


25. The formula for calculating serum osmolality that incorporates a correction for the water content of plasma is:

    a. 2 Na x (Glucose/20) x (BUN/3)
    b. Na + [(2 x Glucose)/20] x (BUN/3)
    c. 2 Na + Glucose/20 + (BUN/3)
    d. 2 Na + Glucose/3 + (BUN/20)


26. Osmolal gap is:

    a. the difference between the ideal and real osmolality values
    b. the difference between the calculated and measured osmolality values
    c. the difference between plasma and water osmolality values
    d. the difference between molality and molarity at 4°C

27. Erroneous ammonia levels can be eliminated by all of the following EXCEPT:

    a. ensuring water and reagents are ammonia-free
    b. separating plasma from cells and performing test analysis as soon as possible
    c. drawing the specimen in a prechilled tube and immersing the tube in ice
    d. storing the specimen protected from light until the analysis is done


28. Which of the following applies to cryoscopic osmometry?

    a. The temperature at equilibrium is a function of the number of particles in solution.
    b. The temperature plateau for a solution is horizontal.
    c. The freezing point of a sample is absolute.
    d. The initial freezing of a sample produces an immediate solid state.


29. The first step to be taken when attempting to repair a piece of electronic equipment is:

    a. check all the electronic connections
    b. reseat all the printed circuit boards
    c. turn the instrument off
    d. replace all the fuses


30. Most of the carbon dioxide present in blood is in the form of:

    a. dissolved $CO_2$
    b. carbonate
    c. bicarbonate ion
    d. carbonic acid


31. The degree to which the kidney concentrates the glomerular filtrate can be determined by:

    a. urine creatine
    b. serum creatinine
    c. creatinine clearance
    d. urine to serum osmolality ratio


32. How many grams of sulfosalicylic acid (MW = 254) are required to prepare 1 L of a 3% (w/v) solution?

    a. 3
    b. 30
    c. 254
    d. 300

33. A physician suspects his patient has pancreatitis. Which test(s) would be most indicative of this disease?

    a. creatinine
    b. LD isoenzymes
    c. β-hydroxybutyrate
    d. amylase


34. The statistical term for the average value is the:

    a. mode
    b. median
    c. mean
    d. coefficient of variation


35. An index of precision is statistically known as the:

    a. median
    b. mean
    c. standard deviation
    d. coefficient of variation


36. The most frequent value in a collection of data is statistically known as the:

    a. mode
    b. median
    c. mean
    d. standard deviation


37. The middle value of a data set is statistically known as the:

    a. mean
    b. median
    c. mode
    d. standard deviation


38. In a specimen collected for plasma glucose analysis, sodium fluoride:

    a. serves as a coenzyme of hexokinase
    b. prevents reactivity of non–glucose reducing substances
    c. precipitates proteins
    d. inhibits glycolysis

39. In the international system of units serum urea is expressed in millimoles per liter. A serum urea nitrogen concentration of 28 mg/dL would be equivalent to what concentration of urea?

    (Urea: $NH_2CONH_2$; atomic wt N = 14, C = 12, O = 16, H = 1)

    a. 4.7 mEq/L
    b. 5.0 mEq/L
    c. 10.0 mEq/L
    d. 20.0 mEq/L

40. The osmolal gap is defined as measured Osm/kg minus the calculated Osm/kg. The average osmolal gap is near:

    a. 0
    b. 2
    c. 4
    d. 6

41. To be analyzed by gas liquid chromatography, a compound must:

    a. be volatile or made volatile
    b. not be volatile
    c. be water-soluble
    d. contain a nitrogen atom

42. The solute that contributes the most to the total serum osmolality is:

    a. glucose
    b. sodium
    c. chloride
    d. urea

43. In automated methods utilizing a bichromatic analyzer, dual wavelengths are employed to:

    a. minimize the effect of interference
    b. improve precision
    c. increase throughput
    d. monitor temperature changes

44. Which of the following electrodes is based on the principle of amperometric measurement?

    a. $PCO_2$ electrode
    b. $PO_2$ electrode
    c. pH electrode
    d. ionized calcium electrode

45. One international unit of enzyme activity is the amount of enzyme that, under specified reaction conditions of substrate concentration, pH, and temperature, causes utilization of substrate at the rate of:

    a.  1 mole/min
    b.  1 millimole/min
    c.  1 micromole/min
    d.  1 nanomole/min

46. The Porter-Silber method (phenylhydrazine in alcohol and sulfuric acid) involves which part of the steroid molecule?

    a.  ketone group
    b.  hydroxyl group
    c.  dihydroxyacetone side chain
    d.  steroid ring

47. Which family of steroid hormones is characterized by an unsaturated A ring?

    a.  progestins
    b.  estrogens
    c.  androgens
    d.  glucocorticoids

48. Which of the following statements about immunoassays using enzyme-labeled antibodies or antigens is correct?

    a.  Inactivation of the enzyme is required.
    b.  The enzyme label is less stable than an isotopic label.
    c.  Quantitation of the label can be carried out with a spectrophotometer.
    d.  The enzyme label is not an enzyme found naturally in serum.

49. Which of the following chemical determinations may be of help in establishing the presence of seminal fluid?

    a.  lactic dehydrogenase (LD)
    b.  isocitrate dehydrogenase (ICD)
    c.  acid phosphatase
    d.  alkaline phosphatase

50. Which of the following serum protein fractions is most likely to be elevated in patients with nephrotic syndrome?

    a.  alpha-1 globulin
    b.  alpha-1 globulin and alpha-2 globulin
    c.  alpha-2 globulin and beta globulin
    d.  beta globulin and gamma globulin

51. Which of the following enzyme substrates for prostatic acid phosphatase determination results in the highest specificity?

    a. phenyl-phosphate
    b. thymolphthalein monophosphate
    c. alpha-naphthyl-phosphate
    d. beta-glycerophosphate

52. The following laboratory results were obtained on arterial blood:

    | | |
    |---|---|
    | Sodium | 136 mEq/L |
    | pH | 7.32 |
    | Potassium | 4.4 mEq/L |
    | $PCO_2$ | 79 mm Hg |
    | Chloride | 92 mEq/L |
    | Bicarbonate | 40 mEq/L |

    These results are most compatible with:

    a. respiratory alkalosis
    b. respiratory acidosis
    c. metabolic alkalosis
    d. metabolic acidosis

53. Increased total serum lactic dehydrogenase (LD) activity, confined to fractions 4 and 5, is most likely to be associated with:

    a. pulmonary infarction
    b. hemolytic anemia
    c. myocardial infarction
    d. acute viral hepatitis

54. Regan isoenzyme has the same properties as alkaline phosphatase that originates in the:

    a. skeleton
    b. kidney
    c. intestine
    d. placenta

55. Assay of transketolase activity in blood is used to detect deficiency of:

    a. thiamine
    b. folic acid
    c. ascorbic acid
    d. riboflavin

56. The substance that is measured to estimate the serum concentration of triglycerides by MOST methods is:

a. phospholipids
b. glycerol
c. fatty acids
d. pre-beta lipoprotein

57. The most sensitive enzymatic indicator for liver damage from ethanol intake is:

a. alanine aminotransferase (ALT)
b. aspartate aminotransferase (AST)
c. gamma-glutamyl transferase (GGT)
d. alkaline phosphatase

58. Refer to the following illustration:

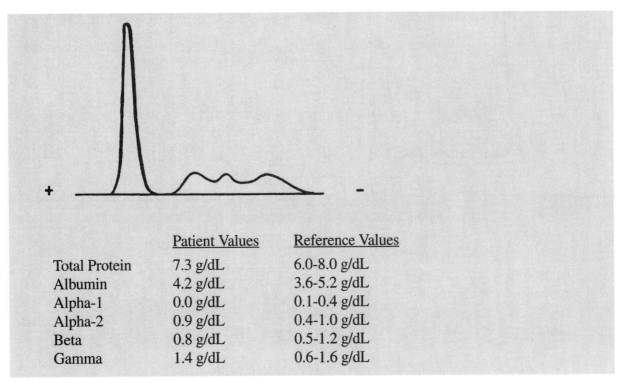

| | Patient Values | Reference Values |
|---|---|---|
| Total Protein | 7.3 g/dL | 6.0-8.0 g/dL |
| Albumin | 4.2 g/dL | 3.6-5.2 g/dL |
| Alpha-1 | 0.0 g/dL | 0.1-0.4 g/dL |
| Alpha-2 | 0.9 g/dL | 0.4-1.0 g/dL |
| Beta | 0.8 g/dL | 0.5-1.2 g/dL |
| Gamma | 1.4 g/dL | 0.6-1.6 g/dL |

This electrophoresis pattern is consistent with:

a. cirrhosis
b. monoclonal gammopathy
c. polyclonal gammopathy (eg, chronic inflammation)
d. alpha-1 antitrypsin deficiency; severe emphysema

59. Patients with Cushing's syndrome exhibit:

    a. decreased plasma 17-hydroxysteroid concentration
    b. decreased urinary 17-hydroxysteroid excretion
    c. serum cortisol concentrations greater than 15 mg/dL
    d. decreased cortisol secretory rate

60. A one molal solution is equivalent to:

    a. a solution containing one mole of solute per kg of solvent
    b. 1000 mL of solution containing one mole of solute
    c. a solution containing one gram-equivalent weight of solute in one liter of solution
    d. a 1-L solution containing 2 moles of solute

61. Refer to the following illustration:

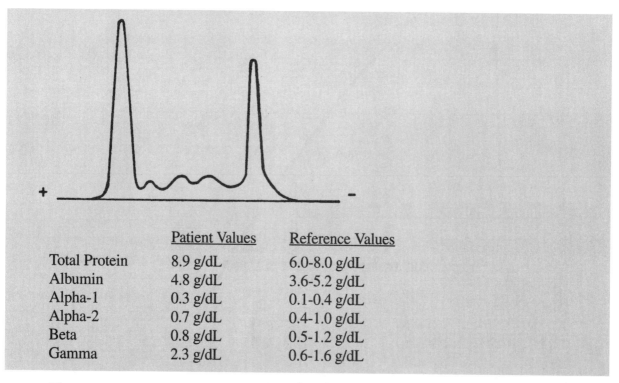

|  | Patient Values | Reference Values |
|---|---|---|
| Total Protein | 8.9 g/dL | 6.0-8.0 g/dL |
| Albumin | 4.8 g/dL | 3.6-5.2 g/dL |
| Alpha-1 | 0.3 g/dL | 0.1-0.4 g/dL |
| Alpha-2 | 0.7 g/dL | 0.4-1.0 g/dL |
| Beta | 0.8 g/dL | 0.5-1.2 g/dL |
| Gamma | 2.3 g/dL | 0.6-1.6 g/dL |

The serum protein electrophoresis pattern is consistent with:

a. cirrhosis
b. acute inflammation
c. monoclonal gammopathy
d. polyclonal gammopathy (eg, chronic inflammation)

62. Refer to the following pattern:

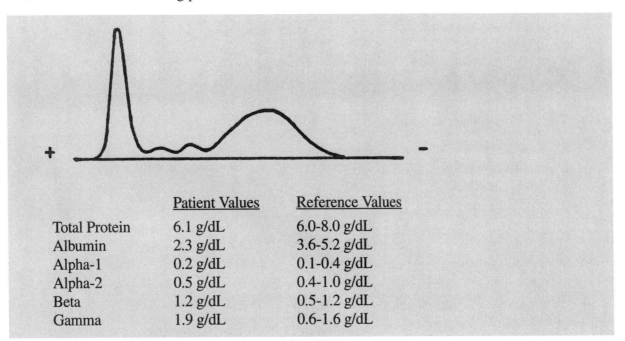

|  | Patient Values | Reference Values |
|---|---|---|
| Total Protein | 6.1 g/dL | 6.0-8.0 g/dL |
| Albumin | 2.3 g/dL | 3.6-5.2 g/dL |
| Alpha-1 | 0.2 g/dL | 0.1-0.4 g/dL |
| Alpha-2 | 0.5 g/dL | 0.4-1.0 g/dL |
| Beta | 1.2 g/dL | 0.5-1.2 g/dL |
| Gamma | 1.9 g/dL | 0.6-1.6 g/dL |

This pattern is consistent with:

a. cirrhosis
b. acute inflammation
c. polyclonal gammopathy (eg, chronic inflammation)
d. alpha-1 antitrypsin deficiency; severe emphysema


63. Given the following results:

| Alkaline phosphatase | Slight increase |
|---|---|
| Aminotransferase | Marked increase |
| Aspartate aminotransferase | Marked increase |
| Alanine gamma-glutamyl transferase | Slight increase |

This is most consistent with:

a. acute hepatitis
b. chronic hepatitis
c. obstructive jaundice
d. liver hemangioma

64. Given the following results:

| | |
|---|---|
| Alkaline phosphatase | Marked increase |
| Aminotransferase | Slight increase |
| Aspartate aminotransferase | Slight increase |
| Alanine gamma-glutamyl transferase | Marked increase |

This is most consistent with:

a. acute hepatitis
b. osteitis fibrosa
c. chronic hepatitis
d. obstructive jaundice

65. Given the following results:

| | |
|---|---|
| Alkaline phosphatase | Slight increase |
| Aminotransferase | Slight increase |
| Aspartate aminotransferase | Slight increase |
| Alanine gamma-glutamyl transferase | Slight increase |

This is most consistent with:

a. acute hepatitis
b. chronic hepatitis
c. obstructive jaundice
d. liver hemangioma

66. Which of the following statements about fluorometry are true?

a. A compound is said to fluoresce when it absorbs light at one wavelength and emits light at a second wavelength.
b. Detectors in fluorometers are placed 180° from the excitation source.
c. It is less sensitive than spectrophotometry.
d. It avoids the necessity for complexing of components because fluorescence is a native property.

67. A benefit of microassays includes:

a. increased analytical reliability
b. reduced reagent requirements
c. increased diagnostic specificity
d. reduced numbers of repeated tests

68. Refer to the following illustration:

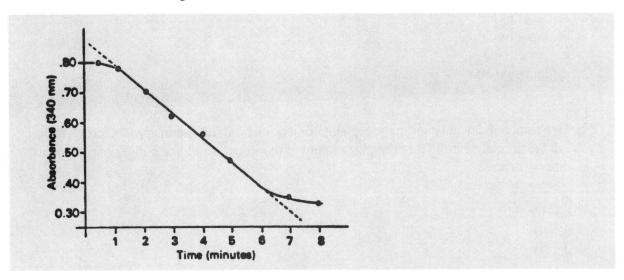

This illustration represents the change in absorbance at 340 nm over a period of 8 minutes in an assay for lactate dehydrogenase. True statements about this figure include:

a. The reaction follows zero order kinetics between 5 and 8 minutes.
b. The reaction is proceeding from lactate to pyruvate.
c. Nonlinearity after 6 minutes is due to substrate exhaustion.
d. The change in absorbance is due to reduction of NAD to NADH.

69. A serum sample drawn in the emergency room from a 42-year-old man yielded the following laboratory results:

CK          185 Units (Normal = 15-160)
AST         123 Units (Normal = 0-48)
CK-MB       6 Units (Normal = 2-12)

Which of the following conditions might account for these values?

a. crush injury to the thigh
b. cerebrovascular accident
c. pulmonary infarction
d. early acute hepatitis

70. In competitive inhibition of an enzyme reaction the:

a. inhibitor binds to the enzyme at the same site as the substrate
b. inhibitor often has a chemical structure different from that of the substrate
c. activity of the reaction can be decreased by increasing the concentration of the substrate
d. activity of the reaction can be increased by decreasing the temperature

71. Kernicterus is an abnormal accumulation of bilirubin in:

   a. heart tissue
   b. brain tissue
   c. liver tissue
   d. kidney tissue

72. Two standard deviations is the acceptable limit of error in the chemistry laboratory. If you run the normal control 100 times, how many of the values would be out of control due to random error?

   a. 1
   b. 5
   c. 10
   d. 20

73. Serum haptoglobin:

   a. is decreased in patients with tissue injury and neoplasia
   b. is increased in patients with prosthetic heart valves
   c. can be separated into distinct phenotypes by starch-gel electrophoresis
   d. binds heme

74. Which of the following serum proteins migrates with the beta-globulins on cellulose acetate at pH 8.6?

   a. ceruloplasmin
   b. hemoglobin
   c. haptoglobin
   d. C3 component of complement

75. Fasting serum phosphate concentration is controlled primarily by the:

   a. pancreas
   b. skeleton
   c. parathyroid glands
   d. small intestine

76. Serum "anion gap" is increased in patients with:

   a. renal tubular acidosis
   b. diabetic alkalosis
   c. metabolic acidosis due to diarrhea
   d. lactic acidosis

77. Increased serum lactic dehydrogenase activity due to elevation of fast fraction (1 and 2) on electrophoretic separation is caused by:

    a. nephrotic syndrome
    b. hemolytic anemia
    c. pancreatitis
    d. hepatic damage

78. The nanometer is used as a measure of:

    a. absorbance
    b. % transmittance
    c. intensity of radiant energy
    d. wavelength of radiant energy

79. Major actions of angiotensin II include:

    a. increased pituitary secretion of renin
    b. increased vasoconstriction
    c. increased parathyroid hormone secretion by the parathyroid
    d. decreased adrenal secretion of aldosterone

80. The presence of increased CK-MB activity on a CK electrophoresis pattern is most likely found in a patient suffering from:

    a. acute muscular stress following strenuous exercise
    b. malignant liver disease
    c. myocardial infarction
    d. severe head injury

81. What is the molarity of a solution that contains 18.7 g of KCl (MW = 74.5) in 500 mL of water?

    a. 0.1
    b. 0.5
    c. 1.0
    d. 5.0

82. In the total bilirubin assay, bilirubin reacts with diazotized sulfanilic acid to form:

    a. diazo bilirubin
    b. biliverdin
    c. azobilirubin
    d. bilirubin glucuronide

83. Total glycosylated hemoglobin levels in a hemolysate reflect the:

    a. average blood glucose levels of the past 2-3 months
    b. average blood glucose levels for the past week
    c. blood glucose level at the time the sample is drawn
    d. hemoglobin $A_1C$ level at the time the sample is drawn


84. The identification of Bence Jones protein is best accomplished by:

    a. a sulfosalicylic acid test
    b. urine reagent strips
    c. immunofixation
    d. electrophoresis


85. The anion gap is useful for quality control of laboratory results for:

    a. amino acids and proteins
    b. blood gas analyses
    c. sodium, potassium, chloride, and total $CO_2$
    d. calcium, phosphorus, and magnesium


86. Which percentage of total serum calcium is nondiffusible protein bound?

    a. 80%-90%
    b. 51%-60%
    c. 40%-50%
    d. 10%-30%


87. The buffering capacity of blood is maintained by a reversible exchange process between bicarbonate and:

    a. sodium
    b. potassium
    c. calcium
    d. chloride


88. Which of the following electrolytes is the chief plasma cation whose main function is maintaining osmotic pressure?

    a. chloride
    b. calcium
    c. potassium
    d. sodium

89. A reciprocal relationship exists between:

   a. sodium and potassium
   b. calcium and phosphorus
   c. chloride and $CO_2$
   d. calcium and magnesium


90. A colorimetric method calls for the use of 0.1 mL serum, 5 mL of reagent and 4.9 mL of water. What is the dilution of the serum in the final solution?

   a. 1:5
   b. 1:10
   c. 1:50
   d. 1:100


91. At blood pH 7.40 what is the ratio between bicarbonate and carbonic acid?

   a. 15:1
   b. 20:1
   c. 25:1
   d. 30:1


92. The bicarbonate and carbonic acid ratio is calculated from an equation by:

   a. Siggaard-Andersen
   b. Gibbs-Donnan
   c. Natelson
   d. Henderson-Hasselbalch


93. Acidosis and alkalosis are best defined as fluctuations in blood pH and $CO_2$ content due to changes in:

   a. Bohr's effect
   b. $O_2$ content
   c. bicarbonate buffer
   d. carbonic anhydrase


94. A common cause of respiratory alkalosis is:

   a. vomiting
   b. starvation
   c. asthma
   d. hyperventilation

95. Metabolic acidosis is described as a(n):

  a. increase in $CO_2$ content and $PCO_2$ with a decreased pH
  b. decrease in $CO_2$ content with an increased pH
  c. increase in $CO_2$ with an increased pH
  d. decrease in $CO_2$ content and $PCO_2$ with a decreased pH

96. Respiratory acidosis is described as a(n):

  a. increase in $CO_2$ content and $PCO_2$ with a decreased pH
  b. decrease in $CO_2$ content with an increased pH
  c. increase in $CO_2$ content with an increased pH
  d. decrease in $CO_2$ content and $PCO_2$ with a decreased pH

97. Normally the bicarbonate concentration is about 24 mEq/L and the carbonic acid concentration is about 1.2; pK = 6.1. Using the equation pH = pK + log[salt]/[acid], calculate the pH.

  a. 7.28
  b. 7.38
  c. 7.40
  d. 7.42

98. The normal range for the pH of arterial blood measured at 37°C is:

  a. 7.28-7.34
  b. 7.33-7.37
  c. 7.35-7.45
  d. 7.45-7.50

99. Unless blood gas measurements are made immediately after sampling, in vitro glycolysis of the blood causes a:

  a. rise in pH and $PCO_2$
  b. fall in pH and a rise in $PO_2$
  c. rise in pH and a fall in $PO_2$
  d. fall in pH and a rise in $PCO_2$

100. Hydrogen ion concentration (pH) in blood is usually determined by means of which of the following electrodes?

  a. silver
  b. glass
  c. platinum
  d. platinum-lactate

101. In the immunoinhibition phase of the CK-MB procedure:

    a. M subunit is inactivated
    b. B subunit is inactivated
    c. MB is inactivated
    d. BB is inactivated

102. The conversion of glucose or other hexoses into lactate or pyruvate is called:

    a. glycogenesis
    b. glycogenolysis
    c. gluconeogenesis
    d. glycolysis

103. The different water content of erythrocytes and plasma makes true glucose concentrations in whole blood a function of the:

    a. hematocrit
    b. leukocyte count
    c. erythrocyte count
    d. erythrocyte indices

104. In the fasting state, the arterial and capillary blood glucose concentration varies from the venous glucose concentration by approximately how many mg/dL?

    a. 2 mg/dL higher
    b. 5 mg/dL higher
    c. 10 mg/dL lower
    d. 12 mg/dL lower

105. Which of the following hemoglobins has glucose-6-phosphate on the amino-terminal valine of the beta chain?

    a. S
    b. C
    c. $A_2$
    d. $A_{1c}$

106. Increased concentrations of ascorbic acid inhibit chromogen production in which of the following glucose methods?

    a. ferricyanide
    b. ortho-toluidine
    c. glucose oxidase (peroxidase)
    d. hexokinase

107. The function of the major lipid components of the very low density lipoproteins (VLDL) is to transport:

    a. cholesterol from peripheral cells to the liver
    b. cholesterol and phospholipids to peripheral cells
    c. exogenous triglycerides
    d. endogenous triglycerides


108. The most widely used support medium for electrophoretic separation of lipoproteins is:

    a. agar gel
    b. starch gel
    c. paper
    d. agarose gel


109. A hospitalized patient is experiencing increased neuromuscular irritability (tetany). Which of the following tests should be ordered immediately?

    a. calcium
    b. phosphorus
    c. BUN
    d. glucose


110. Analysis of CSF for oligoclonal bands is used to screen for which of the following disease states?

    a. multiple myeloma
    b. multiple sclerosis
    c. myasthenia gravis
    d. von Willebrand's disease


111. Sixty to seventy-five percent of the plasma cholesterol is transported by:

    a. chylomicrons
    b. very low density lipoprotein
    c. low density lipoprotein
    d. high density lipoprotein


112. The major fraction of organic iodine in the circulation is in the form of:

    a. thyroglobulin
    b. thyroxine
    c. triiodothyronine
    d. diiodotyrosine

113. Measurement of total $T_4$ by competitive protein binding or displacement is based on the specific binding properties of:

    a. thyroxine-binding prealbumin
    b. albumin
    c. thyroxine-binding globulin
    d. thyroid-stimulating hormone


114. Which of the following methods employs a highly specific antibody to thyroxine?

    a. total $T_4$ by competitive protein binding
    b. $T_4$ by RIA
    c. $T_4$ by column
    d. $T_4$ by equilibrium dialysis


115. A mean value of 100 and a standard deviation of 1.8 mg/dL were obtained from a set of glucose measurements on a control solution. The 95% confidence interval in mg/dL would be:

    a. 94.6-105.4
    b. 96.4-103.6
    c. 97.3-102.7
    d. 98.2-101.8


116. The extent to which measurements agree with the true value of the quantity being measured is known as:

    a. reliability
    b. accuracy
    c. reproducibility
    d. precision


117. When myocardial infarction occurs, the first enzyme to become elevated is:

    a. CK
    b. LD
    c. AST
    d. ALT


118. In the determination of lactate dehydrogenase at 340 nm, using pyruvate as the substrate, one actually measures the:

    a. decrease in pyruvate
    b. decrease in NADH
    c. increase in lactate
    d. increase in NADH

119. In the Jaffe reaction, creatinine reacts with:

    a. alkaline sulfasalazine solution to produce an orange-yellow complex
    b. potassium iodide to form a reddish-purple complex
    c. sodium nitroferricyanide to yield a reddish-brown color
    d. alkaline picrate solution to yield an orange-red complex


120. Which of the following represents the end product of purine metabolism in humans?

    a. AMP and GMP
    b. DNA and RNA
    c. allantoin
    d. uric acid


121. In electrophoresis of proteins, when the sample is placed in an electric field connected to a buffer of pH 8.6, all of the proteins:

    a. have a positive charge
    b. have a negative charge
    c. are electrically neutral
    d. migrate toward the cathode


122. Maple syrup urine disease is characterized by an increase in which of the following urinary amino acids?

    a. phenylalanine
    b. tyrosine
    c. valine, leucine, and isoleucine
    d. cystine and cysteine


123. The hemoglobin that is resistant to alkali (KOH) denaturation is:

    a. A
    b. $A_2$
    c. C
    d. F


124. The parent substance in the biosynthesis of androgens and estrogens is:

    a. cortisol
    b. catecholamines
    c. progesterone
    d. cholesterol

125. The biologically most active, naturally occurring androgen is:

   a. androstenedione
   b. dehydroepiandrosterone
   c. epiandrosterone
   d. testosterone

126. A 24-hour urine specimen (total volume = 1136 mL) is submitted to the laboratory for quantitative urine protein. Calculate the amount of protein excreted per day, if the total protein is 52 mg/dL.

   a. 591 mg
   b. 487 mg
   c. 220 mg
   d. 282 mg

127. Which of the following is secreted by the placenta and used for the early detection of pregnancy?

   a. follicle-stimulating hormone (FSH)
   b. human chorionic gonadotropin (HCG)
   c. luteinizing hormone (LH)
   d. progesterone

128. Decreased serum iron associated with increased TIBC is compatible with which of the following disease states?

   a. anemia of chronic infection
   b. iron deficiency anemia
   c. chronic liver disease
   d. nephrosis

129. A characteristic of the Bence Jones protein that is used to distinguish it from other urinary proteins is its solubility:

   a. in ammonium sulfate
   b. in sulfuric acid
   c. at 40°C-60°C
   d. at 100°C

130. Which of the following is an example of a peptide bond?

131. The principal excretory form of nitrogen is:

a. amino acids
b. creatinine
c. urea
d. uric acid

132. A 45-year-old male of average height and weight was admitted to the hospital for renal function studies. He had the following lab results:

| | |
|---|---|
| Urine creatinine | 120 mg/dL |
| Serum creatinine | 1.5 mg/dL |
| Total urine volume in 24 hours | 1800/mL |

Calculate the creatinine clearance for this patient in mL/min.

a. 100
b. 144
c. 156
d. 225

133. In the Malloy and Evelyn method for the determination of bilirubin, the reagent that is reacted with bilirubin to form a purple azobilirubin is:

a. dilute sulfuric acid
b. diazonium sulfate
c. sulfobromophthalein
d. diazotized sulfanilic acid

134. Bile acid concentrations are useful to assess:

   a. diabetes mellitus
   b. hepatobiliary disease
   c. intestinal malabsorption
   d. kidney function

135. Which of the following enzymes catalyzes the conversion of starch to glucose and maltose?

   a. malate dehydrogenase (MD)
   b. amylase (AMS)
   c. creatine kinase (CK)
   d. isocitric dehydrogenase (ICD)

136. A scanning of a CK isoenzyme fractionation revealed two peaks: a slow cathodic peak (CK-MM) and an intermediate peak (CK-MB). A possible interpretation for this pattern is:

   a. brain tumor
   b. muscular dystrophy
   c. myocardial infarction
   d. viral hepatitis

137. Which of the following enzymes are used in the diagnosis of acute pancreatitis?

   a. amylase (AMS) and lipase (LPS)
   b. aspartate aminotransferase (AST) and alanine aminotransferase (ALT)
   c. 5'-nucleotidase (5'N) and gamma-glutamyl transferase (GGT)
   d. aspartate aminotransferase (AST) and lactate dehydrogenase (LD)

138. Which of the following is a glycolytic enzyme that catalyzes the cleavage of fructose-1, 6-diphosphate to glyceraldehyde-3-phosphate and dihydroxyacetone phosphate?

   a. aldolase
   b. phosphofructokinase
   c. pyruvate kinase
   d. glucose-6-phosphate dehydrogenase

139. The greatest activities of serum AST and ALT are seen in:

   a. acute hepatitis
   b. primary biliary cirrhosis
   c. metastatic hepatic carcinoma
   d. alcoholic cirrhosis

140. An electrophoretic separation of lactate dehydrogenase isoenzymes that demonstrates an elevation in LD-1 and LD-2 in a "flipped" pattern is consistent with:

   a. myocardial infarction
   b. viral hepatitis
   c. pancreatitis
   d. renal failure

141. Which of the following is a characteristic shared by lactate dehydrogenase, malate dehydrogenase, isocitrate dehydrogenase, and hydroxybutyrate dehydrogenase?

   a. They are liver enzymes.
   b. They are cardiac enzymes.
   c. They catalyze oxidation-reduction reactions.
   d. They are class III enzymes.

142. The protein portion of an enzyme complex is called the:

   a. apoenzyme
   b. coenzyme
   c. holoenzyme
   d. proenzyme

143. The most heat labile fraction of alkaline phosphatase is obtained from:

   a. liver
   b. bone
   c. intestine
   d. placenta

144. Refer to the following illustration:

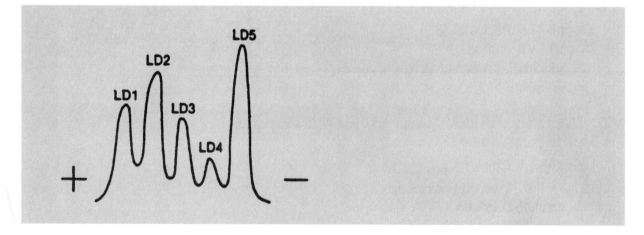

Which of the following is the most likely interpretation of the LD isoenzyme scan illustrated on the previous page?

a. myocardial infarction
b. megaloblastic anemia
c. acute pancreatitis
d. viral hepatitis

145. Blood specimens for digoxin assays should be obtained between 8 hours or more after drug administration because:

a. tissue and serum levels need to reach equilibrium
b. serum digoxin concentration will be falsely low prior to 6 hours
c. all of the digoxin is in the cellular fraction prior to 6 hours
d. digoxin protein-binding interactions are minimal prior to 6 hours

146. Bioavailability of a drug refers to the:

a. availability for therapeutic administration
b. availability of the protein-bound fraction of the drug
c. drug transformation
d. the fraction of the drug absorbed into the systemic circulation

147. The cyclic antidepressants are classified as:

a. basic drugs
b. neutral drugs
c. acidic drugs
d. structurally cycloparaffinic

148. Zinc protoporphyrin or free erythrocyte protoporphyrin measurements are useful to assess blood concentrations of:

a. lead
b. mercury
c. arsenic
d. beryllium

149. Gas chromatography with the nitrogen/phosphorus detector is the most commonly used technique for the analysis of:

a. digoxin
b. acetylsalicylic acid
c. ethyl alcohol
d. cyclic antidepressants

150. The most widely employed screening technique for drug abuse is:

    a. high-performance liquid chromatography
    b. gas-liquid chromatography
    c. thin layer chromatography
    d. UV spectrophotometry

151. Malic dehydrogenase is added to the aspartate aminotransaminase (AST) reaction to catalyze the conversion of:

    a. alpha-ketoglutarate to aspartate
    b. alpha-ketoglutarate to malate
    c. aspartate to oxalacetate
    d. oxalacetate to malate

152. Phenobarbital is a metabolite of:

    a. primidone
    b. phenytoin
    c. amobarbital
    d. secobarbital

153. Increased serum albumin concentrations are seen in which of the following conditions?

    a. nephrotic syndrome
    b. acute hepatitis
    c. chronic inflammation
    d. dehydration

154. Which of the following amino acids is associated with a sulfhydryl group?

    a. cysteine
    b. glycine
    c. serine
    d. tyrosine

155. Beriberi is associated with deficiency of:

    a. vitamin A
    b. vitamin C
    c. niacin
    d. thiamine

156. Night blindness is associated with deficiency of which of the following vitamins?

   a. A
   b. C
   c. niacin
   d. thiamine


157. Scurvy is associated with deficiency of which of the following vitamins?

   a. A
   b. C
   c. niacin
   d. thiamine


158. Pellagra is associated with deficiency of which of the following vitamins?

   a. A
   b. $B_1$
   c. thiamine
   d. niacin


159. Rickets is associated with deficiency of which of the following vitamins?

   a. $B_1$
   b. C
   c. niacin
   d. D


160. The regulation of calcium and phosphorus metabolism is accomplished by which of the following glands?

   a. thyroid
   b. parathyroid
   c. adrenal glands
   d. pituitary


161. Lithium therapy is widely used in the treatment of:

   a. hypertension
   b. hyperactivity
   c. aggression
   d. manic-depression

162. The anticonvulsant used to control tonic-clonic (grand mal) seizures is:

    a. digoxin
    b. acetaminophen
    c. lithium
    d. phenytoin


163. A drug that relaxes the smooth muscles of the bronchial passages is:

    a. acetaminophen
    b. lithium
    c. phenytoin
    d. theophylline


164. A cardiac glycoside that is used in the treatment of congenital heart failure and arrhythmias by increasing the force and velocity of myocardial contraction is:

    a. digoxin
    b. acetaminophen
    c. lithium
    d. phenytoin


165. A carbonate salt used to control manic-depressive disorders is:

    a. digoxin
    b. acetaminophen
    c. lithium
    d. phenytoin


166. In which of the following disease states is conjugated bilirubin a major serum component?

    a. biliary obstruction
    b. hemolysis
    c. neonatal jaundice
    d. erythroblastosis fetalis


167. Spectrophotometers isolate a narrow band pass by means of:

    a. filters and prisms
    b. prisms and grating
    c. barrier layer cells and filters
    d. gratings and lanier layer cells

168. Refer to the following illustration:

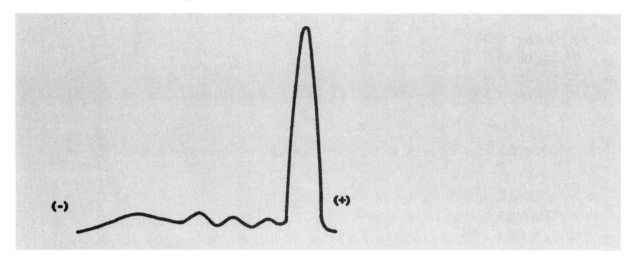

The serum protein electrophoresis pattern shown below was obtained on cellulose acetate at pH 8.6. Identify the serum protein fraction on the far right of the illustration.

a. gamma globulin
b. albumin
c. alpha-1 globulin
d. alpha-2 globulin

169. The creatinine clearance (mL/min) is equal to:

a. urinary creatinine (mg/L)/[volume of urine (mL/min) x plasma creatinine (mg/L)]
b. [urinary creatinine (mg/L) x volume (mL/min)]/plasma creatinine (mg/L)
c. urinary creatinine (mg/L)/[volume of urine (mL/hour) x plasma creatinine (mg/L)]
d. [urinary creatinine (mg/L) x volume (mL/hour)]/plasma creatinine (mg/L)

170. A solution contains 20 g of solute dissolved in 0.5 L of water. What is the percentage of this solution?

a. 2%
b. 4%
c. 6%
d. 8%

171. Which of the following is the formula for calculating the unknown concentration based on Beer's law (A = absorbance, C = concentration)?

a. (A unknown/A standard) x C standard
b. C standard x A unknown
c. A standard x A unknown
d. (C standard)/(A standard) x 100

172. Which of the following is the formula for calculating absorbance given the percent transmittance (%T) of a solution?

    a.  1 – log of %T
    b.  log of %T/2
    c.  2 x log of %T
    d.  2 – log of %T

173. Which of the following is the formula for calculating the amount of moles of a chemical?

    a.  g/GMW
    b.  g x GMW
    c.  GMW/g
    d.  (g x 100)/GMW

174. How many milliliters of a 3% solution can be made if 6 g of solute are available?

    a.  100 mL
    b.  200 mL
    c.  400 mL
    d.  600 mL

175. Which of the following is the formula for calculating the gram equivalent weight of a chemical?

    a.  MW x oxidation number
    b.  MW/oxidation number
    c.  MW + oxidation number
    d.  MW – oxidation number

176. Which of the following is the formula for calculating the dilution of a solution (V = volume, C = concentration)?

    a.  V1 + C1 = V2 + C2
    b.  V1 + C2 = V2 + C1
    c.  V1 x C1 = V2 x C2
    d.  V1 x V2 = V1 x C2

177. Which of the following is the Henderson-Hasselbalch equation?

    a.  pKa = pH + log(acid/salt)
    b.  pKa = pH + log(salt/acid)
    c.  pH = pKa + log(acid/salt)
    d.  pH = pKa + log(salt/acid)

178. Which of the following is the formula for calculating a percent (w/v) solution?

    a. grams of solute/volume of solvent x 100
    b. grams of solute x volume of solvent x 100
    c. volume of solvent/grams of solute x 100
    d. (grams of solute x volume of solvent)/100

179. Which of the following is the formula for coefficient of variation?

    a. (standard deviation x 100)/standard error
    b. (mean x 100)/standard deviation
    c. (standard deviation x 100)/mean
    d. (variance x 100)/mean

180. Given the following values:

    100
    120
    150
    140
    130

What is the mean?

    a. 100
    b. 128
    c. 130
    d. 640

181. Which of the following is the formula for arithmetic mean?

    a. square root of the sum of values
    b. sum of values x number of values
    c. number of values/sum of values
    d. sum of values/number of values

182. Which of the following is the formula for calculating the molarity of a solution?

    a. number of moles of solute/L of solution
    b. number of moles of solute x 100
    c. 1 GEW of solute x 10
    d. 1 GEW of solute/L of solution

183. The following results were obtained:

| | |
|---|---|
| Urine creatinine | 90 mg/100 mL |
| Serum creatinine | 0.90 mg/100 mL |
| Patient's total body surface | 1.73 m² (average = 1.73 m²) |
| Total urine volume in 24 hours | 1500 mL |

Given the above data, calculate the patient's creatinine clearance in mL/min.

a. 104
b. 124
c. 144
d. 150

184. 25 g of NaOH (MW = 40) is added to 0.5 L of water. What is the molarity of this solution if an additional 0.25 L of water is added to this solution?

a. 0.25 M
b. 0.50 M
c. 0.75 M
d. 0.83 M

185. 4 mL of water is added to 1 mL of serum. This represents which of the following serum dilutions?

a. 1:3
b. 1:4
c. 1:5
d. 1:6

186. 80 g of NaOH (MW = 40) is how many gram-equivalents?

a. 1
b. 2
c. 3
d. 4

187. How many grams of $H_2SO_4$ (MW = 98) are in 750 mL of 3 N $H_2SO_4$?

a. 36 g
b. 72 g
c. 110 g
d. 146 g

188. What is the normality of a solution that contains 280 g of NaOH (MW = 40) in 2000 mL of solution?

   a. 3.5 N
   b. 5.5 N
   c. 7.0 N
   d. 8.0 N

189. A serum potassium is 19.5 mg/100 mL. This value is equal to how many mEq/L (MW of K = 39)?

   a. 3.9
   b. 4.2
   c. 5.0
   d. 8.9

190. How many milliliters of 0.25 N NaOH are needed to make 100 mL of a 0.05 N solution of NaOH?

   a. 5 mL
   b. 10 mL
   c. 15 mL
   d. 20 mL

191. An arterial blood specimen submitted for blood gas analysis was obtained at 8:30 AM but was not received in the laboratory until 11:00 AM. The technologist should:

   a. perform the test immediately upon receipt
   b. perform the test only if the specimen was submitted in ice water
   c. request a venous blood specimen
   d. request a new arterial specimen be obtained

192. A potassium level of 6.8 mEq/L is obtained. Before reporting the results, the first step the technologist should take is to:

   a. check the serum for hemolysis
   b. rerun the test
   c. check the age of the patient
   d. do nothing, simply report the result

193. Specimens for blood gas determination should be drawn into a syringe containing:

   a. no preservative
   b. heparin
   c. EDTA
   d. oxalate

194. A patient has the following test results:

Increased serum calcium levels
Decreased serum phosphorus levels
Increased levels of parathyroid hormone

This patient most likely has:

a. hyperparathyroidism
b. hypoparathyroidism
c. nephrosis
d. steatorrhea

195. If the total bilirubin is 4.3 mg/dL and the conjugated bilirubin is 2.1 mg/dL, the unconjugated bilirubin is:

a. 1.1 mg/dL
b. 2.2 mg/dL
c. 4.2 mg/dL
d. 6.3 mg/dL

196. The measurement of light scattered by particles in the sample is the principle of:

a. spectrophotometry
b. fluorometry
c. nephelometry
d. atomic absorption

197. The measurement of the amount of electricity passing between two electrodes in an electrochemical cell is the principle of:

a. electrophoresis
b. amperometry
c. nephelometry
d. coulometry

198. Coulometry is used to measure:

a. chloride
b. pH
c. bicarbonate
d. ammonia

199. Which of the following lipid results would be expected to be falsely elevated on a serum specimen from a nonfasting patient?

a. cholesterol
b. triglyceride
c. HDL
d. LDL

200. Turbidity in serum suggests elevation of:

a. cholesterol
b. total protein
c. chylomicrons
d. albumin

201. Which of the following would be an example of a glucose-specific colorimetric method?

a. alkaline ferricyanide
b. glucose oxidase
c. hexokinase
d. o-toluidine

202. The relative migration rate of proteins on cellulose acetate is based on:

a. molecular weight
b. concentration
c. ionic charge
d. particle size

203. As part of a hyperlipidemia screening program, the following results were obtained on a 25-year-old woman 6 hours after eating:

| Triglycerides | 260 mg/dL |
| Cholesterol | 120 mg/dL |

Which of the following is the BEST interpretation of these results?

a. Both results are normal and not affected by the recent meal.
b. The cholesterol is normal but the triglycerides are elevated, which may be attributed to the recent meal.
c. Both results are elevated, indicating a metabolic problem in addition to the nonfasting state.
d. Both results are below normal despite the recent meal, indicating a metabolic problem.

204. Enzyme-multiplied immunoassay techniques (EMIT) differ from all other types of enzyme immunoassays in that:

a. lysozyme is the only enzyme used to label the hapten molecule
b. no separation of bound and free antigen is required
c. inhibition of the enzyme label is accomplished with polyethyleneglycol
d. antibody absorption to polystyrene tubes precludes competition to labeled and unlabeled antigen

205. Refer to the following graph:

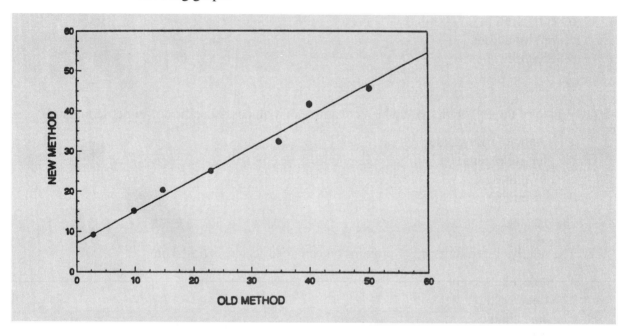

A new methodology for amylase has been developed and compared with the existing method as illustrated in the graph shown above. The new method can be described as:

a. poor correlation with constant bias
b. good correlation with constant bias
c. poor correlation with no bias
d. good correlation with no bias

206. A 48-year-old woman with mild jaundice has the following serum enzyme results:

| | |
|---|---|
| Alkaline phosphatase (untreated) | 600 U/L (adult: 0-150 U/L) |
| Gamma-glutamyl transferase | 230 U/L (normal: 0-55 U/L) |
| Alkaline phosphatase after 10 minutes' incubation at 56°C | 300 U/L (50% of original activity) |
| AST | 400 U/L (normal: 0-50 U/L) |

Which of the following sources most contributes to the patient's serum alkaline phosphatase activity?

a. bone
b. liver
c. placenta
d. Regan isoenzyme

207. A potentiometric electrode that measures an analyte that passes through a selectively permeable membrane and rapidly enters into an equilibrium with an electrolyte solution is:

a. pH
b. $PCO_2$
c. $PO_2$
d. $HCO_3^-$

208. Ion selective electrodes are called selective rather than specific because they actually measure the:

a. activity of one ion only
b. concentration of one ion
c. activity of one ion much more than other ions present
d. concentration and activity of one ion only

209. An automated method for measuring chloride that generates silver ions in the reaction is:

a. coulometry
b. mass spectroscopy
c. chromatography
d. polarography

210. A patient's values are as follows:

|  | Patient | Reference Range |
|---|---|---|
| $T_4$ (RIA) | 4 µg/dL | 5-12 µg/dL |
| $T_3$ Uptake (RIA) | 40% | 25%-35% |

What is the patient's free thyroxine index?

a. 0.1
b. 1.6
c. 10.0
d. 36.0

211. A person suspected of having metabolic alkalosis would have which of the following laboratory findings?

    a. $CO_2$ content and $PCO_2$ elevated, pH decreased
    b. $CO_2$ content decreased and pH elevated
    c. $CO_2$ content, $PCO_2$, and pH decreased
    d. $CO_2$ content and pH elevated

212. Refer to the following graph:

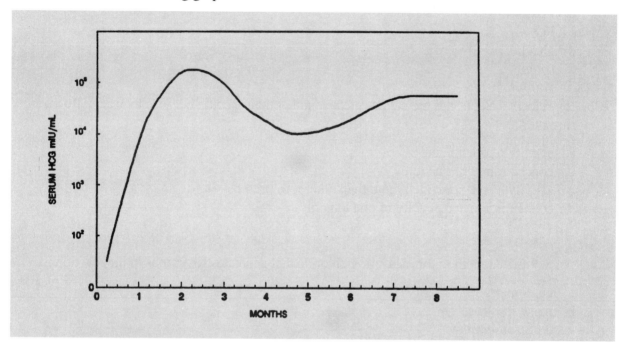

The HCG levels shown in the above graph most probably represent:

    a. hydatidiform mole following miscarriage at 4 months
    b. normal pregnancy
    c. development of hydatidiform mole
    d. miscarriage at 2 months with retained placenta

213. Fluctuation of the needle on a coulometric type titrator is most probably due to:

    a. common ion effect
    b. lack of indicator
    c. faulty reference voltage
    d. dirty electrodes

214. Iodine 125 has a physical half-life of 60.0 days. A sample tested today had activity of 10,000 CPM/mL. How many days from today will the count be 1250 CPM/mL?

a. 60
b. 180
c. 240
d. 1250


215. Which of the following is most likely to be ordered in addition to serum calcium to determine the cause of tetany?

a. magnesium
b. phosphorus
c. sodium
d. vitamin D


216. A 9-month-old boy from Israel has gradually lost the ability to sit up and develops seizures. He has an increased amount of a phospholipid called $GM_2$-ganglioside in his neurons, and he lacks the enzyme hexosaminidase A in his leukocytes. These findings suggest:

a. Neimann-Pick disease
b. Tay-Sachs disease
c. phenylketonuria
d. Hurler's syndrome


217. An adult diabetic with renal complications has the following results:

| | |
|---|---|
| Sodium | 133 mEq/L |
| BUN | 84 mg/dL |
| Glucose | 487 mg/dL |
| Creatinine | 5 mg/dL |

On the basis of these results, the calculated serum osmolality is:

a. 266 mOsm/kg
b. 290 mOsm/kg
c. 304 mOsm/kg
d. 709 mOsm/kg


218. The formation of estriol in a pregnant woman is dependent on:

a. maternal ovarian function
b. fetal and placental function
c. fetal adrenal function
d. maternal liver function

219. Arterial blood collected in a heparinized syringe but exposed to room air would cause which of the following changes in the specimen?

| | PO$_2$ | PCO$_2$ | pH |
|---|---|---|---|
| a. | elevated | decreased | elevated |
| b. | decreased | elevated | decreased |
| c. | unchanged | elevated | unchanged |
| d. | decreased | decreased | decreased |

220. Magnesium carbonate is added in an iron binding capacity determination in order to:

a. allow color to develop
b. precipitate protein
c. bind with hemoglobin iron
d. remove excess unbound iron

221. An elevated serum iron with normal iron binding capacity is most likely associated with:

a. iron deficiency anemia
b. renal damage
c. pernicious anemia
d. septicemia

222. A patient's blood was drawn at 8 AM for a serum iron determination. The result was 85 μg/dL. A repeat specimen was drawn at 8 PM; the serum was stored at 4°C and run the next morning. The result was 40 μg/dL. These results are most likely due to:

a. iron deficiency anemia
b. improper storage of the specimen
c. possible liver damage
d. the time of day the second specimen was drawn

223. A patient with glomerulonephritis would present the following serum results:

a. creatinine decreased
b. calcium increased
c. phosphorus decreased
d. BUN increased

224. Absorption of vitamin B$_{12}$ requires the presence of:

a. intrinsic factor
b. gastrin
c. secretin
d. folic acid

225. Refer to the following illustration:

The above symbol posted in an area would indicate which of the following hazards?

a. flammable
b. electrical
c. radiation
d. biohazard

226. A 68-year-old man arrives in the emergency room with a glucose level of 722 mg/dL and serum acetone of 4+ undiluted. An arterial blood gas from this patient is likely to indicate which of the following?

a. low pH
b. high pH
c. low $PO_2$
d. high $PO_2$

227. What battery of tests is most useful in evaluating an anion gap of 22 mEq/L?

a. $Ca^{++}$, $Mg^{++}$, $PO^{-4}$, and pH
b. BUN, creatinine, salicylate, and methanol
c. AST, ALT, LD, and amylase
d. glucose, CK, myoglobin, and cryoglobulin

228. Serum levels that define hypoglycemia in preterm or low birth weight infants are:

a. the same as in adults
b. lower than in adults
c. the same as in a normal full-term infant
d. higher than in a normal full-term infant

229. Oligoclonal bands are present on electrophoresis of concentrated CSF and also on concurrently tested serum of the same patient. The proper interpretation is:

    a. diagnostic for primary CNS tumor
    b. diagnostic for multiple sclerosis
    c. CNS involvement by acute leukemia
    d. nondiagnostic for multiple sclerosis

230. In developing the reference for a new EIA for CEA, the range for the normal population was broader than that published by the vendor. Controls are acceptable with a narrow coefficient of variation. This may be explained by:

    a. positive interference by another tumor marker
    b. population skewed to a younger age
    c. improper temperature control during assay
    d. inclusion of nonsmokers and smokers in the study population

231. Most automated blood gas analyzers directly measure:

    a. pH, $HCO_3^-$, and % $O_2$ saturation
    b. pH, $PCO_2$, and $PO_2$
    c. $HCO_3^-$, $PCO_2$, and $PO_2$
    d. pH, $PO_2$, and % $O_2$ saturation

232. In the assay of lactate dehydrogenase (LD), the reaction is dependent on which of the following coenzyme systems?

    a. NAD/NADH
    b. ATP/ADP
    c. $Fe^{++}/Fe^{+++}$
    d. $Cu/Cu^{++}$

233. Creatinine clearance is used to estimate the:

    a. tubular secretion of creatinine
    b. glomerular secretion of creatinine
    c. renal glomerular and tubular mass
    d. glomerular filtration rate

234. A pH of 7.0 represents a $H^+$ concentration of:

    a. 70 mEq/L
    b. 10 μmol/L
    c. 7 nmol/L
    d. 100 nmol/L

235. The chemical composition of HDL-cholesterol corresponds to:

| | Triglyceride | Cholesterol | Protein |
|---|---|---|---|
| a. | 60% | 15% | 10% |
| b. | 10% | 45% | 25% |
| c. | 5% | 15% | 50% |
| d. | 85% | 5% | 2% |

236. The principle of the tablet test for bilirubin in urine or feces is:

    a. the reaction between bile and 2,4-dichloronitrobenzene to a yellow color
    b. the liberation of oxygen by bile to oxidize orthotolidine to a blue-purple color
    c. chemical coupling of bile with a diazonium salt to form a brown color
    d. chemical coupling of bilirubin with a diazonium salt to form a purple color

237. To make up 1 L of 1.000 N NaOH from a 1.025 N NaOH solution, how many milliliters of the NaOH should be used?

    a. 950.0
    b. 975.6
    c. 997.5
    d. 1025.0

238. If 0.5 mL of a 1:300 dilution contains 1 antigenic unit, 2 antigenic units would be contained in 0.5 mL of a dilution of:

    a. 1:150
    b. 1:450
    c. 1:500
    d. 1:600

239. If the $pK_a$ is 6.1, the $CO_2$ content is 25 mmol/L, the salt equals the total $CO_2$ content minus the carbonic acid, the carbonic acid equals 0.03 x $PCO_2$, and $PCO_2$ is 40 mm Hg, it may be concluded that:

    a. $pH = 6.1 + \log [(40 - 0.03)/(0.03)]$
    b. $pH = 6.1 + \log [(25 - 0.03)/(0.03)]$
    c. $pH = 6.1 + \log [(25 - 1.2)/(1.2)]$
    d. $pH = 6.1 + \log [(1.2)/(1.2 - 25)]$

240. Blood was collected in a serum separator tube from a patient who had been fasting since midnight. The time of collection was 7:00 AM. The laboratory test that should be re-collected is:

    a. triglycerides
    b. iron
    c. LD
    d. sodium

241. The cellulose acetate electrophoresis at pH 8.6 of serum proteins will show an order of migration beginning with the fastest migration as follows:

    a. albumin, alpha-1 globulin, alpha-2 globulin, beta globulin, gamma globulin
    b. alpha-1 globulin, alpha-2 globulin, beta globulin, gamma globulin, albumin
    c. albumin, alpha-2 globulin, alpha-1 globulin, beta globulin, gamma globulin
    d. gamma globulin, beta globulin, alpha-2 globulin, alpha-1 globulin, albumin

242. The TRH (thyrotropin-releasing hormone) stimulation test is useful in assessing which of the following?

    a. TRH concentration
    b. iodine deficiency
    d. depression
    d. hyperthyroidism

243. A patient has the following results:

|  | Patient Values | Reference Values |
|---|---|---|
| Serum iron | 250 µg/dL | 60-150 µg/dL |
| TIBC | 350 µg/dL | 300-350 µg/dL |

The best conclusion is that this patient has:

    a. normal iron status
    b. iron deficiency anemia
    c. chronic disease
    d. iron hemachromatosis

244. Which of the following elevates carboxyhemoglobin?

    a. nitrite poisoning
    b. exposure to carbon monoxide
    c. sulfa drug toxicity
    d. sickle cell anemia

245. A patient is admitted to the emergency room in a state of metabolic alkalosis. Which of the following would be consistent with this diagnosis?

    a. high $TCO_2$, increased $HCO_3$
    b. low $TCO_2$, increased $HCO_3$
    c. high $TCO_2$, decreased $H_2CO_3$
    d. low $TCO_2$, decreased $H_2CO_3$

246. For the past 3 weeks serum estriol levels in a pregnant woman have been steadily increasing. This is consistent with:

a. a normal pregnancy
b. hemolytic disease of the newborn
c. fetal death
d. congenital cytomegalovirus infection

247. In the atomic absorption method for calcium, lanthanum is used:

a. as an internal standard
b. to bind calcium
c. to eliminate protein interference
d. to prevent phosphate interference

248. A patient has the following thyroid profile:

| | |
|---|---|
| Total $T_4$ | Increased |
| Free thyroxine index | Normal |
| $T_3$ uptake | Decreased |
| TSH | Normal |

This patient most probably:

a. is hyperthyroid
b. is hypothyroid
c. has a pituitary adenoma
d. has increased protein-bound $T_4$

249. The following data were calculated on a series of 30 determinations of serum uric acid control: mean = 5.8 mg/dL, 1 standard deviation = 0.15 mg/dL. If confidence limits are set at ± 2 standard deviations, which of the following represents the allowable limits for the control?

a. 5.65-5.95 mg/dL
b. 5.35-6.25 mg/dL
c. 5.50-6.10 mg/dL
d. 5.70-5.90 mg/dL

250. The reason carbon monoxide is so toxic is because it:

a. is a protoplasmic poison
b. combines with cytochrome oxidase
c. has 200 times the affinity of oxygen for hemoglobin binding sites
d. sensitizes the myocardium

251. Clinical assays for tumor markers are most important for:

a. screening for the presence of cancer
b. monitoring the course of a known cancer
c. confirming the absence of disease
d. identifying patients at risk for cancer

252. Estrogen and progesterone receptor assays are useful in assessing prognosis in which of the following?

a. ovarian cancer
b. breast cancer
c. endometriosis
d. amenorrhea

253. A chemiluminescent EIA:

a. measures absorption of light
b. is less sensitive than radioisotopic reactions
c. is monitored by the use of a gamma counter
d. is quantitated by the amount of light produced by the reaction

254. The selectivity of an ion-selective electrode is determined by the:

a. properties of the membrane used
b. solution used to fill the electrode
c. magnitude of the potential across the membrane
d. internal reference electrode

255. Valinomycin enhances the selectivity of the electrode used to quantitate:

a. sodium
b. chloride
c. potassium
d. calcium

256. A 45-year-old woman has a fasting serum glucose concentration of 95 mg/dL and a 2-hour postprandial glucose concentration of 105 mg/dL. The statement that best describes this patient's fasting serum glucose concentration is:

a. normal, reflecting glycogen breakdown by the liver
b. normal, reflecting glycogen breakdown by skeletal muscle
c. abnormal, indicating diabetes mellitus
d. abnormal, indicating hypoglycemia

257. An HPLC operator notes that the column pressure is too high, is rising too rapidly, and the recorder output is not producing normal peaks. The most probable cause of the problem is:

 a. not enough sample injected
 b. bad sample detector
 c. effluent line obstructed
 d. strip chart motor hanging-up

258. An infant with diarrhea is being evaluated for a carbohydrate intolerance. His stool yields a positive copper reduction test and a pH of 5.0. It should be concluded that:

 a. further tests are indicated
 b. results are inconsistent, repeat both tests
 c. the diarrhea is not due to carbohydrate intolerance
 d. the tests provided no useful information

259. In a centrifugal analyzer, centrifugal force is used to:

 a. add reagents to the rotor
 b. transfer liquids from the inner disc to the outer cuvette
 c. measure changes in optical density in the centrifugal force field
 d. counteract the tendency of precipitates to settle in the cuvette

260. A fasting serum sample from an asymptomatic 43-year-old woman is examined visually and chemically with the following results:

Initial appearance of serum: Milky
Appearance of serum after overnight refrigeration: Cream layer over turbid serum
Triglyceride level: 2000 mg/dL
Cholesterol level: 550 mg/dL

This sample contains predominantly:

 a. chylomicrons alone
 b. chylomicrons and very-low-density lipoproteins (VLDL)
 c. very-low-density lipoproteins (VLDL) and low-density lipoproteins (LDL)
 d. high-density lipoproteins (HDL)

261. Factors that contribute to a $PCO_2$ electrode's requiring 60-120 seconds to reach equilibrium include the:

 a. diffusion characteristics of the membrane
 b. actual blood $PO_2$
 c. type of calibrating standard (ie, liquid or humidified gas)
 d. potential of the polarizing mercury cell

262. In which of the following conditions would a NORMAL level of creatine kinase be found?

    a. acute myocardial infarct
    b. hepatitis
    c. progressive muscular dystrophy
    d. intramuscular injection


263. The direction in which albumin migrates (ie, toward anode or cathode) during electrophoretic separation of serum proteins, at pH 8.6, is determined by:

    a. the ionization of the amine groups, yielding a net positive charge
    b. the ionization of the carboxyl groups, yielding a net negative charge
    c. albumin acting as a zwitterion
    d. the density of the gel layer


264. In a double-beam photometer, the additional beam is used to:

    a. compensate for variation in wavelength
    b. correct for variations in light source intensity
    c. correct for changes in light path
    d. compensate for variation in slit widths


265. Gel filtration chromatography is used to separate:

    a. polar and nonpolar compounds
    b. compounds on the basis of molecular weight and size
    c. isomers of the same compound
    d. compounds on the basis of different functional groups


266. Aminotransferase enzymes catalyze the:

    a. exchange of amino groups and sulfhydryl groups between alpha-amino and sulfur-containing acids
    b. exchange of amino and keto groups between alpha-amino and alpha-keto acids
    c. hydrolysis of amino acids and keto acids
    d. reversible transfer of hydrogen from amino acids to coenzyme


267. Ninety percent of the copper present in plasma is bound to:

    a. transferrin
    b. ceruloplasmin
    c. albumin
    d. immunoglobulin


268. In lipoprotein phenotyping, chylomicrons are present in the plasma of persons with which of the following lipoprotein phenotypes?

    a. I and IIa
    b. I and IIb
    c. II and III
    d. I and V

269. A 600 mg/dL glucose solution is diluted 1:30. The concentration of the final solution in mg/dL is:

    a. 2
    b. 20
    c. 180
    d. 1800


270. Monitoring long-term glucose control in patients with adult onset diabetes mellitus can best be accomplished by measuring:

    a. weekly fasting 7 AM serum glucose
    b. glucose tolerance testing
    c. 2-hour postprandial serum glucose
    d. hemoglobin $A_{1c}$


271. Of the following diseases, the one most often associated with elevations of lactate dehydrogenase isoenzymes 4 and 5 on electrophoresis is:

    a. liver disease
    b. hemolytic anemia
    c. myocardial infarction
    d. pulmonary edema


272. The following five sodium control values (mEq/L) were obtained:

    140, 135, 138, 140, 142

    Calculate the coefficient of variation.

    a. 1.9%
    b. 2.7%
    c. 5.6%
    d. 6.1%


273. A spectrophotometer is being considered for purchase by a small laboratory. Which of the following specifications reflects the spectral purity of the instrument?

    a. photomultiplier tube
    b. dark current
    c. band width
    d. galvanometer

274. An LD1 greater than LD2 fraction of lactic dehydrogenase is most often associated with:

   a. alcoholic hepatitis
   b. pulmonary disease
   c. myocardial infarction
   d. muscular dystrophy

275. How many milliliters of 30% bovine albumin are needed to make 6 mL of a 10% albumin solution?

   a. 1
   b. 2
   c. 3
   d. 4

276. Which of the following substrates provides the best specificity for prostatic acid phosphatase?

   a. D-isocitrate
   b. thymolphthalein monophosphate
   c. 2-oxoglutarate
   d. butyrylthiocholine ion

277. A lipemic serum is separated and frozen at $-20°C$ for assay at a later date. One week later, prior to performing an assay for triglycerides, the specimen should be:

   a. warmed to 37°C and mixed thoroughly
   b. warmed to 15°C and centrifuged
   c. transferred to a glycerated test tube
   d. discarded and a new specimen obtained

278. In the proper use of cobalt-treated anhydrous $CaCl_2$, the desiccant should be:

   a. changed when it turns pink
   b. changed when it turns blue
   c. kept in the dark
   d. kept in the cold

279. A serum sample was assayed for bilirubin at 10 AM and the result was 12 mg/dL. The same sample was retested at 3 PM. The result now is 8 mg/dL. The most likely explanation for this discrepancy is:

   a. the reagent has deteriorated
   b. the sample was exposed to light
   c. a calculation error in the first assay
   d. the sample was not refrigerated

280. To prepare a physiologic saline solution, dissolve:

    a. 85 g NaCl in 1 L $H_2O$
    b. 8.5 g NaCl in 1 L $H_2O$
    c. 0.85 g NaCl in 1 L $H_2O$
    d. 85 mg NaCl in 100 mL $H_2O$

281. A chemistry assay utilizes a bichromatic analysis. This means that absorbance readings are taken at:

    a. two wavelengths so that two compounds can be measured at the same time
    b. two wavelengths to correct for spectral interference from another compound
    c. the beginning and end of a time interval to measure the absorbance change
    d. two times and then are averaged to obtain a more accurate result

282. Serial bilirubin determinations are charted below with the best explanation for the results due to:

| Day | Collected | Assayed | Result |
| --- | --- | --- | --- |
| 1 | 7 AM | 8 AM | 14.0 mg/dL |
| 2 | 7 AM | 6 PM | 9.0 mg/dL |
| 3 | 6 AM | 8 AM | 15.0 mg/dL |

    a. sample hemolysis and hemoglobin deterioration
    b. sample exposure to light
    c. sample left in warm location
    d. reagent deterioration

283. In familial hypercholesterolemia, the hallmark finding is an elevation of:

    a. low-density lipoproteins
    b. chylomicrons
    c. high-density lipoproteins
    d. apolipoprotein AI

284. Pregnant women with symptoms of thirst, frequent urination, or unexplained weight loss should have which of the following tests performed?

    a. tolbutamide test
    b. lactose tolerance test
    c. epinephrine tolerance test
    d. glucose tolerance test

285. The most consistent analytical error involved in the routine determination of HDL-cholesterol is caused by:

    a. incomplete precipitation of LDL-cholesterol
    b. coprecipitation of HDL and LDL-cholesterol
    c. inaccurate protein estimation of HDL-cholesterol
    d. a small concentration of APO-B containing lipoproteins after precipitation

286. Nephelometers measure light:

    a. scattered at a right angle to the light path
    b. absorbed by suspended particles
    c. transmitted by now-particulate mixtures
    d. reflected back to the source from opaque suspensions

287. What substance gives feces its normal color?

    a. uroerythrin
    b. urochrome
    c. urobilin
    d. urobilinogen

288. Premature atherosclerosis can occur when which of the following becomes elevated?

    a. chylomicrons
    b. prostaglandins
    c. low density lipoproteins
    d. high density lipoproteins

289. If the LDL-cholesterol is to be calculated by the Friedenwald formula, what are the two measurements that need to be carried out by the same chemical procedure?

    a. total cholesterol and HDL-cholesterol
    b. total cholesterol and triglyceride
    c. triglyceride and chylomicrons
    d. apolipoprotein A and apolipoprotein B

290. High levels of which lipoprotein class are associated with decreased risk of accelerated atherosclerosis?

    a. chylomicrons
    b. VLDL
    c. LDL
    d. HDL

291. Following overnight fasting, hypoglycemia in adults is defined as a glucose of:

    a. ≤ 70 mg/dL
    b. ≤ 60 mg/dL
    c. ≤ 55 mg/dL
    d. ≤ 45 mg/dL

292. The first step in the quantitation of serum iron is:

    a. direct reaction with appropriate chromogen
    b. iron saturation of transferrin
    c. free iron precipitation
    d. separation of iron from transferrin

293. The principle of the occult blood test depends on the:

    a. coagulase ability of blood
    b. oxidative power of atmospheric oxygen
    c. hydrogen peroxide in hemoglobin
    d. peroxidase-like activity of hemoglobin

294. In an internal standard flame photometer, the internal standard is used to:

    a. correct for errors in making dilutions
    b. help in separating the sodium and potassium signals
    c. correct for variations in flame and atomizer characteristics
    d. give a direct reading in concentration

295. Which of the following wavelengths is within the ultraviolet range?

    a. 340 nm
    b. 450 nm
    c. 540 nm
    d. 690 nm

296. A glucose determination was read on a spectrophotometer. The absorbance reading of the standard was 0.30. The absorbance reading of the unknown was 0.20. The value of the unknown is:

    a. two thirds of the standard
    b. three fifths of the standard
    c. the same as the standard
    d. one and a half times the standard

297. Aspartate aminotransferase (AST) is characteristically elevated in diseases of the:

   a. liver
   b. kidney
   c. intestine
   d. pancreas

298. The enzyme that exists chiefly in skeletal muscle, heart, and brain; is grossly elevated in active muscular dystrophy; and rises early in myocardial infarction is:

   a. lipase
   b. transaminase
   c. lactate dehydrogenase
   d. creatine kinase

299. The primary function of serum albumin in the peripheral blood is to:

   a. maintain colloidal osmotic pressure
   b. increase antibody production
   c. increase fibrinogen formation
   d. maintain blood viscosity

300. Most chemical methods for determining total protein utilize which of the following reactions?

   a. molybdenum blue
   b. ferri-ferrocyanide
   c. resorcinol-HCl
   d. biuret

301. The mean value of a series of hemoglobin controls was found to be 15.2 g/dL, and the standard deviation was calculated at 0.20. Acceptable control range for the laboratory is ± 2 standard deviations. Which of the following represents the allowable limits for the control?

   a. 14.5-15.5 g/dL
   b. 15.0-15.4 g/dL
   c. 15.2-15.6 g/dL
   d. 14.8-15.6 g/dL

302. The presence of C-reactive protein in the blood is an indication of:

   a. a recent streptococcal infection
   b. recovery from a pneumococcal infection
   c. an inflammatory process
   d. a state of hypersensitivity

303. Chromatography is based on the principle of:

   a. differential solubility
   b. gravity
   c. vapor pressure
   d. temperature

304. The $T_3$-uptake test is based on:

   a. binding of $T_4$ to charcoal
   b. stimulation of the thyroid by TSH
   c. stimulation of the thyroid by $T_3$
   d. relative binding of $T_3$ and $T_4$ to globulin

305. The most specific method for the assay of glucose utilizes:

   a. hexokinase
   b. glucose oxidase
   c. glucose-6-phosphatase
   d. glucose dehydrogenase

306. The enzyme present in almost all tissues that may be separated by electrophoresis into five components is:

   a. lipase
   b. transaminase
   c. creatine kinase
   d. lactate dehydrogenase

307. In quality control, ± 2 standard deviations from the mean includes what percent of the sample population?

   a. 50
   b. 75
   c. 95
   d. 98

308. The term used to describe reproducibility is:

   a. sensitivity
   b. specificity
   c. accuracy
   d. precision

309. When 0.25 mL is diluted to 20 mL, the resulting dilution is:

 a. 1:20
 b. 1:40
 c. 1:60
 d. 1:80


310. The extent to which measurements agree with or approach the true value of the quantity being measured is referred to as:

 a. accuracy
 b. precision
 c. reproducibility
 d. reliability


311. A breakdown product of hemoglobin is:

 a. lipoprotein
 b. bilirubin
 c. hematoxylin
 d. Bence Jones protein


312. When the exact concentration of the solute of a solution is known and is used to evaluate the concentration of an unknown solution, the known solution is:

 a. standard
 b. normal
 c. control
 d. baseline


313. A serum glucose sample was too high to read, so a 1:5 dilution using saline (dilution A) was made. Dilution A was tested and was again too high to read. A further 1:2 dilution was made using saline (dilution B). To calculate the result, the dilution B value must be multiplied by:

 a. 5
 b. 8
 c. 10
 d. 20


314. In performing a spinal fluid protein determination, the specimen is diluted 1 part spinal fluid to 3 parts saline to obtain a result low enough to measure. To calculate the protein concentration the result must be:

 a. multiplied by 3
 b. multiplied by 4
 c. divided by 3
 d. divided by 4

315. In order to prepare 100 mL of 15 mg/dL BUN working standard from a stock standard containing 500 mg/dL of urea nitrogen, the amount of stock solution used is:

    a. 3 mL
    b. 5 mL
    c. 33 mL
    d. 75 mL

316. In monitoring glomerular function, which of the following tests has the highest sensitivity?

    a. urine sodium
    b. BUN/creatinine ratio
    c. creatinine clearance
    d. urea clearance

317. An automated CK assay gives a reading that is above the limits of linearity. A dilution of the serum sample is made by adding 1 mL of serum to 9 mL of water. The instrument now reads 350 U/L. The correct report on the undiluted serum should be:

    a. 2850 U/L
    b. 3150 U/L
    c. 3500 U/L
    d. 3850 U/L

318. Blood received in the laboratory for blood gas analysis must meet which of the following requirements?

    a. on ice, thin fibrin strands only, no air bubbles
    b. on ice, no clots, fewer than four air bubbles
    c. on ice, no clots, no air bubbles
    d. room temperature, no clots, no air bubbles

319. An electrode has a silver/silver chloride anode and a platinum wire cathode. It is suspended in KCl solution and separated from the blood to be analyzed by a selectively permeable membrane. Such an electrode is used to measure which of the following?

    a. pH
    b. $PCO_2$
    c. $PO_2$
    d. $HCO_3^-$

320. Which blood gas electrode is composed of calomel and glass?

    a. $PO_2$
    b. pH
    c. $CO_2$
    d. $HCO_3^-$

321. A thick white turbid specimen was received in the laboratory labeled as pericardial fluid. A microscopic examination was performed, and the differential included 90% PMNs. The fluid is:

    a. serous
    b. purulent
    c. milky
    d. fibrinous

322. In the assay of lactate dehydrogenase, which of the following products is actually measured?

    a. NADH
    b. ATP
    c. lactic acid
    d. pyruvic acid

323. The sodium content (in grams) in 100 g of NaCl (atomic weights: Na = 23.0, Cl = 35.5) is approximately:

    a. 10
    b. 20
    c. 40
    d. 60

324. Bromcresol purple at a pH of 5.2 is used in a colorimetric method to measure:

    a. albumin
    b. globulin
    c. Bence Jones protein
    d. immunoprotein

325. In spectrophotometry, the device that allows for a narrow band of wavelengths is the:

    a. hollow cathode lamp
    b. monochromator
    c. refractometer
    d. photodetector

326. The following results were obtained from a set of automated white blood cell counts performed on 40 samples:

| Standard deviation | 153.2/$\mu$L |
| Mean value | 12,450/$\mu$L |

Calculate the coefficient of variation.

a. 0.01%
b. 1.2%
c. 2.5%
d. 8.1%

327. If a fasting glucose were 90 mg/dL, which of the following 2-hour postprandial glucose results would most closely represent normal glucose metabolism?

a. 55 mg/dL
b. 100 mg/dL
c. 180 mg/dL
d. 260 mg/dL

328. The following bilirubin results are obtained on a patient:

Day 1: 4.3 mg/dL          Day 4: 2.2 mg/dL
Day 2: 4.6 mg/dL          Day 5: 4.4 mg/dL
Day 3: 4.5 mg/dL          Day 6: 4.5 mg/dL

Given that the controls were within range each day, what is a probable explanation for the result on day 4?

a. no explanation necessary
b. serum, not plasma, was used for testing
c. specimen had prolonged exposure to light
d. specimen was hemolyzed

329. In flame emission photometry, an excited orbital electron returns to ground state and emits:

a. a photon of light with a specific wavelength for the element being measured
b. a measurable current proportional to the concentration of the element being measured
c. a total charge proportional to the energy used in the reduction of the element being measured
d. a constant potential equal to the concentration of the element being measured

330. The first procedure to be followed if the blood gas instrument is out of control for all parameters is:

a. recalibrate, then repeat control
b. repeat control on the next shift
c. replace electrodes, then repeat control
d. report patient results after duplicate testing

331. Which of the following methods for quantitation of high-density lipoprotein is most suited for clinical laboratory use?

   a. Gomori procedure
   b. precipitation
   c. column chromatography
   d. agarose gel electrophoresis

332. Urobilinogen is formed in the:

   a. kidney
   b. spleen
   c. liver
   d. intestine

333. A healthy person with a blood glucose of 80 mg/dL would have a simultaneously determined cerebrospinal fluid glucose value of:

   a. 25
   b. 50
   c. 100
   d. 150

334. Upon completion of a run of cholesterol tests, the technician recognizes that the controls are not within the two standard deviations confidence range. What is the appropriate course of action?

   a. report the results without any other action
   b. run a new set of controls
   c. run a new set of controls and repeat specimens
   d. recalibrate instrument and run controls

335. A technician is asked by the supervisor to prepare a standard solution from the stock standard. What is the glassware of choice for this solution?

   a. graduated cylinder
   b. volumetric flask
   c. acid-washed beaker
   d. graduated flask

336. Slight hemolysis can cause erroneous laboratory results in which serum analyte?

   a. $Ca^{++}$
   b. $Na^{+}$
   c. $K^{+}$
   d. $Cl^{-}$

337. The volume of 25% stock sulfosalicylic acid needed to prepare 100 mL of 5% working solution is:

    a.  1.25 mL
    b.  5 mL
    c.  20 mL
    d.  50 mL

338. A stool specimen that appears black and tarry should be tested for the presence of:

    a.  occult blood
    b.  fecal fat
    c.  trypsin
    d.  excess mucus

339. In bilirubin determinations, the purpose of adding a concentrated caffeine solution or methyl alcohol is to:

    a.  allow indirect bilirubin to react with color reagent
    b.  dissolve conjugated bilirubin
    c.  precipitate protein
    d.  prevent any change in pH

340. To prepare 25 mL of 3% acetic acid, how much glacial acetic acid is needed?

    a.  7.5 mL
    b.  3.0 mL
    c.  1.5 mL
    d.  0.75 mL

341. How many grams of sodium chloride are needed to prepare 1 L of 0.9% normal saline?

    a.  0.9
    b.  1.8
    c.  9.0
    d.  18.0

342. The first step in analyzing a 24-hour urine specimen for quantitative urine protein is:

    a.  subculture the urine for bacteria
    b.  add the appropriate preservative
    c.  screen for albumin using a dipstick
    d.  measure the total volume

343. How many milliliters of reagent are needed to prepare 5 mL of a 1:25 dilution?

   a. 0.1
   b. 0.2
   c. 0.25
   d. 0.5

344. What is the first step in preparing a spectrophotometer for an assay?

   a. adjust wavelength selector
   b. zero with deionized water
   c. read standard absorbance
   d. place a cuvette in the well

345. A 25-year-old man became nauseated and vomited 90 minutes after receiving a standard 75-g carbohydrate dose for an oral glucose tolerance test. The best course of action is:

   a. give the patient a glass of orange juice and continue the test
   b. start the test over immediately with a 50-g carbohydrate dose
   c. draw blood for glucose and discontinue test
   d. place the patient in a recumbent position, reassure him, and continue the test

346. A common cause of a falsely increased LD1 fraction of lactic dehydrogenase is:

   a. specimen hemolysis
   b. liver disease
   c. congestive heart failure
   d. drug toxicity

347. The presence of which of the following isoenzymes indicates acute myocardial damage?

   a. CK-MM
   b. CK-MB
   c. CK-BB
   d. none of the above

348. Cerebrospinal fluid for glucose assay should be:

   a. refrigerated
   b. analyzed immediately
   c. heated to 56°C
   d. stored at room temperature after centrifugation

349. The preparation of a patient for standard glucose tolerance testing should include:

   a. high carbohydrate diet for 3 days
   b. low carbohydrate diet for 3 days
   c. fasting for 48 hours prior to testing
   d. bed rest for 3 days

350. Measurement of the serum acid phosphatase is used to detect neoplastic disease of the:

   a. liver
   b. lung
   c. ovary
   d. prostate

351. A serum sample demonstrates an elevated result when tested with the Jaffe reaction. This indicates:

   a. prolonged hypothermia
   b. renal functional impairment
   c. pregnancy
   d. arrhythmia

352. An increase in serum acetone is indicative of a defect in the metabolism of:

   a. carbohydrates
   b. fat
   c. urea nitrogen
   d. uric acid

353. To prepare 40 mL of a 3% working solution, a technician would use what volume of stock solution?

   a. 0.9 mL
   b. 1.2 mL
   c. 1.5 mL
   d. 3.0 mL

354. A technician is preparing a 75% solution. What volume of stock solution should be used to prepare 8 mL?

   a. 4.5 mL
   b. 6.0 mL
   c. 7.5 mL
   d. 9.4 mL

355. The following results are from a 21-year-old patient with a back injury who appears otherwise healthy:

| | |
|---|---|
| Whole blood glucose | 77 mg/dL |
| Serum glucose | 88 mg/dL |
| CSF glucose | 56 mg/dL |

The best interpretation of these results is that:

a. the whole blood and serum values are expected but the CSF value is elevated
b. the whole blood glucose value should be higher than the serum value
c. all values are consistent with a normal healthy individual
d. the serum and whole blood values should be identical

356. The nanometer is a measurement of:

a. wavelength of radiant energy
b. specific gravity
c. density
d. intensity of light

357. If the total bilirubin is 3.1 mg/dL and the conjugated bilirubin is 2.0 mg/dL, the unconjugated bilirubin is:

a. 0.5 mg/dL
b. 1.1 mg/dL
c. 2.2 mg/dL
d. 5.1 mg/dL

358. The ability of a procedure to measure only the component(s) it claims to measure is called:

a. specificity
b. sensitivity
c. precision
d. reproducibility

359. The most widely used methods for bilirubin measurement are those based on the:

a. Jaffe reaction
b. Schales and Schales method
c. 8-hydroxyquinoline reaction
d. Jendrassik Grof method

360. After a difficult venipuncture requiring prolonged application of the tourniquet, the serum $K^+$ was found to be 6.8 mEq/L. The best course of action is to:

a. repeat the test using the same specimen
b. adjust the value based on the current serum $Na^+$
c. repeat the test using freshly drawn serum
d. cancel the test

361. A serum sample for acid phosphatase determination is best prepared for room temperature storage by:

a. centrifuging for 30 minutes
b. adding an acid stabilizer
c. alkalizing the serum
d. adding NaF

362. Serum from a patient with metastatic carcinoma of the prostate was separated from the clot and stored at room temperature. The following results were obtained:

|  | Patient | Reference Range |
|---|---|---|
| Calcium | 10.8 mg/dL | 8.8-10.3 mg/dL |
| LD | 420 U/L | 50-150 U/L |
| Acid phosphatase | 0.1 U/L | 0-5.5 U/L |

The technician should repeat the:

a. LD using diluted serum
b. acid phosphatase with freshly drawn serum
c. LD with fresh serum
d. tests using plasma

363. When performing a manual protein analysis on a xanthochromic spinal fluid, the technician should:

a. perform the test as usual
b. make a patient blank
c. centrifuge the specimen
d. dilute the specimen with deionized water

364. Which of the following 2-hour postprandial glucose values demonstrates unequivocal hyperglycemia diagnostic for diabetes mellitus?

a. 160 mg/dL
b. 170 mg/dL
c. 180 mg/dL
d. 200 mg/dL

365. The glycosylated hemoglobin value represents a time average of glucose concentration during the preceding:

    a. 1-3 weeks
    b. 4-5 weeks
    c. 8-12 weeks
    d. 16-20 weeks

366. To ensure an accurate ammonia level result, the specimen should be:

    a. incubated at 37°C prior to testing
    b. spun and separated immediately, tested as routine
    c. spun, separated, iced, and tested immediately
    d. stored at room temperature until tested

367. The most specific enzyme test for acute pancreatitis is:

    a. acid phosphatase
    b. trypsin
    c. amylase
    d. lipase

*The remaining questions (\*) have been identified as more appropriate for the entry level medical technologist.*

*368. The procedure used to determine the presence of neural tube defects is:

    a. lecithin/sphingomyelin ratio
    b. amniotic fluid creatinine
    c. measurement of absorbance at 450 nm
    d. alpha-fetoprotein

*369. The normal concentration of proteins in cerebrospinal fluid, relative to serum protein, is:

    a. <1%
    b. 5%-10%
    c. 25%-30%
    d. 50%-60%

*370. The serum glucose concentration of a diabetic patient undergoing a 2-hour glucose tolerance test should return to the baseline (fasting level) after a minimum of:

a. 30 minutes
b. 60 minutes
c. 90 minutes
d. 120 minutes

*371. The urea nitrogen concentration of a serum sample was measured as 15 mg/dL (atomic weights: carbon = 12, oxygen = 16, nitrogen = 14, hydrogen = 1). The urea concentration of the same sample, in mg/dL, is:

a. 15
b. 24
c. 32
d. 40

*372. In thin layer chromatography, the $R_f$ value for a compound is given by the:

a. ratio of distance moved by compound to distance moved by solvent
b. rate of movement of compound through the adsorbent
c. distance between the compound spot and solvent front
d. distance moved by compound from the origin

*373. Below are the results of a protein electrophoresis:

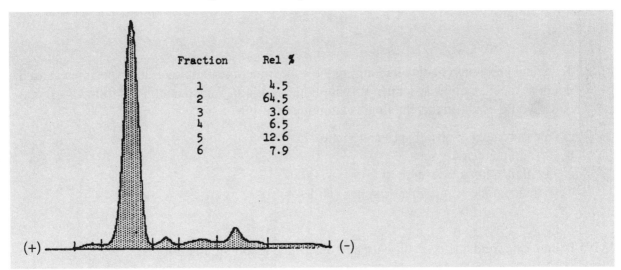

| Fraction | Rel % |
|----------|-------|
| 1 | 4.5 |
| 2 | 64.5 |
| 3 | 3.6 |
| 4 | 6.5 |
| 5 | 12.6 |
| 6 | 7.9 |

These results are consistent with a(n):

a. normal serum protein pattern
b. normal CSF protein pattern
c. abnormal serum protein pattern
d. abnormal CSF protein pattern

*374. At a pH of 8.6 the gamma globulins move toward the cathode, despite the fact that they are negatively charged. What is this phenomenon called?

a. reverse migration
b. molecular sieve
c. endosmosis
d. migratory inhibition factor

*375. Which of the following is a regulatory hormone?

a. thyroxine
b. estriol
c. parathyroid hormone
d. growth hormone

*376. In respiratory acidosis, a compensatory mechanism is the increase in:

a. respiration rate
b. ammonia formation
c. blood $PCO_2$
d. plasma bicarbonate concentration

*377. In amniotic fluid, the procedure used to detect Rh isosensitization is:

a. human amniotic placental lactogen (HPL)
b. alpha-fetoprotein
c. measurement of absorbance at 450 nm
d. creatinine

*378. Technical problems encountered during the collection of an amniotic fluid specimen caused doubt as to whether the specimen was amniotic in origin. Which one of the following procedures would establish that the fluid is amniotic in origin?

a. measurement of absorbance at 450 nm
b. creatinine measurement
c. lecithin/sphingomyelin ratio
d. human amniotic placental lactogen (HPL)

*379. In amniotic fluid, the procedure used to determine fetal lung maturity is:

a. lecithin/sphingomyelin ratio
b. creatinine
c. measurement of absorbance at 450 nm
d. alpha-fetoprotein

*380. In amniotic fluid, the procedure most closely related to fetoplacental function is:

    a. measurement of absorbance at 450 nm
    b. creatinine
    c. lecithin/sphingomyelin ratio
    d. estriol

*381. The method of choice for diagnosis of a protracted attack of porphyria is:

    a. screening a fresh morning urine for porphobilinogen
    b. analysis of delta-aminolevulinic acid in a morning urine
    c. screening a fresh morning urine for porphyrin
    d. HPLC analysis of porphobilinogen on a 24-hour urine

*382. The buffer pH most effective at allowing amphoteric proteins to migrate toward the cathode in an electrophoretic system would be:

    a. 4.5
    b. 7.5
    c. 8.6
    d. 9.5

*383. The protein that has the highest dye-binding capacity is:

    a. albumin
    b. alpha globulin
    c. beta globulin
    d. gamma globulin

*384. When the clinical response does not agree with total drug concentration, free drug levels may be of clinical use in all of the following cases, EXCEPT:

    a. uremia
    b. hypoalbuminemia
    c. ingestion of other drugs
    d. patient noncompliance

*385. In an electrophoretic separation, the zones appear artifactually crescent-shaped. The most likely cause is:

    a. insufficient amount of sample
    b. overload of sample
    c. use of phosphate-borate buffer
    d. inadequate fixation prior to staining

*386. In electrophoresis of serum proteins, artifacts at the application point are most frequently caused by:

    a. endosmosis
    b. prestaining with tracer dye
    c. overloading of serum sample
    d. dirty applicators


*387. On electrophoresis, distorted zones of protein separation are usually due to:

    a. presence of therapeutic drugs in serum sample
    b. dirty applicators
    c. overloading of serum sample
    d. prestaining with tracer dye


*388. On electrophoresis, transient bisalbuminemia is associated with:

    a. dirty applicators
    b. presence of therapeutic drugs in serum sample
    c. endosmosis
    d. prestaining with tracer dye


*389. Fecal porphyrin analysis by talc thin-layer chromatography will reveal:

    a. hereditary coproporphyria
    b. carrier state of acute intermittent porphyria
    c. erythrocytic protoporphyria
    d. acute porphyric attack


*390. Analysis of erythrocytes for uroporphyrinogen I synthetase detects:

    a. acute porphyric attack
    b. lead poisoning
    c. hereditary coproporphyria
    d. acute intermittent porphyria


*391. The wavelength used for porphyrin analyses is:

    a. 399 nm
    b. 420 nm
    c. 540 nm
    d. 680 nm

*392. A fresh urine sample is received for analysis for "porphyrins" or "porphyria" without further information or specifications. Initial analysis should include:

    a. porphyrin screen and quantitative total porphyrin
    b. quantitative total porphyrin and porphobilinogen screen
    c. porphyrin and porphobilinogen screen
    d. porphobilinogen screen and ion-exchange analysis for porphobilinogen


*393. A test request slip indicates that an acute porphyric attack is suspected clinically. Analysis should include:

    a. quantitative delta-aminolevulinic acid
    b. porphyrin screen
    c. quantitative 24-hour porphobilinogen
    d. porphobilinogen screen


*394. Testing for the diagnosis of lead poisoning should include:

    a. ion-exchange analysis of urine for porphobilinogen
    b. analysis of morning urine for delta-aminolevulinic acid
    c. analysis of feces for porphyrin
    d. ion-exchange analysis of feces for protoporphyrin


*395. Detection of carriers of hereditary coproporphyria should include analysis of:

    a. 24-hour urine for porphobilinogen
    b. fresh morning urine for delta-aminolevulinic acid
    c. erythrocyte protoporphyrin
    d. 24-hour urine for porphyrin


*396. The fast hemoglobin fraction is:

    a. Hgb A
    b. Hgb $A_2$
    c. Hgb $A_1$
    d. Hgb F


*397. A patient with hemolytic anemia will:

    a. show a decrease in glycosylated Hgb value
    b. show an increase in glycosylated Hgb value
    c. show little or no change in glycosylated Hgb value
    d. demonstrate an elevated Hgb $A_1$

*398. The main reason for suboptimal drug levels in therapeutic drug monitoring is:

    a. renal failure
    b. liver failure
    c. improper dosage prescribed
    d. patient noncompliance with dosage regimen


*399. In using ion-exchange chromatographic methods, falsely increased levels of Hgb $A_{1c}$ will be demonstrated in the presence of:

    a. Hgb F
    b. pernicious anemia
    c. thalassemias
    d. Hgb S


*400. A sweat chloride result of 55 mEq/L and a sweat sodium of 52 mEq/L were obtained on a patient who has a history of respiratory problems. The best interpretation of these results is:

    a. normal
    b. normal sodium and an abnormal chloride test should be repeated
    c. abnormal results
    d. borderline results, the test should be repeated


*401. Currently the most common method for specific identification and quantitation of serum barbiturates is:

    a. immunoassay
    b. thin-layer chromatography
    c. gas-liquid chromatography
    d. ultraviolet absorption spectroscopy


*402. A critically ill patient becomes comatose. The physician believes the coma is due to hepatic failure. The assay most helpful in this diagnosis is:

    a. ammonia
    b. ALT
    c. AST
    d. GGT


*403. A cholesterol QC chart has the following data for the normal control:

| | |
|---|---|
| x = mean of data | |
| x = 137 mg/dL | $\Sigma x$ = 1,918 mg/dL |
| 2 SD = 6 mg/dL | N = 14 |

The coefficient of variation for this control is:

a. 1.14%
b. 2.19%
c. 4.38%
d. 9.49%

*404. If the correlation coefficient (r) of two variables is zero:

a. there is complete correlation between the variables
b. there is an absence of correlation
c. as one variable increases, the other decreases
d. as one variable decreases, the other increases

*405. Refer to the following illustration:

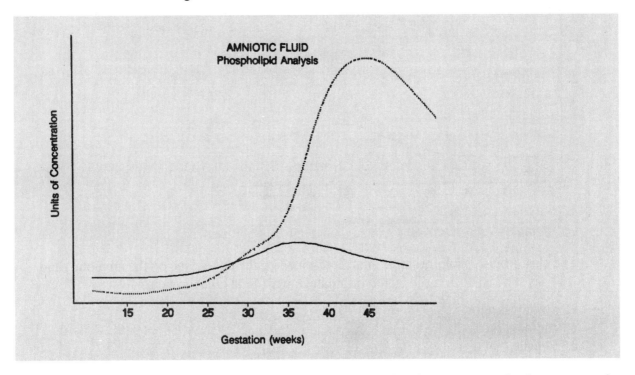

Which class of phospholipid surfactants associated with pulmonary maturity is represented by the dotted line on the amniotic fluid analysis shown above?

a. sphingomyelin
b. choline
c. lecithin
d. phosphatidic acid

*406. Most drugs and intracellular metabolites measured by radioimmunoassay have molecular weights between 200 and 1000 and can be made immunogenic by:

a. attaching them to protein molecules
b. frequent injections of the compound mixed with Freund's adjuvant
c. sensitizing the animal with another antigen first
d. treating the animals with glucocorticoids


*407. Refer to the following illustration:

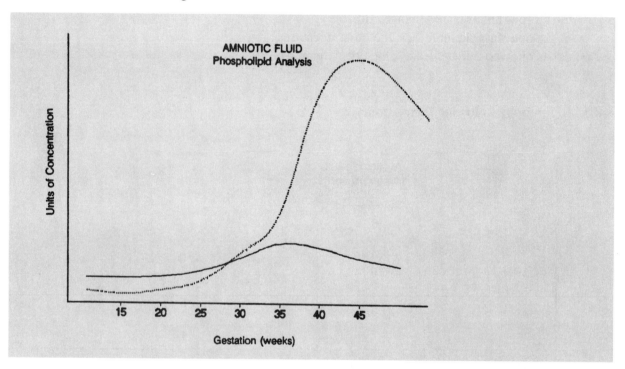

The class of phospholipid surfactants represented by the dotted line on the amniotic fluid analysis shown above is thought to originate in what fetal organ system?

a. cardiovascular
b. pulmonary
c. hepatic
d. placental

*408. The illustration below represents a Lineweaver-Burk plot of 1/v versus 1/[S] in an enzyme reaction and the following assumptions should be made:

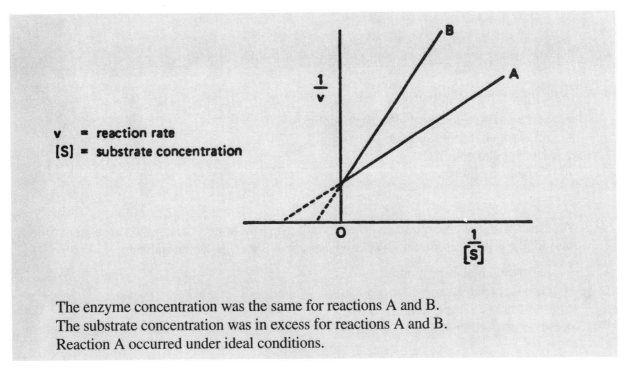

v = reaction rate
[S] = substrate concentration

The enzyme concentration was the same for reactions A and B.
The substrate concentration was in excess for reactions A and B.
Reaction A occurred under ideal conditions.

Which of the following statements about reaction B is true?

a. It illustrates noncompetitive inhibition.
b. It illustrates competitive inhibition.
c. It illustrates neither competitive nor noncompetitive inhibition.
d. It could be the result of heavy metal contamination.

*409. The concentration of serum carotene is affected MOST by which of the following?

a. diet
b. hepatic function
c. drawing time of specimen
d. age

*410. The following laboratory results were obtained:

|  | Calcium | Phosphate | Alkaline Phosphatase |
|---|---|---|---|
| Serum | Increased | Decreased | Normal or increased |
| Urine | Increased | Increased | |

These results are most compatible with:

a. multiple myeloma
b. milk-alkali syndrome
c. sarcoidosis
d. primary hyperparathyroidism

*411. A 4-year-old girl has edema that is most obvious in her eyelids. Laboratory studies reveal:

| | |
|---|---|
| Serum albumin | 1.8 g/dL |
| Serum cholesterol | 450 mg/dL |
| Serum urea nitrogen | 20 mg/dL |
| Urinalysis | Protein 4+; hyaline, granular, and fatty casts |

This is most compatible with:

a. acute poststreptococcal glomerulonephritis
b. minimal change glomerular disease
c. acute pyelonephritis
d. diabetes mellitus

*412. A patient with malabsorption receives 25 g of d-xylose orally; during the subsequent 5-hour period, the urine excretion of d-xylose is less than 3 g. This would indicate:

a. pancreatic malabsorption
b. chronic pancreatitis
c. intestinal malabsorption
d. absence of disease

*413. The most common type of congenital adrenal hyperplasia associated with increased plasma concentrations of 17 $\alpha$-hydroxyprogesterone and increased urinary excretion of pregnanetriol is:

a. 17 $\alpha$-hydroxylase deficiency
b. 11 $\beta$-hydroxylase deficiency
c. 21-hydroxylase deficiency
d. 18-hydroxysteroid dehydrogenase deficiency

*414. A patient has signs and symptoms suggestive of acromegaly. The diagnosis would be confirmed if the patient had which of the following?

a. an elevated serum phosphate concentration
b. a decreased serum growth hormone releasing factor concentration
c. no decrease in serum growth hormone concentration 90 minutes after oral glucose administration
d. an increased serum somatostatin concentration

*415. In a normal individual, injection of thyrotropin-releasing hormone (TRH) causes an increase in blood concentrations of which of the following hormones?

a. growth hormone
b. prolactin
c. ACTH
d. insulin

*416. The thyrotropin-releasing hormone (TRH) stimulation test rules out the diagnosis of mild or subclinical hyperthyroidism if TRH infusion causes:

a. a rise in plasma TSH
b. no rise in plasma TSH
c. a rise in plasma growth hormone concentration
d. no rise in plasma growth hormone concentration

*417. A 2-year-old child with a decreased serum $T_4$ is described as being somewhat dwarfed, stocky, overweight, and having coarse features. Of the following, the most informative additional laboratory test would be the serum:

a. thyroxine-binding globulin (TBG)
b. thyroid-stimulating hormone (TSH)
c. triiodothyronine ($T_3$)
d. cholesterol

*418. The test for adrenal cortical hyperfunction that has the greatest diagnostic sensitivity is measurement of:

a. urinary free cortisol
b. plasma cortisol
c. urinary 17-hydroxycorticosteroids
d. plasma corticosterone

*419. The definitive diagnosis of primary adrenal insufficiency requires demonstration of:

a. decreased urinary 17-keto- and 17-hydroxysteroids
b. decreased cortisol production
c. impaired response to ACTH stimulation
d. increased urinary cortisol excretion after metyrapone

*420. Urinary estrogen in pregnant women consists chiefly of:

a. estradiol
b. estriol
c. estrone
d. pregnanediol

*421. Which of the following determinations is useful in prenatal diagnosis of open neural tube defects?

a. amniotic fluid alpha-fetoprotein
b. amniotic fluid estriol
c. maternal serum estradiol
d. maternal serum estrone

*422. Biochemical profile:

|  | Patient Values | Reference Range |
| --- | --- | --- |
| Total protein | 7.3 g/dL | 6.0-8.0 g/dL |
| Albumin | 4.1 g/dL | 3.5-5.0 g/dL |
| Calcium | 9.6 mg/dL | 8.5-10.5 mg/dL |
| Phosphorus | 3.3 mg/dL | 2.5-4.5 mg/dL |
| Glucose | 95 mg/dL | 65-110 mg/dL |
| BUN | 16 mg/dL | 10-20 mg/dL |
| Uric acid | 6.0 mg/dL | 2.5-8.0 mg/dL |
| Creatinine | 1.2 mg/dL | 0.7-1.4 mg/dL |
| Total bilirubin | 3.7 mg/dL | 0.2-0.9 mg/dL |
| Alkaline phosphatase | 275 U/L | 30-80 U/L |
| Lactate dehydrogenase | 185 U/L | 100-225 U/L |
| AST | 75 U/L | 10-40 U/L |

The results of the biochemical profile are most consistent with:

a. viral hepatitis
b. hemolytic anemia
c. common bile duct stone
d. chronic active hepatitis

*423. Refer to the following illustration:

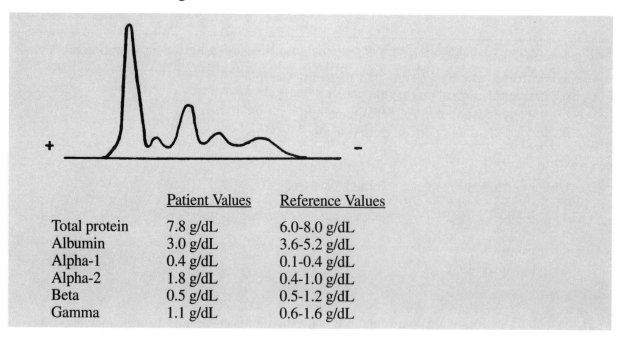

|  | Patient Values | Reference Values |
| --- | --- | --- |
| Total protein | 7.8 g/dL | 6.0-8.0 g/dL |
| Albumin | 3.0 g/dL | 3.6-5.2 g/dL |
| Alpha-1 | 0.4 g/dL | 0.1-0.4 g/dL |
| Alpha-2 | 1.8 g/dL | 0.4-1.0 g/dL |
| Beta | 0.5 g/dL | 0.5-1.2 g/dL |
| Gamma | 1.1 g/dL | 0.6-1.6 g/dL |

The serum protein electrophoresis pattern is consistent with:

a. cirrhosis
b. acute inflammation
c. polyclonal gammopathy (eg, chronic inflammation)
d. alpha-1-antitrypsin deficiency; severe emphysema

*424. A low concentration of serum phosphorus is commonly found in:

a. patients who are receiving carbohydrate hyperalimentation
b. chronic renal disease
c. hypoparathyroidism
d. patients with pituitary tumors

*425. Serum concentrations of vitamin B$_{12}$ are elevated in:

a. pernicious anemia in relapse
b. patients on chronic hemodialysis
c. chronic granulocytic leukemia
d. Hodgkin's disease

*426. The urinary excretion of porphobilinogen is increased in patients with:

a. erythropoietic protoporphyria
b. porphyria cutanea tarda
c. hemolytic anemia
d. acute intermittent porphyria

*427. Refer to the following illustration:

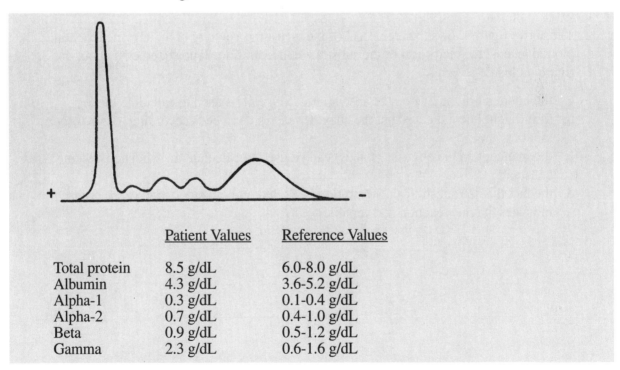

| | Patient Values | Reference Values |
| --- | --- | --- |
| Total protein | 8.5 g/dL | 6.0-8.0 g/dL |
| Albumin | 4.3 g/dL | 3.6-5.2 g/dL |
| Alpha-1 | 0.3 g/dL | 0.1-0.4 g/dL |
| Alpha-2 | 0.7 g/dL | 0.4-1.0 g/dL |
| Beta | 0.9 g/dL | 0.5-1.2 g/dL |
| Gamma | 2.3 g/dL | 0.6-1.6 g/dL |

The above serum protein electrophoresis pattern is consistent with:

a. cirrhosis
b. monoclonal gammopathy
c. polyclonal gammopathy (eg, chronic inflammation)
d. alpha-1-antitrypsin deficiency; severe emphysema

*428. A true statement about high performance liquid chromatography (HPLC) is that it:

    a. utilizes a flame ionization detector
    b. requires derivation of nonvolatile compounds
    c. can be used to separate gases, liquids, or soluble solids
    d. can be used for adsorption, partition, ion exchange, and gel permeation chromatography

*429. Refer to the following illustration:

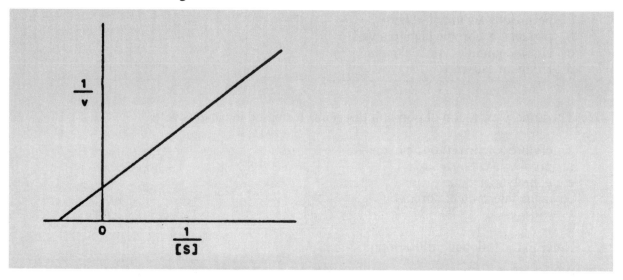

The above figure shows the reciprocal of the measured velocity of an enzyme reaction plotted against the reciprocal of the substrate concentration. True statements about this figure include:

    a. the intercept of the line on the abscissa (x-axis) can be used to calculate the $V_{max}$
    b. the straight line indicates that the enzyme reaction proceeds according to zero order kinetics
    c. the intercept on the abscissa (x-axis) can be used to calculate the Michaelis-Menten constant
    d. the fact that the substrate concentration is plotted on both sides of the zero point indicates that the reaction is reversible

*430. Refer to the following illustration:

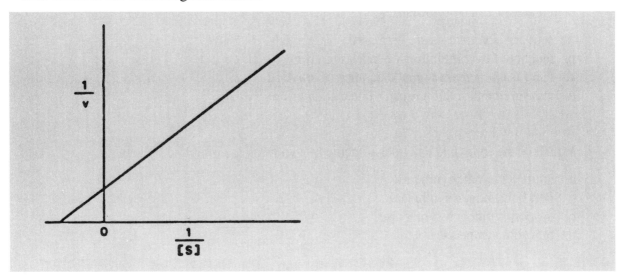

The figure above shows the reciprocal of the measured velocity of an enzyme reaction plotted against the reciprocal of the substrate concentration. True statements about this figure include:

a. the intercept of the line on the ordinate (y-axis) can be used to calculate the $V_{max}$
b. the straight line indicates that the enzyme reaction proceeds according to zero order kinetics
c. the intercept on the ordinate (y-axis) can be used to calculate the Michaelis-Menten constant
d. the fact the substrate concentration is plotted on both sides of the zero point indicates that the reaction is reversible


*431. Characteristics of malabsorption syndrome due to pancreatic insufficiency include:

a. fecal fat excretion greater than 10 g/day
b. urinary excretion of 2.0 g of d-xylose within 5 hours after the patient has received 24 g orally
c. marked changes of secretion into the duodenum following injection of secretin
d. normal or elevated serum carotene concentration


*432. When taken by a euthyroid individual, oral contraceptives containing estrogens will have which of the following effects on the thyroid function studies?

a. increase total circulating $T_4$
b. increase $T_3$ resin uptake
c. decrease thyroxine-binding globulin
d. decrease circulating $T_3$

*433. In acute pancreatitis, the relative increase in urinary amylase activity is greater than that of serum amylase activity because:

    a. salivary isoamylases are increased
    b. there are fewer inhibitors of amylase in urine
    c. there is an increased renal clearance of amylase
    d. measurements exhibit greater linearity in urine

*434. Which of the following enzymes of heme biosynthesis are inhibited by lead?

    a. aminolevulinate synthetase
    b. porphobilinogen synthetase
    c. uroporphyrinogen synthetase
    d. bilirubin synthetase

*435. Which of the following calcium procedures utilizes lanthanum chloride to eliminate interfering substances?

    a. o-cresolphthalein complex one
    b. precipitation with chloranilic acid
    c. chelation with EDTA
    d. atomic absorption spectrophotometry

*436. A patient in her 33rd week of pregnancy is hospitalized with toxemia. Her doctor would like to deliver the baby early because the toxemia is becoming more severe. The baby's best chance of delivery without respiratory distress due to lung immaturity is if:

    a. the L/S ratio is greater than 3.5
    b. the L/S ratio is greater than 2.5
    c. PG is absent
    d. creatinine is 1.3 mg/dL

*437. Which of the following diseases results from a familial absence of high-density lipoprotein?

    a. Krabbe's
    b. Gaucher's
    c. Tangier
    d. Tay-Sachs

*438. Diagnostic specificity is defined as the percentage of individuals:

    a. with a given disease who have a positive result by a given test
    b. without a given disease who have a negative result by a given test
    c. with a given disease who have a negative result by a given test
    d. without a given disease who have a positive result by a given test

*439. A blood gas sample was sent to the lab on ice, and a bubble was present in the syringe. The blood had been exposed to room air for at least 30 minutes. The following change in blood gases occurred:

    a. $CO_2$ content increased/$PCO_2$ decreased
    b. $CO_2$ content and $PO_2$ increased/pH increased
    c. $CO_2$ content and $PCO_2$ decreased/pH decreased
    d. $PO_2$ increased/$HCO_3^-$ decreased


*440. In the Bessey-Lowry-Brock method for determining alkaline phosphatase activity, the substrate used is:

    a. monophosphate
    b. phenylphosphate
    c. disodium phenylphosphate
    d. para-nitrophenylphosphate


*441. In which of the following conditions does decreased activity of glucuronyl transferase result in increased unconjugated bilirubin and kernicterus in neonates?

    a. Gilbert's disease
    b. Rotor's syndrome
    c. Dubin-Johnson syndrome
    d. Crigler-Najjar syndrome


*442. The predictive value of a positive test is defined as:

    a. (true positives + true negatives)/true positives x 100
    b. true positives/(true positives + false positives) x 100
    c. (true positives + true negatives)/true negatives x 100
    d. true negatives/(true negatives + false positives) x 100


*443. A 10-year-old child was admitted to pediatrics with an initial diagnosis of skeletal muscle disease. The best confirmatory tests would be:

    a. creatine kinase and isocitrate dehydrogenase
    b. gamma-glutamyl transferase and alkaline phosphatase
    c. aldolase and creatine kinase
    d. lactate dehydrogenase and malate dehydrogenase


*444. The general types of interference in atomic absorption spectrophotometry:

    a. are chemical, ionization, and matrix
    b. only occur in organic solvents
    c. can all be overcome by the addition of certain competing cations
    d. significantly hinder method specificity

*445. About 90% of phenytoin is excreted in the urine as:

   a. phenobarbital
   b. para-hydroxyphenyl phenylhydantoin
   c. dibenzazepine-5-carboxamide
   d. N-acetylprocainamide


*446. Certain enzymes are activated to metabolize drugs as a result of another drug action. This is referred to as:

   a. substrate depletion
   b. enzyme depletion
   c. enzyme induction
   d. enzyme inhibition


*447. Nortriptyline is a metabolite of:

   a. amitriptyline
   b. protriptyline
   c. butriptyline
   d. norbutriptyline


*448. Cocaine is metabolized to:

   a. carbamazepine
   b. codeine
   c. hydrocodone
   d. benzoylecgonine


*449. If a drug has a half-life of 7 hours, how many doses given at 7-hour intervals does it usually take to achieve a steady state or plateau level?

   a. one
   b. three
   c. five
   d. eight


*450. Reverse phase high-performance liquid chromatography is being increasingly utilized in therapeutic drug monitoring. The term reverse phase implies that the column eluant is:

   a. pumped up the column
   b. more polar than the stationary phase
   c. always nonpolar
   d. less polar than the stationary phase

*451. Serum and urine copper levels are assayed on a hospital patient with the following results:

|  | Patient's Values | Reference Values |
|---|---|---|
| Serum Cu | 58 µg/dL | 70-140 µg/dL |
| Urine Cu | 83 µg/dL | < 40 µg/dL |

This is most consistent with:

a. normal copper levels
b. Wilms' tumor
c. Wilson's disease
d. Addison's disease

*452. Refer to the following diagram:

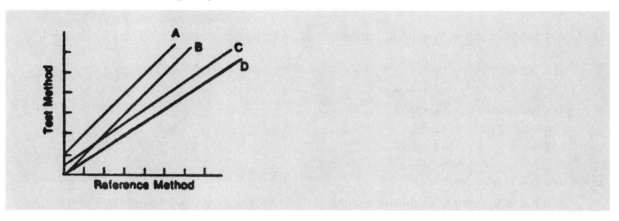

The line that demonstrates a proportional error relationship is:

a. line A
b. line B
c. line C
d. line D

*453. In gas-liquid chromatography (GLC), actual separation of compounds occurs in the column by the:

a. inert phase
b. solid phase
c. liquid phase
d. mobile phase

*454. An analgesic that alleviates pain without causing loss of consciousness is:

a. digoxin
b. acetaminophen
c. lithium
d. phenytoin

*455. In spectrophotometric determination, which of the following is the formula for calculating the absorbance of a solution?

a. (absorptivity x light path)/concentration
b. (absorptivity x concentration)/light path
c. absorptivity x light path x concentration
d. (light path x concentration)/absorptivity


*456. Which of the following is the formula for standard deviation?

a. square root of the mean
b. square root of (sum of squared differences)/(N-1)
c. square root of the variance
d. square root of (mean)/(sum of squared differences)


*457. A 1-year-old girl with hyperlipoproteinemia and a lipase deficiency has the following lipid profile:

| | |
|---|---|
| Cholesterol | 300 mg/dL |
| Triglycerides | 200 mg/dL |
| Chylomicrons | Present |
| LDL | Increased |
| HDL | Decreased |

A serum specimen from this patient that was refrigerated overnight would most likely be:

a. clear
b. cloudy
c. creamy layer over cloudy serum
d. creamy layer over clear serum


*458. Thin-layer chromatography is of particular use in the identification of:

a. lipids
b. drugs
c. inorganic ions
d. enzyme inhibitors


*459. Which of the following is used to verify wavelength settings for narrow band width spectrophotometers?

a. didymium filter
b. prisms
c. holmium oxide glass
d. diffraction gratings

*460. A psychiatric patient was experiencing severe depression, but responded to treatment with amitriptyline with no apparent side effects. A blood sample was sent to the laboratory for therapeutic monitoring. Which of the following drug levels would be MOST reflective of this patient's condition?

    a. amitriptyline = 237 μg/L
    b. amitriptyline = 104 μg/L
    c. protriptyline = 76 μg/L
    d. imipramine = 103 μg/L

*461. Which of the following sets of results would be consistent with macroamylasemia?

    a. normal serum amylase and elevated urine amylase values
    b. increased serum amylase and normal urine amylase values
    c. increased serum and urine amylase values
    d. normal serum and urine amylase values

*462. In the hexokinase method for glucose determination, the actual end product measured is the:

    a. amount of hydrogen peroxide produced
    b. NADH produced from the reduction of NAD
    c. amount of glucose combined with bromcresol purple
    d. condensation of glucose with an aromatic amine

*463. A 21-year-old man with nausea, vomiting, and jaundice has the following laboratory findings:

| | |
|---|---|
| Total serum bilirubin level | 8.5 mg/dL (normal, 0-1.0) |
| Conjugated serum bilirubin level | 6.1 mg/dL (normal, 0-0.5) |
| Urine urobilinogen | Increased |
| Fecal urobilinogen | Decreased |
| Urine bilirubin | Positive |
| AST | 300 U/L (normal, 0-50 U/L) |
| Alkaline phosphatase | 170 U/L (normal, 0-150 U/L) |

These can best be explained as representing:

    a. unconjugated hyperbilirubinemia, probably due to hemolysis
    b. unconjugated hyperbilirubinemia, probably due to toxic liver damage
    c. conjugated hyperbilirubinemia, probably due to biliary tract disease
    d. conjugated hyperbilirubinemia, probably due to hepatocellular obstruction

*464. Macroenzymes are occasionally seen as persistent aberrant bands on electrophoresis with larger molecular weight than their corresponding normal form. They generally represent:

    a. production of large enzyme molecules
    b. enzymes bound to immunoglobulins
    c. media artifact seen on cellulose acetate electrophoresis
    d. autosomal recessive variants

*465. The glucose level in normal peritoneal fluid should be:

    a.  near zero
    b.  the same as the plasma glucose
    c.  twice the plasma glucose
    d.  ten times the plasma glucose

*466. A course of instruction is being planned to teach laboratory employees to correct simple malfunctions in selected laboratory instruments. In writing the objectives for this course, which one of the following would be most appropriate?

    a.  learn how to repair 9 of 10 simple instrument malfunctions
    b.  correctly answer 9 of 10 test questions dealing with simple instrument malfunctions
    c.  be able to detect 9 of 10 simple instrument malfunctions
    d.  document corrective action procedure for 9 of 10 simple instrument malfunctions

*467. Which of the following methods offers the greatest sensitivity for HBsAg testing?

    a.  counterimmunoelectrophoresis
    b.  enzyme immunoassay
    c.  spectrophotometry
    d.  nephelometry

*468. A blood creatinine value of 5.0 mg/dL is most likely to be found with which of the following blood values?

    a.  osmolality      292 mOsm/kg
    b.  uric acid         8 mg/dL
    c.  urea nitrogen   80 mg/dL
    d.  ammonia       80 μg/dL

*469. Ninety percent of the copper present in the blood is bound to:

    a.  transferrin
    b.  ceruloplasmin
    c.  albumin
    d.  cryoglobulin

*470. Refer to the following illustration:

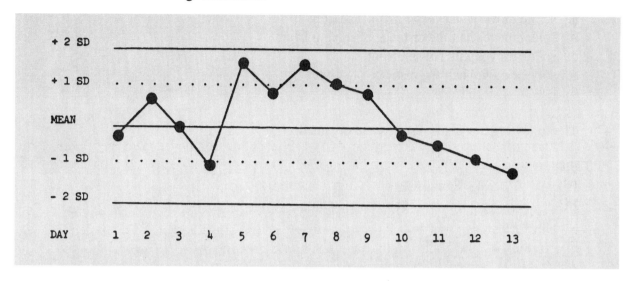

Shown above is a Levy-Jennings quality control chart that represents control values for 13 consecutive analyses for a particular serum constituent. If the 14th value is below the – 2 SD limit, which of the following should be done?

a. The control should be repeated to see if it will fall within the established interval.
b. The analysis system should be checked for a deteriorating component.
c. The analysis system should be checked for a change in reagent lot number.
d. It is not necessary to take any action.

*471. A blood sample was received from the emergency room with a request for narcotic analysis. The request slip indicated that the patient (a known heroin addict) responded to naloxone administration. The serum was negative for morphine by EIA. What other tests should be performed in assessing suspected opiate abuse?

a. heroin
b. salicylate
c. alcohol
d. methadone

*472. Blood samples were collected at the beginning of an exercise class and after 30 minutes of aerobic activity. Which of the following would be most consistent with the postexercise sample?

a. normal lactic acid, low pyruvate
b. low lactic acid, elevated pyruvate
c. elevated lactic acid, low pyruvate
d. elevated lactic acid, elevated pyruvate

*473. An $R_f$ value of 0.5 in thin-layer chromatography means:

    a. solute moves twice as far as solvent front
    b. solute moves half the distance of solvent front
    c. solute moves with solvent front
    d. solvent moves half the distance of solute

*474. The following blood gas results were obtained:

| | |
|---|---|
| pH | 7.18 |
| $PO_2$ | 86 mm Hg |
| $PCO_2$ | 60 mm Hg |
| $O_2$ saturation | 92% |
| $HCO_3^-$ | 21 mEq/L |
| $TCO_2$ | 23 mEq/L |
| Base excess | –8.0 mEq/L |

The patient's results are compatible with which of the following?

    a. fever
    b. uremia
    c. emphysema
    d. dehydration

*475. After adding 8 drops of 10% ferric chloride to 5 mL of urine, the mixture develops a stable deep red color. This is presumptive evidence of:

    a. lead
    b. bromide
    c. salicylates
    d. quinidine

*476. While performing a serum lithium determination on a flame photometer with cesium as the internal standard, the technologist noticed that there was a flickering flame. The most probable cause of this problem is:

    a. changes in the fuel reaching the instrument
    b. incorrect internal standard for this type of determination
    c. a surging line voltage
    d. faulty monochromator

*477. Upon development of a thin layer chromatogram for drug analysis, all drug spots (including the standards) had migrated with the solvent front. The most probable cause for this would be:

a. environmental temperature too warm
b. incorrect aqueous to nonaqueous solvent mixture
c. too much sample applied
d. chromatogram dried too quickly

*478. Amniotic fluid submitted for a lecithin/sphingomyelin (L/S) ratio has been left in a brown container since the night before. Which of the following would you expect?

a. decreased lecithin
b. decreased sphingomyelin
c. no phosphatidylglycerol (PG) present
d. no phosphatidylethanolamine (PE) present

*479. A patient is admitted with biliary cirrhosis. If a serum protein electrophoresis is performed, which of the following globulin fractions will be most elevated?

a. alpha-1
b. alpha-2
c. beta
d. gamma

*480. One method to enhance the differentiation of bone from liver alkaline phosphatase isoenzyme is to pretreat an aliquot of the serum specimen:

a. with tartaric acid
b. by heating at 56°C
c. with bovine albumin
d. by polyethylene glycol precipitation

*481. A patient had the following serum results:

| | |
|---|---|
| $Na^+$ | 140 mEq/L |
| $K^+$ | 4.0 mEq/L |
| Glucose | 95 mg/dL |
| BUN | 10 mg/dL |

Which osmolality is consistent with these results?

a. 188
b. 204
c. 270
d. 390

*482. Three consecutive serum amylases were elevated to the same degree. A 24-hour urine amylase was within the reference range, within the same time period. The technologist should:

    a. perform a serum lipase and trypsinogen
    b. obtain another serum and urine amylase in three weeks
    c. repeat serum amylase after polyethylene glycol precipitation
    d. report the results with no further testing

*483. A 45-year-old woman complains of fatigue, heat intolerance, and hair loss. Serum thyroxine and $^{125}$I-T$_3$ resin uptake are abnormally low. What test would confirm that this is a pituitary deficiency?

    a. free T$_3$
    b. free T$_4$
    c. thyroglobulin
    d. TSH

*484. Given the following results, calculate the molar absorptivity:

| | |
|---|---|
| Absorbance | 0.500 |
| Light path | 1.0 cm |
| Concentration | 0.2 M/L |

    a. 0.4
    b. 0.7
    c. 1.6
    d. 2.5

*485. A new method is being evaluated. A recovery experiment is performed with the following results:

| | |
|---|---|
| 0.9 mL serum sample + 0.1 mL H$_2$O | 89 mEq/L |
| 0.9 mL serum sample + 0.1 mL analyte standard at 800 mEq/L | 161 mEq/L |

The percent recovery of the added analyte standard is:

    a. 55%
    b. 81%
    c. 90%
    d. 180%

*486. An emphysema patient suffering from fluid accumulation in the alveolar spaces is likely to be in what metabolic state?

a. respiratory acidosis
b. respiratory alkalosis
c. metabolic acidosis
d. metabolic alkalosis

*487. A patient with myeloproliferative disorder has the following values:

| | |
|---|---|
| Hgb | 13 g/dL |
| Hct | 38% |
| WBC | 30 x 10³/µL |
| Platelets | 1000 x 10³/µL |
| Serum Na⁺ | 140 mEq/L |
| Serum K⁺ | 7 mEq/L |

The serum K⁺ should be confirmed by:

a. repeat testing of the original serum
b. testing freshly drawn serum
c. testing heparinized plasma
d. atomic absorption spectrometry

*488. The following data were obtained on amniotic fluid from a gestation of 36 weeks' duration by menstrual dates:

L/S = 2
Phosphatidyl glycerol not present

Which of the following can be concluded from these data?

a. The fetus may be safely delivered because it is mature by history.
b. The fetus is in severe distress because of cessation of PG synthesis.
c. The fetus is at risk for respiratory distress if delivered immediately.
d. The fetus may be safely delivered because its lungs are mature by L/S criteria.

*489. Stray light can be detected in a spectrophotometer by utilizing a:

a. mercury vapor lamp
b. helium oxide glass
c. potassium dichromate solution
d. sharp cutoff filter

*490. A technologist is asked to write a procedure to measure the Evans blue concentration on a spectrophotometer. The technologist is given four standard solutions of Evans blue:

Std A = 0.8 mg/dL
Std B = 1.6 mg/dL
Std C = 2.4 mg/dL
Std D = 4.0 mg/dL

The first step is to:

a. calculate the slope of the calibration curve
b. determine the absorbance of the four standards
c. find the wavelength of the greatest % transmittance for Evans blue
d. find the wavelength of the greatest absorbance for Evans blue


*491. Hemoglobin S can be separated from hemoglobin D by:

a. electrophoresis on a different medium and acidic pH
b. hemoglobin $A_2$ quantitation
c. electrophoresis at higher voltage
d. Kleihauer-Betke acid elution


*492. A patient with type I insulin-dependent diabetes mellitus has the following results:

|  | Patient | Reference Range |
|---|---|---|
| Fasting blood glucose | 150 mg/dL | 70-110 mg/dL |
| Hemoglobin $A_{1c}$ | 25% | 6.0%-19.5% |
| Fructosamine | 3.0 mmol/L | 2.0-5.3 mmol/L |

After reviewing these test results, the technologist concluded that the patient is in a:

a. "steady state" of metabolic control
b. state of flux, progressively worsening metabolic control
c. improving state of metabolic control, as indicated by fructosamine
d. state of flux, as indicated by the fasting glucose level


*493. The methodology based on the amount of energy absorbed by a substance as a function of its concentration and using a specific source of the same material as the substance analyzed is:

a. flame emission photometry
b. atomic absorption spectrophotometry
c. emission spectrography
d. x-ray fluorescence spectrometry

*494. One means of checking a spectrophotometer wavelength calibration in the visible range is by using a:

a. quartz filter
b. diffraction grating
c. quartz prism
d. didymium filter

*495. When separating serum proteins by cellulose acetate electrophoresis using veronal buffer at pH 8.6, beta globulin migrates:

a. faster than albumin
b. slower than gamma globulin
c. faster than gamma globulin
d. faster than alpha-2 globulin

*496. An acid cleaning solution for glassware consists of:

a. 10% hydrochloric acid
b. potassium dichromate in concentrated sulfuric acid
c. potassium chlorate in concentrated sulfuric acid
d. concentrated sulfuric acid

*497. Before unconjugated bilirubin can react with Ehrlich's diazo reagent, which of the following must be added?

a. acetone
b. ether
c. distilled water
d. methyl alcohol

*498. The following data were obtained from a cellulose acetate protein electrophoresis scan:

| | |
|---|---|
| Albumin area | 75 units |
| Gamma globulin area | 30 units |
| Total area | 180 units |
| Total protein | 6.5 g/dL |

The gamma globulin content in g/dL is:

a. 1.1
b. 2.7
c. 3.8
d. 4.9

*499. Four children are admitted with malaise, anorexia, and abdominal pain. Further evaluations reveal mild anemia, erythrocyte basophilic stippling, and profound pica habits. Poisoning by which heavy metal is most likely responsible?

    a. arsenic
    b. iron
    c. mercury
    d. lead

*500. Of the following diseases, which one is associated with the greatest elevation of lactate dehydrogenase isoenzyme 1?

    a. pneumonia
    b. glomerulonephritis
    c. pancreatitis
    d. $B_{12}$ deficiency

*501. Isoenzyme assays are performed to improve:

    a. precision
    b. accuracy
    c. sensitivity
    d. specificity

*502. In a pleural effusion caused by *Streptococcus pneumoniae*, the protein value of the pleural fluid compared with the serum value would probably be:

    a. decreased by 2
    b. decreased by one half
    c. increased by one half
    d. equal

*503. Hemoglobin S can be separated from hemoglobin D by which of the following methods?

    a. agar gel electrophoresis at pH 5.9
    b. thin layer chromatography
    c. alkali denaturation
    d. ammonium precipitation

*504. What specimen preparation is commonly used to perform the alkaline phosphatase isoenzyme determination?

    a. Serum is divided into two aliquots, one is frozen and the other is refrigerated.
    b. Serum is divided into two aliquots, one is heated at 56°C and the other is unheated.
    c. No preparation is necessary since the assay uses EDTA plasma.
    d. Protein-free filtrate is prepared first.

*505. What is the proper pH for the buffered solution used to perform serum protein electrophoresis?

    a. 5.6
    b. 7.6
    c. 8.6
    d. 9.6

*506. The expected blood gas results for a patient in chronic renal failure would match the pattern of:

    a. metabolic acidosis
    b. respiratory acidosis
    c. metabolic alkalosis
    d. respiratory alkalosis

*507. Which of the following tests must have clinically appropriate methods suitable for stat use?

    a. triglyceride
    b. amylase
    c. gamma-glutamyl transferase
    d. lactate dehydrogenase isoenzymes

*508. The most important buffer pair in plasma is the:

    a. phosphate/biphosphate pair
    b. hemoglobin/imidazole pair
    c. bicarbonate/carbonic acid pair
    d. sulfate/bisulfate pair

*509. The unit of measure for a standard solution is:

    a. g/L
    b. %
    c. mg/%
    d. mg/mL

*510. TSH is produced by the:

    a. hypothalamus
    b. pituitary gland
    c. adrenal cortex
    d. thyroid

*511. Severe diarrhea causes:

    a.  metabolic acidosis
    b.  metabolic alkalosis
    c.  respiratory acidosis
    d.  respiratory alkalosis

*512. Select the test that evaluates renal tubular function.

    a.  IVP
    b.  creatinine clearance
    c.  osmolarity
    d.  microscopic urinalysis

*513. Quantitation of $NA^+$ and $K^+$ by ion-selective electrode is more rapid than flame photometry because:

    a.  dilution is required for flame photometry
    b.  there is no lipoprotein interference
    c.  whole blood can be used
    d.  of the absence of an internal standard

# Chemistry **Answer Key**

| | | | | |
|---|---|---|---|---|
| 1. d | 42. b | 83. a | 124. d | 165. c |
| 2. c | 43. a | 84. c | 125. d | 166. a |
| 3. c | 44. b | 85. c | 126. a | 167. b |
| 4. a | 45. c | 86. c | 127. b | 168. b |
| 5. d | 46. c | 87. d | 128. b | 169. b |
| 6. d | 47. b | 88. d | 129. d | 170. b |
| 7. b | 48. c | 89. b | 130. b | 171. a |
| 8. c | 49. c | 90. d | 131. c | 172. d |
| 9. c | 50. c | 91. b | 132. a | 173. a |
| 10. a | 51. b | 92. d | 133. d | 174. b |
| 11. d | 52. b | 93. c | 134. b | 175. b |
| 12. b | 53. d | 94. d | 135. b | 176. c |
| 13. b | 54. d | 95. d | 136. c | 177. d |
| 14. b | 55. a | 96. a | 137. a | 178. a |
| 15. b | 56. b | 97. c | 138. a | 179. c |
| 16. a | 57. c | 98. c | 139. a | 180. b |
| 17. b | 58. d | 99. d | 140. a | 181. d |
| 18. a | 59. c | 100. b | 141. c | 182. a |
| 19. d | 60. a | 101. a | 142. a | 183. a |
| 20. c | 61. c | 102. d | 143. b | 184. d |
| 21. c | 62. a | 103. a | 144. d | 185. c |
| 22. b | 63. a | 104. b | 145. a | 186. b |
| 23. d | 64. d | 105. d | 146. d | 187. c |
| 24. b | 65. b | 106. c | 147. a | 188. a |
| 25. c | 66. a | 107. d | 148. a | 189. c |
| 26. b | 67. b | 108. d | 149. d | 190. d |
| 27. d | 68. c | 109. a | 150. c | 191. d |
| 28. a | 69. a | 110. b | 151. d | 192. a |
| 29. c | 70. a | 111. c | 152. a | 193. b |
| 30. c | 71. b | 112. b | 153. d | 194. a |
| 31. d | 72. b | 113. c | 154. a | 195. b |
| 32. b | 73. c | 114. b | 155. d | 196. c |
| 33. d | 74. d | 115. b | 156. a | 197. d |
| 34. c | 75. c | 116. b | 157. b | 198. a |
| 35. d | 76. d | 117. a | 158. d | 199. b |
| 36. a | 77. b | 118. b | 159. d | 200. c |
| 37. b | 78. d | 119. d | 160. b | 201. b |
| 38. d | 79. b | 120. d | 161. d | 202. c |
| 39. c | 80. c | 121. b | 162. d | 203. b |
| 40. a | 81. b | 122. c | 163. d | 204. b |
| 41. a | 82. c | 123. d | 164. a | 205. b |

| | | | | |
|---|---|---|---|---|
| 206. b | 252. b | 298. d | 344. a | 390. d |
| 207. b | 253. d | 299. a | 345. c | 391. a |
| 208. c | 254. a | 300. d | 346. a | 392. c |
| 209. a | 255. c | 301. d | 347. b | 393. d |
| 210. b | 256. a | 302. c | 348. b | 394. b |
| 211. d | 257. c | 303. a | 349. a | 395. b |
| 212. b | 258. a | 304. d | 350. d | 396. c |
| 213. d | 259. b | 305. a | 351. b | 397. a |
| 214. b | 260. b | 306. d | 352. a | 398. d |
| 215. a | 261. a | 307. c | 353. b | 399. d |
| 216. b | 262. b | 308. d | 354. b | 400. d |
| 217. c | 263. b | 309. d | 355. c | 401. c |
| 218. b | 264. b | 310. a | 356. a | 402. a |
| 219. a | 265. b | 311. b | 357. b | 403. b |
| 220. d | 266. b | 312. a | 358. a | 404. b |
| 221. c | 267. b | 313. c | 359. d | 405. c |
| 222. d | 268. d | 314. b | 360. c | 406. a |
| 223. d | 269. b | 315. a | 361. b | 407. b |
| 224. a | 270. d | 316. c | 362. b | 408. b |
| 225. a | 271. a | 317. c | 363. b | 409. a |
| 226. a | 272. a | 318. c | 364. d | 410. d |
| 227. b | 273. c | 319. c | 365. c | 411. b |
| 228. b | 274. c | 320. c | 366. c | 412. c |
| 229. d | 275. b | 321. b | 367. d | 413. c |
| 230. d | 276. b | 322. a | 368. d | 414. c |
| 231. b | 277. a | 323. c | 369. a | 415. b |
| 232. a | 278. a | 324. a | 370. d | 416. a |
| 233. d | 279. b | 325. b | 371. c | 417. b |
| 234. d | 280. b | 326. b | 372. a | 418. a |
| 235. c | 281. b | 327. b | 373. b | 419. c |
| 236. d | 282. b | 328. c | 374. c | 420. b |
| 237. b | 283. a | 329. a | 375. c | 421. a |
| 238. a | 284. d | 330. a | 376. d | 422. c |
| 239. c | 285. d | 331. b | 377. c | 423. b |
| 240. a | 286. a | 332. d | 378. b | 424. a |
| 241. a | 287. c | 333. b | 379. a | 425. c |
| 242. d | 288. c | 334. c | 380. d | 426. d |
| 243. d | 289. a | 335. b | 381. d | 427. c |
| 244. b | 290. d | 336. c | 382. a | 428. d |
| 245. a | 291. d | 337. c | 383. a | 429. c |
| 246. a | 292. d | 338. a | 384. d | 430. a |
| 247. d | 293. d | 339. a | 385. b | 431. a |
| 248. d | 294. c | 340. d | 386. d | 432. a |
| 249. c | 295. a | 341. c | 387. c | 433. c |
| 250. c | 296. a | 342. d | 388. b | 434. b |
| 251. b | 297. a | 343. b | 389. c | 435. d |

| 436. a | 452. d | 468. c | 484. d | 500. d |
| 437. c | 453. c | 469. b | 485. c | 501. d |
| 438. b | 454. b | 470. b | 486. a | 502. b |
| 439. d | 455. c | 471. d | 487. c | 503. a |
| 440. d | 456. b | 472. d | 488. c | 504. b |
| 441. d | 457. d | 473. b | 489. d | 505. c |
| 442. b | 458. b | 474. c | 490. d | 506. a |
| 443. c | 459. c | 475. c | 491. a | 507. b |
| 444. a | 460. b | 476. a | 492. c | 508. c |
| 445. b | 461. b | 477. b | 493. b | 509. d |
| 446. c | 462. b | 478. a | 494. d | 510. b |
| 447. a | 463. d | 479. c | 495. c | 511. a |
| 448. d | 464. b | 480. b | 496. b | 512. c |
| 449. c | 465. b | 481. c | 497. d | 513. c |
| 450. b | 466. c | 482. c | 498. a | |
| 451. c | 467. b | 483. d | 499. d | |

# CHAPTER 11

# *Hematology*

*The following items have been identified as appropriate for both entry level medical technologists and medical laboratory technicians.*

1. Which of the following is the standard calibration method for hematology instrumentation against which other methods must be verified?

   a. latex particles of known dimension
   b. stabilized red cell suspensions
   c. stabilized 7 parameter reference controls
   d. normal whole blood

2. The most common form of childhood leukemia is:

   a. acute lymphocytic
   b. acute granulocytic
   c. acute monocytic
   d. chronic granulocytic

3. Which of the following measures platelet function?

   a. bleeding time
   b. prothrombin time
   c. thrombin time
   d. partial thromboplastin time

4. The values below were obtained on an automated blood count system performed on a blood sample from a 25-year-old man:

|      | Patient | Normal |
|------|---------|--------|
| WBC  | 5.1 x 10³/μL | 5.0-10.0 x 10³/μL |
| RBC  | 2.94 x 10⁶/μL | 4.6-6.2 x 10⁶/μL |
| Hgb  | 13.8 g/dL | 14-18 g/dL |
| Hct  | 35.4% | 40%-54% |
| MCV  | 128 fL | 82-90 fL |
| MCH  | 46.7 pg | 27-31 pg |
| MCHC | 40% | 32%-36% |

These results are most consistent with which of the following?

a. megaloblastic anemia
b. hereditary spherocytosis
c. a high titer of cold agglutinins
d. an elevated reticulocyte count


5. A blood smear shows 80 nucleated red cells per 100 leukocytes. The total leukocyte count is 18 x 10³/μL. The true white cell count expressed in SI units is:

a. 17.2 x 10³/μL
b. 9.0 x 10³/μL
c. 10.0 x 10³/μL
d. 13.4 x 10³/μL


6. The following results were obtained on an electronic particle counter:

|      |      |
|------|------|
| WBC  | ++++ |
| RBC  | 2.01 x 10⁶/μL |
| Hgb  | 7.7 g/dL |
| Hct  | 28.2% |
| MCV  | 141 fL |
| MCH  | 38.5 pg |
| MCHC | 23.3% |

What step should be taken before recycling the sample?

a. clean the apertures
b. warm the specimen
c. replace the lysing agent
d. dilute the specimen

7. Of the following, the disease most closely associated with granulocyte hyposegmentation is:

   a. May-Hegglin anomaly
   b. Pelger-Huët anomaly
   c. Chédiak-Higashi syndrome
   d. Gaucher's disease


8. The most appropriate screening test for detecting hemoglobin F is:

   a. osmotic fragility
   b. dithionite solubility
   c. Kleihauer-Betke
   d. heat instability test


9. The most appropriate screening test for hemoglobin H is:

   a. dithionite solubility
   b. osmotic fragility
   c. sucrose hemolysis
   d. heat instability test


10. The most appropriate screening test for hemoglobin S is:

    a. Kleihauer-Betke
    b. dithionite solubility
    c. osmotic fragility
    d. sucrose hemolysis


11. The most appropriate screening test for hereditary spherocytosis is:

    a. osmotic fragility
    b. sucrose hemolysis
    c. heat instability test
    d. Kleihauer-Betke


12. The most appropriate screening test for paroxysmal nocturnal hemoglobinuria is:

    a. heat instability test
    b. sucrose hemolysis
    c. osmotic fragility
    d. dithionite solubility

13. The characteristic morphologic feature in multiple myeloma is:

    a. cytotoxic T cells
    b. rouleaux formation
    c. spherocytosis
    d. macrocytosis


14. A characteristic morphologic feature in hemoglobin C disease is:

    a. macrocytosis
    b. spherocytosis
    c. rouleaux formation
    d. target cells


15. Hematology standards include:

    a. stabilized red blood cell suspension
    b. latex particles
    c. stabilized avian red blood cells
    d. certified cyanmethemoglobin solution


16. The following results were obtained on an electronic particle counter:

| | |
|---|---|
| WBC | $6.5 \times 10^3/\mu L$ |
| RBC | $4.55 \times 10^6/\mu L$ |
| Hgb | 18.0 g/dL |
| Hct | 41.5% |
| MCV | 90.1 fL |
| MCH | 39.6 pg |
| MCHC | 43.4% |

The first step in obtaining valid results is to:

    a. perform a microhematocrit
    b. correct the hemoglobin for lipemia
    c. dilute the blood
    d. replace the lysing agent


17. Which of the following tests is used to monitor red cell production?

    a. packed cell volume
    b. total iron-binding capacity
    c. Schilling test
    d. reticulocyte count

18. A differential was performed on an asymptomatic patient. The differential included 60% neutrophils: 55 of which had 2 lobes and 5 had 3 lobes. There were no other abnormalities. This is consistent with which of the following anomalies?

   a. Pelger-Huët
   b. May-Hegglin
   c. Alder-Reilly
   d. Chédiak-Higashi

19. The following results were obtained on an electronic particle counter:

| | |
|---|---|
| WBC | $61.3 \times 10^3/\mu L$ |
| RBC | $1.19 \times 10^6/\mu L$ |
| Hgb | 9.9 g/dL |
| Hct | 21% |
| MCV | 125 fL |
| MCHC | 54.1% |

   What action should be taken to obtain accurate results?

   a. dilute the specimen and recount
   b. warm the specimen and recount
   c. check the tube for clots
   d. clean the aperture tubes and recount

20. Thalassemias are characterized by:

   a. structural abnormalities in the hemoglobin molecule
   b. absence of iron in hemoglobin
   c. decreased rate of heme synthesis
   d. decreased rate of globin synthesis

21. Phagocytosis is a function of:

   a. erythrocytes
   b. granulocytes
   c. lymphocytes
   d. thrombocytes

22. Cells involved in hemostasis are:

   a. erythrocytes
   b. granulocytes
   c. lymphocytes
   d. thrombocytes

23. Cells for the transport of $O_2$ and $CO_2$ are:

  a. erythrocytes
  b. granulocytes
  c. lymphocytes
  d. thrombocytes


24. Cells that produce antibodies and lymphokines are:

  a. erythrocytes
  b. granulocytes
  c. lymphocytes
  d. thrombocytes


25. In polycythemia vera, the hemoglobin, hematocrit, red blood cell count, and red cell mass are:

  a. elevated
  b. normal
  c. decreased


26. In polycythemia vera, the platelet count is:

  a. elevated
  b. normal
  c. decreased


27. 50%-90% myeloblasts in a peripheral blood sample is typical of which of the following?

  a. chronic granulocytic leukemia
  b. myelofibrosis with myeloid metaplasia
  c. erythroleukemia
  d. acute granulocytic leukemia


28. Auer rods are most likely present in which of the following?

  a. chronic granulocytic leukemia
  b. myelofibrosis with myeloid metaplasia
  c. erythroleukemia
  d. acute granulocytic leukemia


29. All stages of neutrophils are most likely to be seen in the peripheral blood of a patient with:

  a. chronic granulocytic leukemia
  b. myelofibrosis with myeloid metaplasia
  c. erythroleukemia
  d. acute granulocytic leukemia

30. Erythropoietin acts to:

    a.  shorten the replication time of the granulocytes
    b.  stimulate RNA synthesis of erythroid cells
    c.  increase colony-stimulating factors produced by the B-lymphocytes
    d.  decrease the release of marrow reticulocytes


31. In the French-American-British (FAB) classification, acute lymphocytic leukemia is divided into groups according to:

    a.  prognosis
    b.  immunology
    c.  cytochemistry
    d.  morphology


32. The specimen of choice for preparation of blood films for manual differential leukocyte counts is whole blood collected in:

    a.  EDTA
    b.  oxalate
    c.  citrate
    d.  heparin


33. When platelets concentrate at the edges and feathered end of a blood smear, it is usually due to:

    a.  abnormal proteins
    b.  inadequate mixing of blood and anticoagulant
    c.  hemorrhage
    d.  poorly made wedge smear


34. Irregular clumping of platelets is usually due to:

    a.  inadequate mixing of blood and anticoagulant
    b.  hemorrhage
    c.  poorly made wedge smear
    d.  hypersplenism


35. Platelet satellitosis is usually due to:

    a.  abnormal proteins
    b.  inadequate mixing of blood and anticoagulant
    c.  hemorrhage
    d.  poorly made wedge smear

36. Elevation of the granulocyte percentage above 75% is termed:

    a. absolute lymphocytosis
    b. leukocytosis
    c. relative neutrophilic leukocytosis
    d. absolute neutrophilic leukocytosis

37. Elevation of the lymphocyte percentage above 47% is termed:

    a. relative lymphocytosis
    b. absolute lymphocytosis
    c. leukocytosis
    d. absolute neutrophilic leukocytosis

38. Elevation of the total granulocyte count above $9.0 \times 10^3/\mu L$ is termed:

    a. relative lymphocytosis
    b. leukocytosis
    c. relative neutrophilic leukocytosis
    d. absolute neutrophilic leukocytosis

39. Elevation of the total white cell count above $12 \times 10^9/\mu L$ is termed:

    a. relative lymphocytosis
    b. absolute lymphocytosis
    c. leukocytosis
    d. relative neutrophilic leukocytosis

40. The chamber counting method of platelet enumeration:

    a. allows direct visualization of the particles being counted
    b. has a high degree of precision
    c. has a high degree of reproducibility
    d. is the method of choice for the performance of 50-60 counts per day

41. Specific (secondary) granules of the neutrophilic granulocyte:

    a. appear first at the myelocyte stage
    b. contain lysosomal enzymes
    c. are formed on the mitochondria
    d. are derived from azurophil (primary) granules

42. The anemia of chronic infection is characterized by:

    a. decreased iron stores in the reticuloendothelial system
    b. decreased serum iron levels
    c. macrocytic erythrocytes
    d. increased serum iron-binding capacity

43. Which of the following are characteristic of polycythemia vera?

    a. elevated urine erythropoietin levels
    b. increased oxygen affinity of hemoglobin
    c. "teardrop" poikilocytosis
    d. decreased or absent bone marrow iron stores

44. Factors commonly involved in producing anemia in patients with chronic renal disease include:

    a. marrow hypoplasia
    b. ineffective erythropoiesis
    c. vitamin $B_{12}$ deficiency
    d. increased erythropoietin production

45. Thrombocytopenia is a characteristic of:

    a. classic von Willebrand's disease
    b. hemophilia A
    c. Glanzmann's thrombasthenia
    d. May-Hegglin anomaly

46. A leukocyte count and differential on a 40-year-old Caucasian man revealed:

| | |
|---|---|
| WBC | $5.4 \times 10^3/\mu L$ |
| **Differential** | |
| Segs | 20% |
| Lymphs | 58% |
| Monos | 20% |
| Eos | 2% |

These data represent:

    a. relative lymphocytosis
    b. absolute lymphocytosis
    c. relative neutrophilia
    d. leukopenia

47. A leukocyte count and differential on a 40-year-old white man revealed:

| WBC | 5.4 x 10³/μL |
|-----|--------------|

Differential

| | |
|---|---|
| Segs | 20% |
| Lymphs | 58% |
| Monos | 20% |
| Eos | 2% |

These data represent:

a. absolute lymphocytosis
b. relative neutrophilia
c. absolute neutropenia
d. leukopenia

48. Which of the following platelet responses is most likely associated with classic von Willebrand's disease?

a. decreased platelet aggregation to ristocetin
b. normal platelet aggregation to ristocetin
c. absent aggregation to epinephrine, ADP, and collagen
d. decreased amount of ADP in platelets

49. The majority of the iron in an adult is found as a constituent of:

a. hemoglobin
b. hemosiderin
c. myoglobin
d. transferrin

50. A patient has the following blood values:

| RBC | 6.5 x 10⁶/μL |
|-----|--------------|
| Hgb | 14.0 g/dL |
| Hct | 42.0% |
| MCV | 65 fL |
| MCH | 21.5 pg |
| MCHC | 33% |

These results are compatible with:

a. iron deficiency
b. pregnancy
c. thalassemia minor
d. beta thalassemia major

51. A 60-year-old man has a painful right knee and a slightly enlarged spleen. Hematology results include:

Hemoglobin                          15 g/dL
Absolute neutrophil count           10.0 x 10³/μL
Platelet count                      900 x 10³/μL
Uncorrected retic count             1%
Normal red cell morphology and indices
A slight increase in bands
Rare metamyelocyte and myelocyte
Giant and bizarre-shaped platelets

These results are most compatible with:

a. congenital spherocytosis
b. rheumatoid arthritis with reactive thrombocytosis
c. myelofibrosis
d. idiopathic thrombocythemia


52. A 50-year-old woman who has been receiving busulfan for 3 years for chronic myelogenous leukemia becomes anemic. Laboratory tests reveal:

Thrombocytopenia
Many peroxidase-negative blast cells in the peripheral blood
Bone marrow hypercellular in blast transformation
Markedly increased bone marrow TdT

Which of the following complications is this patient most likely to have?

a. acute lymphocytic leukemia
b. acute myelocytic leukemia
c. acute myelomonocytic leukemia
d. busulfan toxicity


53. Which of the following is the most common cause of an abnormality in hemostasis?

a. decreased plasma fibrinogen level
b. decreased Factor VIII level
c. decreased Factor IX level
d. quantitative abnormality of platelets


54. A hemophiliac male and a normal female can produce a:

a. female carrier
b. male carrier
c. male hemophiliac
d. normal female

55. A patient has a normal prothrombin time and a prolonged activated partial thromboplastin time (APTT) using a kaolin activator. The APTT corrects to normal when the incubation time is increased. These results suggest that the patient has:

a. hemophilia A (Factor VIII deficiency)
b. Hageman factor (XII) deficiency
c. Fletcher factor deficiency (prekallikrein)
d. Factor V deficiency

56. Acute disseminated intravascular coagulation is characterized by:

a. hypofibrinogenemia
b. thrombocytosis
c. negative D-dimer
d. shortened thrombin time

57. Coagulation factors affected by coumarin drugs are:

a. VIII, IX, and X
b. I, II, V, and VII
c. II, VII, IX, and X
d. II, V, and VII

58. The following data were obtained on a patient:

| | |
|---|---|
| PT | 20 sec |
| Thrombin time | 13 sec |
| APTT | 55 sec |
| APTT plus aged serum | Corrected |
| APTT plus adsorbed plasma | Not corrected |
| Circulatory inhibitor | None present |

Which of the following coagulation factors is deficient?

a. Factor V
b. Factor VIII
c. Factor X
d. Factor XI

59. Which of the following laboratory procedures is most helpful in differentiating severe liver disease and accompanying secondary fibrinolysis from disseminated intravascular coagulation?

a. presence of fibrin split products
b. increased APTT
c. Factor VIII activity
d. fibrinogen level

60. Which of the following laboratory findings is associated with Factor XIII deficiency?

   a. prolonged activated partial thromboplastin time
   b. clot solubility in a 5 molar urea solution
   c. prolonged thrombin time
   d. prolonged prothrombin time

61. An automated leukocyte count is 22.5 x $10^3$/μL. The differential reveals 200 normoblasts/ 100 leukocytes. What is the actual leukocyte count per microliter?

   a. 7500/μL
   b. 11,500/μL
   c. 14,400/μL
   d. 22,300/μL

62. On Monday a patient's hemoglobin determination was 11.3 g/dL and on Tuesday it measured 11.8 g/dL. The standard deviation of the method used is ± 0.2 g/dL. What can be concluded about the hemoglobin values given?

   a. One value probably resulted from laboratory error.
   b. There is poor precision; daily quality control charts should be checked.
   c. The second value is out of range and should be repeated.
   d. There is no significant change in the patient's hemoglobin concentration.

63. A patient has a high cold agglutinin titer. Automated cell counter results reveal an elevated MCV, MCH, and MCHC. Individual erythrocytes appear normal on a stained smear, but agglutinates are noted. The appropriate course of action would be to:

   a. perform the RBC, Hgb, and Hct determinations using manual methods
   b. perform the RBC determination by a manual method; use the automated results for the Hgb and Hct
   c. repeat the determinations using a microsample of diluted blood
   d. repeat the determinations using a prewarmed microsample of diluted blood

64. The anticoagulant of choice for routine coagulation procedures is:

   a. sodium oxalate
   b. sodium citrate
   c. heparin
   d. sodium fluoride

65. The most common cause of error when using automated cell counters is:

   a. contamination of the diluent
   b. inadequate mixing of the sample prior to testing
   c. variation in voltage of the current supply
   d. a calibrating error

66. Which of the following is associated with May-Hegglin anomaly?

    a. membrane defect of lysosomes
    b. Döhle bodies and giant platelets
    c. chronic myelogenous leukemia
    d. mucopolysaccharidosis


67. Which of the following is associated with Chédiak-Higashi syndrome?

    a. membrane defect of lysosomes
    b. Döhle bodies and giant platelets
    c. two-lobed neutrophils
    d. mucopolysaccharidosis


68. Which of the following is associated with pseudo–Pelger-Huët anomaly?

    a. aplastic anemia
    b. iron deficiency anemia
    c. myelogenous leukemia
    d. Chédiak-Higashi syndrome


69. Which of the following is associated with Alder-Reilly inclusions?

    a. membrane defect of lysosomes
    b. Döhle bodies and giant platelets
    c. two-lobed neutrophils
    d. mucopolysaccharidosis


70. Many microspherocytes and schistocytes and budding off of spherocytes can be seen on peripheral blood smears of patients with:

    a. hereditary spherocytosis
    b. disseminated intravascular coagulation (DIC)
    c. acquired autoimmune hemolytic anemia
    d. extensive burns


71. Muramidase (lysozyme) is present in:

    a. granulocytes and their precursors
    b. monocytes and their precursors
    c. granulocytes, monocytes, and their precursors
    d. lymphocytes and their precursors

72. Hemolysis in paroxysmal nocturnal hemoglobinuria (PNH) is:

    a. temperature-dependent
    b. complement-independent
    c. antibody-mediated
    d. caused by a red cell membrane defect

73. In order for hemoglobin to combine reversibly with oxygen, the iron must be:

    a. complexed with haptoglobin
    b. freely circulating in the cytoplasm
    c. attached to transferrin
    d. in the ferrous state

74. Heinz bodies are:

    a. readily identified with polychrome stains
    b. rarely found in glucose-6-phosphate dehydrogenase deficient erythrocytes
    c. closely associated with spherocytes
    d. denatured hemoglobin inclusions that are readily removed by the spleen

75. Which of the following sets of laboratory findings is consistent with hemolytic anemia?

    a. normal or slightly increased erythrocyte survival; normal osmotic fragility
    b. decreased erythrocyte survival; increased catabolism of heme
    c. decreased serum lactate dehydrogenase activity; normal catabolism of heme
    d. normal concentration of haptoglobin; marked hemoglobinuria

76. Evidence indicates that the genetic defect in thalassemia usually results in:

    a. the production of abnormal globin chains
    b. a quantitative deficiency in RNA resulting in decreased globin chain production
    c. a structural change in the heme portion of the hemoglobin
    d. an abnormality in the alpha or beta chain binding or affinity

77. Hemoglobin H disease results from:

    a. absence of 3 of 4 alpha genes
    b. absence of 2 of 4 alpha genes
    c. absence of 1 of 4 alpha genes
    d. absence of all 4 alpha genes

78. Which of the following represents characteristic features of iron metabolism in patients with anemia of a chronic disorder?

   a. serum iron is normal, transferrin saturation is normal, TIBC is normal
   b. serum iron is increased, transferrin saturation is increased, TIBC is normal or slightly increased
   c. serum iron is normal, transferrin saturation is markedly increased, TIBC is normal
   d. serum iron is decreased, transferrin saturation is decreased, TIBC is normal or decreased

79. A patient with polycythemia vera who is treated by phlebotomy is most likely to develop a deficiency of:

   a. iron
   b. vitamin $B_{12}$
   c. folic acid
   d. erythropoietin

80. Hemorrhage in polycythemia vera is the result of:

   a. increased plasma viscosity
   b. persistent thrombocytosis
   c. splenic sequestration of platelets
   d. abnormal platelet function

81. In chronic myelocytic leukemia, blood histamine concentrations tend to reflect the:

   a. number of platelets present
   b. serum uric acid concentrations
   c. number of basophils present
   d. total number of granulocytes

82. Which of the following anomalies is an autosomal dominant disorder characterized by irregularly sized inclusions in polymorphonuclear neutrophils, abnormal giant platelets, and often thrombocytopenia?

   a. Pelger-Huët
   b. Chédiak-Higashi
   c. Alder-Reilly
   d. May-Hegglin

83. The bone marrow in the terminal stage of erythroleukemia is often indistinguishable from that seen in:

   a. myeloid metaplasia
   b. polycythemia vera
   c. acute myelocytic leukemia
   d. aplastic anemia

84. Which of the following is a significant feature of erythroleukemia (Di Guglielmo's syndrome)?

    a. persistently increased M:E ratio
    b. megaloblastoid erythropoiesis
    c. marked thrombocytosis
    d. decreased stainable iron in the marrow


85. In which of the following disease states are teardrop cells and abnormal platelets most characteristically seen?

    a. chronic myelocytic leukemia
    b. multiple myeloma
    c. thalassemia
    d. myeloid metaplasia


86. In the French-American-British (FAB) classification, myelomonocytic leukemia would be:

    a. M1 and M2
    b. M3
    c. M4
    d. M5


87. Which of the following is characteristic of platelet disorders?

    a. deep muscle hemorrhages
    b. retroperitoneal hemorrhages
    c. mucous membrane hemorrhages
    d. severely prolonged clotting times


88. Which of the following is a true statement about acute idiopathic thrombocytopenic purpura (ITP)?

    a. It is found primarily in adults.
    b. Spontaneous remission usually occurs within several weeks.
    c. Women are more commonly affected.
    d. Peripheral destruction of platelets is decreased.


89. Which of the following is most useful in differentiating hemophilias A and B?

    a. pattern of inheritance
    b. clinical history
    c. activated partial thromboplastin time
    d. mixing studies (substitution studies)

90. A 56-year-old woman was admitted to the hospital with a history of a moderate to severe bleeding tendency of several years' duration. Epistaxis and menorrhagia were reported. Prolonged APTT was corrected with fresh normal plasma, adsorbed plasma, and aged serum. Deficiency of which of the following is most likely?

    a. Factor XII
    b. Factor VIII
    c. Factor XI
    d. Factor IX

91. A patient has a history of mild hemorrhagic episodes. Laboratory results include a prolonged prothrombin time and activated partial thromboplastin time. The abnormal prothrombin time was corrected by normal and adsorbed plasma, but not aged serum. Which of the following coagulation factors is deficient?

    a. prothrombin
    b. Factor V
    c. Factor X
    d. Factor VII

92. A bone marrow slide shows foam cells ranging from 20 to 100 µm in size with vacuolated cytoplasm containing sphingomyelin and is faintly PAS positive. This cell type is most characteristic of:

    a. Gaucher's disease
    b. myeloma with Russell bodies
    c. Di Guglielmo disease
    d. Niemann-Pick disease

93. Patients with chronic granulomatous disease suffer from frequent pyogenic infections owing to the inability of:

    a. lymphocytes to produce bacterial antibodies
    b. eosinophils to degranulate in the presence of bacteria
    c. neutrophils to kill phagocytized bacteria
    d. basophils to release histamine in the presence of bacteria

94. A 40-year-old man had an erythrocyte count of 2.5 x 10$^6$/µL, hematocrit of 22%, and a reticulocyte count of 2.0%. Which of the following statements best describes his condition?

    a. The absolute reticulocyte count is 50 x 10$^3$/µL, indicating that the bone marrow is not adequately compensating for the anemia.
    b. The reticulocyte count is greatly increased, indicating an adequate bone marrow response for this anemia.
    c. The absolute reticulocyte count is 500 x 10$^3$/µL, indicating that the bone marrow is adequately compensating for the anemia.
    d. The reticulocyte count is slightly increased, indicating an adequate response to the slight anemia.

95. In an electronic or laser particle cell counter, clumped platelets may interfere with which of the following parameters?

    a. white blood cell count
    b. red blood cell count
    c. hemoglobin
    d. hematocrit


96. When using an electronic cell counter, which of the following results can occur in the presence of a cold agglutinin?

    a. increased MCV and decreased RBC
    b. increased MCV and normal RBC
    c. decreased MCV and increased MCHC
    d. decreased MCV and RBC


97. A properly functioning electronic cell counter obtains the following results:

| | |
|---|---|
| WBC | 5.1 x 10³/μL |
| RBC | 4.87 x 10⁶/μL |
| Hgb | 16.1 g/dL |
| Hct | 39.3% |
| MCV | 82.0 fL |
| MCH | 33.1 pg |
| MCHC | 41.3% |

   What is the most likely cause of these results?

    a. lipemia
    b. cold agglutinins
    c. increased WBC
    d. rouleaux


98. Blood collected in EDTA undergoes which of the following changes if kept at room temperature for 6-24 hours?

    a. increased hematocrit and MCV
    b. increased ESR and MCV
    c. increased MCHC and MCV
    d. decreased reticulocyte count and hematocrit


99. On setting up the electronic particle counter in the morning, one of the controls is slightly below the range for the MCV. Which of the following is indicated?

    a. call for service
    b. adjust the MCV up slightly
    c. shut down the instrument
    d. repeat the control

100. Which of the following is associated with Glanzmann's thrombasthenia?

    a. normal bleeding time
    b. normal ADP aggregation
    c. abnormal initial wave ristocetin aggregation
    d. absence of clot retraction

101. Which of the following is a characteristic of Factor XII deficiency?

    a. negative bleeding history
    b. normal clotting times
    c. decreased risk of thrombosis
    d. epistaxis

102. Which of the following is characteristic of Bernard-Soulier syndrome?

    a. giant platelets
    b. normal bleeding time
    c. abnormal aggregation with ADP
    d. increased platelet count

103. Which of the following will not cause erroneous results when using a phase optical system for enumerating platelets?

    a. incipient clotting
    b. decreased hematocrit
    c. Howell-Jolly bodies
    d. leukocyte cytoplasmic fragments

Questions 104-108 refer to the following illustration:

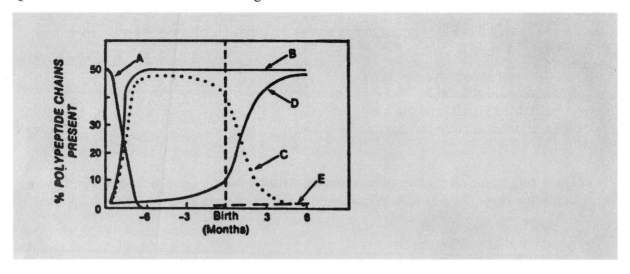

104. Which curve represents the production of alpha polypeptide chains of hemoglobin?

    a. A
    b. B
    c. C
    d. D


105. Which curve represents the production of beta polypeptide chains of hemoglobin?

    a. B
    b. C
    c. E
    d. D


106. Which curve represents the production of gamma polypeptide chains of hemoglobin?

    a. A
    b. B
    c. C
    d. D


107. Which curve represents the production of delta polypeptide chains of hemoglobin?

    a. B
    b. C
    c. D
    d. E


108. Which curve represents the production of epsilon polypeptide chains of hemoglobin?

    a. A
    b. B
    c. C
    d. D


109. Decreased to normal erythropoietin production is most likely to be associated with:

    a. polycythemia vera
    b. polycythemia, secondary to hypoxia
    c. relative polycythemia associated with dehydration
    d. polycythemia associated with renal disease

110. A patient has a tumor that concentrates erythropoietin. He is most likely to have which of the following types of polycythemia?

    a. polycythemia vera
    b. polycythemia, secondary to hypoxia
    c. benign familial polycythemia
    d. polycythemia associated with renal disease


111. Which of the following types of polycythemia is a severely burned patient most likely to have?

    a. polycythemia vera
    b. polycythemia, secondary to hypoxia
    c. relative polycythemia associated with dehydration
    d. polycythemia associated with renal disease


112. Which of the following types of polycythemia is most often associated with emphysema?

    a. polycythemia vera
    b. polycythemia, secondary to hypoxia
    c. relative polycythemia associated with dehydration
    d. polycythemia associated with renal disease


113. Which of the following is most closely associated with idiopathic hemochromatosis?

    a. iron overload in tissue
    b. target cells
    c. basophilic stippling
    d. ringed sideroblasts


114. Which of the following is most closely associated with iron deficiency anemia?

    a. iron overload in tissue
    b. target cells
    c. basophilic stippling
    d. chronic blood loss


115. Which of the following is seen most often in thalassemia?

    a. chronic blood loss
    b. target cells
    c. basophilic stippling
    d. ringed sideroblasts

116. Which of the following is most likely to be seen in lead poisoning?

    a. iron overload in tissue
    b. codocytes
    c. basophilic stippling
    d. ringed sideroblasts


117. Which of the following is most closely associated with chronic myelogenous leukemia?

    a. ringed sideroblasts
    b. disseminated intravascular coagulation
    c. micromegakaryocytes
    d. Philadelphia chromosome


118. Which of the following is most closely associated with chronic myelomonocytic leukemia?

    a. Philadelphia chromosome
    b. disseminated intravascular coagulation
    c. micromegakaryocytes
    d. lysozymuria


119. Which of the following is most closely associated with erythroleukemia?

    a. ringed sideroblasts
    b. disseminated intravascular coagulation
    c. micromegakaryocytes
    d. lysozymuria


120. Which of the following is most closely associated with acute promyelocytic leukemia?

    a. ringed sideroblasts
    b. disseminated intravascular coagulation
    c. micromegakaryocytes
    d. Philadelphia chromosome


121. Which of the following may be used to stain neutral fats, phospholipids, and sterols?

    a. peroxidase
    b. Sudan black B
    c. periodic acid–Schiff (PAS)
    d. Prussian blue

122. Which of the following is vitamin K dependent?

   a. Factor XII
   b. fibrinogen
   c. antithrombin III
   d. Factor VII


Questions 123-126 refer to the following illustration:

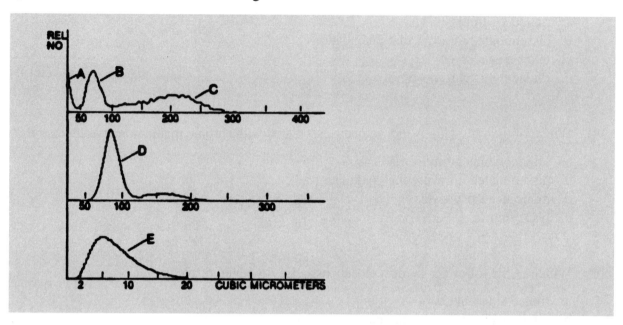

123. Which area of the automated cell counter histogram indicates the nonlymphocyte curve?

   a. B
   b. C
   c. D
   d. E


124. Which area of the automated cell counter histogram indicates the lymphocyte curve?

   a. A
   b. B
   c. C
   d. D


125. Which area in the automated cell counter histogram represents the RBC distribution curve?

   a. A
   b. B
   c. C
   d. D

126. Which area of the automated cell counter histogram represents the platelet distribution curve?

    a. A
    b. B
    c. C
    d. E

127. The following results were obtained on a 55-year-old man complaining of headaches and blurred vision:

| WBC | 19.0 x 10³/µL | Differential | |
|---|---|---|---|
| RBC | 7.2 x 10⁶/µL | Segs | 84% |
| Platelets | 1056 x 10³/µL | Bands | 10% |
| Uric acid | 13.0 mg/dL | Lymphs | 3% |
| O₂ saturation | 93% | Monos | 2% |
| | | Eos | 1% |

Rh¹            Negative
Red cell volume   3911 mL (normal, 1600)

These results are consistent with:

    a. neutrophilic leukemoid reaction
    b. polycythemia vera
    c. chronic granulocytic leukemia
    d. leukoerythroblastosis in myelofibrosis

128. The following results were obtained on a 45-year-old man complaining of chills and fever:

| WBC   23.0 x 10³/µL | Differential | |
|---|---|---|
| | Segs | 60% |
| | Bands | 21% |
| | Lymphs | 11% |
| | Monos | 3% |
| | Metamyelos | 2% |
| | Myelos | 3% |

Toxic granulation, Döhle bodies, and vacuoles

LAP                      200
Philadelphia chromosome   Negative

These results are consistent with:

    a. neutrophilic leukemoid reaction
    b. polycythemia vera
    c. chronic granulocytic leukemia
    d. leukoerythroblastosis in myelofibrosis

129. The following results were obtained:

| WBC | 5.0 x 10³/µL | Differential | |
|---|---|---|---|
| RBC | 1.7 x 10⁶/µL | Segs | 16% |
| MCV | 84 µm³ | Bands | 22% |
| Platelets | 89 x 10³/µL | Lymphs | 28% |
| | | Monos | 16% |
| | | Eos | 1% |
| | | Basos | 1% |
| | | Metamyelos | 4% |
| | | Myelos | 3% |
| | | Promyelos | 4% |
| | | Blasts | 5% |

1 megakaryoblast; 30 nucleated erythrocytes; teardrops; schistocytes; polychromasia; giant, bizarre platelets noted

| LAP | 142 |
|---|---|
| Philadelphia chromosome | Negative |

These results are consistent with:

a. idiopathic thrombocythemia
b. polycythemia vera
c. chronic granulocytic leukemia
d. leukoerythroblastosis in myelofibrosis

130. The following results were obtained on a 35-year-old woman complaining of fatigue and weight loss:

| WBC | 1.8 x 10³/µL | Differential | |
|---|---|---|---|
| RBC | 4.6 x 10⁶/µL | Segs | 30% |
| Platelets | 903 x 10³/µL | Bands | 17% |
| Uric acid | 6.4 x ng/dL | Lymphs | 13% |
| | | Monos | 3% |
| | | Eos | 4% |
| | | Basos | 6% |
| | | Metamyelos | 3% |
| | | Myelos | 20% |
| | | Promyelos | 3% |
| | | Blasts | 1% |

| LAP | 0 |
|---|---|
| Philadelphia chromosome | Positive |

These results are consistent with:

a. neutrophilic leukemoid reaction
b. idiopathic thrombocythemia
c. chronic granulocytic leukemia
d. leukoerythroblastosis in myelofibrosis

131. The following results were obtained:

| | | | |
|---|---|---|---|
| WBC | $1.8 \times 10^3/\mu L$ | Differential | |
| Hgb | 8.9 g/dL | Segs | 70% |
| Hct | 27.4% | Bands | 10% |
| Platelets | $2300 \times 10^3/\mu L$ | Lymphs | 18% |
| | | Monos | 2% |

Giant, bizarre platelets, rare megakaryocytes
3+ poikilocytosis, 2+ anisocytosis, 1+ schizocytosis

LAP    90

These results are consistent with:

a. neutrophilic leukemoid reaction
b. polycythemia vera
c. leukoerythroblastosis in myelofibrosis
d. idiopathic thrombocythemia

132. Which of the following conditions is NOT associated with a high incidence of leukemia?

a. paroxysmal nocturnal hemoglobinuria
b. Fanconi's anemia
c. aplastic anemia
d. megaloblastic anemia

133. Laboratory findings in hereditary spherocytosis do NOT include:

a. decreased osmotic fragility
b. increased autohemolysis corrected by glucose
c. reticulocytosis
d. shortened erythrocyte survival

134. Patients with (A–) type G-6-PD deficiency are LEAST likely to have hemolytic episodes in which of the following situations?

a. following the administration of oxidizing drugs
b. the neonatal period
c. during infections
d. spontaneously

135. In most cases of hereditary persistence of fetal hemoglobin (HPFH):

   a. Hgb F is unevenly distributed throughout the erythrocytes
   b. the black heterozygote has 75% Hgb F
   c. beta and gamma chain synthesis is decreased
   d. gamma chain production equals alpha chain production


136. Which of the following is typical of polycythemia vera?

   a. increased serum iron concentration
   b. decreased thrombocyte count
   c. increased erythropoietin
   d. increased leukocyte alkaline phosphatase activity


137. Auer rods are:

   a. a normal aggregation of lysosomes or primary (azurophilic) granules
   b. predominantly found in acute myelogenous leukemia
   c. peroxidase negative
   d. alkaline phosphatase positive


138. The absence of the Philadelphia chromosome in granulocytic leukemia suggests:

   a. rapid progression of the disease
   b. a polyclonal origin to the disease
   c. excellent response to therapy
   d. conversion from another myeloproliferative disorder


139. Multiple myeloma is generally characterized by:

   a. plasmacytic satellitosis in the bone marrow
   b. many plasma cells in the peripheral blood
   c. many Mott cells in the peripheral blood
   d. rouleaux formation


140. Morphologic variants of plasma cells do NOT include:

   a. flame cells
   b. morula cells
   c. grape cells
   d. Gaucher's cells


141. Platelet aggregation is dependent in vitro on the presence of:

   a. calcium ions
   b. sodium citrate
   c. fibrinogen
   d. potassium

142. Factor VIII activity following cryoprecipitate therapy of patients with von Willebrand's disease is best described by which of the following statements?

    a. The activity is higher than would be predicted.
    b. An immediate response is seen.
    c. The activity disappears quickly.
    d. The pattern is similar to that seen in hemophiliacs.


143. On an electronic cell counter, hemoglobin determinations may be falsely elevated owing to the presence of:

    a. lipemia or elevated bilirubin concentration
    b. a decreased WBC or lipemia
    c. an elevated bilirubin concentration or rouleaux
    d. rouleaux or lipemia


144. A blood sample from a patient with a high-titer cold agglutinin, analyzed at room temperature with an electronic particle counter, would cause an error in the:

    a. hemoglobin and MCV
    b. MCHC and WBC
    c. WBC and RBC
    d. MCV and MCHC


145. Pluripotent stem cells are capable of producing:

    a. daughter cells of only one cell line
    b. only T-lymphocytes and B-lymphocytes
    c. erythropoietin, thrombopoietin, and leukopoietin
    d. lymphoid and myeloid stem cells


146. All of the following conditions are myeloproliferative disorders EXCEPT:

    a. granulocytic leukemia
    b. lymphocytic leukemia
    c. polycythemia vera
    d. idiopathic thrombocythemia


147. The anemia found in myeloproliferative disorders is usually:

    a. microcytic, hypochromic
    b. macrocytic, normochromic
    c. normocytic, normochromic
    d. microcytic, normochromic

148. A term that means varying degrees of leukocytosis with a shift to the left and occasional nucleated red cells in the peripheral blood is:

a. polycythemia vera
b. erythroleukemia
c. leukoerythroblastosis
d. megaloblastoid


149. Which of the following is true of acute lymphoblastic leukemia (ALL)?

a. occurs most commonly in children 1-2 years of age
b. patient is asymptomatic
c. massive accumulation of primitive lymphoid-appearing cells in bone marrow occurs
d. children under 1 year of age have a good prognosis


150. The most frequent type of acute lymphocytic leukemia (ALL) is:

a. T-cell childhood
b. common childhood
c. B-cell childhood
d. undifferentiated childhood


151. Chronic lymphocytic leukemia is defined as:

a. a malignancy of the thymus
b. an accumulation of prolymphocytes
c. an accumulation of hairy cells in the spleen
d. an accumulation of monoclonal B cells with a block in cell maturation


152. Which one of the following factors typically shows an increase in liver disease?

a. Factor VII
b. Factor VIII
c. Factor IX
d. Factor X


153. Which one of the following statements concerning vitamin K is NOT true?

a. There are two sources of vitamin K: vegetable and bacterial.
b. Vitamin K converts precursor molecules into functional coagulation factors.
c. Heparin inhibits the action of vitamin K.
d. Vitamin K is fat soluble.

154. The most characteristic morphologic features of atypical lymphocytes include:

   a. coarse nuclear chromatin and basophilic cytoplasm
   b. blue-gray cytoplasm, fine nuclear chromatin
   c. nucleoli and deep blue RNA-rich cytoplasm
   d. a stretched nucleus and cytoplasmic indentations


155. In comparison with malignant lymphoma cells, reactive lymphocytes:

   a. have a denser nuclear chromatin
   b. are known to be T cells
   c. have more cytoplasm and more mitochondria
   d. are morphologically more variable throughout the smear


156. The disease most frequently present in patients with atypical lymphocytosis and persistently negative tests is:

   a. toxoplasmosis
   b. cytomegalovirus (CMV) infection
   c. herpes virus infection
   d. viral hepatitis


157. In an uncomplicated case of infectious mononucleosis, which of the following cells are affected?

   a. erythrocytes
   b. lymphocytes
   c. monocytes
   d. thrombocytes


158. Hairy cell leukemia (leukemic reticuloendotheliosis) is:

   a. an acute myelocytic leukemia
   b. a chronic leukemia of myelocytic origin
   c. a chronic leukemia of lymphocytic origin
   d. an acute myelocytic monocytic-type leukemia


159. Which of the following is NOT a characteristic usually associated with hairy cell leukemia?

   a. pancytopenia
   b. mononuclear cells with ruffled edges
   c. splenomegaly
   d. increased resistance to infection

160. Which of the following cell types is characteristic of Pelger-Huët anomaly?

a. band form
b. pince-nez form
c. normal neutrophil
d. myelocyte

161. Anemia secondary to uremia characteristically is:

a. microcytic, hypochromic
b. hemolytic
c. normocytic, normochromic
d. macrocytic

162. The cytoplasmic abnormality of the white blood cell of Alder-Reilly anomaly is found in the:

a. endoplasmic reticulum
b. lysosomes
c. mitochondria
d. ribosomes

163. Increased levels of TdT activity are indicative of:

a. Burkitt's lymphoma
b. acute granulocytic leukemia
c. acute lymphocytic leukemia
d. eosinophilia

164. A 53-year-old man was in recovery following a triple bypass operation. Oozing was noted from his surgical wound. The following laboratory data were obtained:

| | |
|---|---|
| Hgb | 12.5 g/dL |
| Hct | 37% |
| Prothrombin time | 12.3 sec |
| APTT | 34 sec |
| Platelet count | $40.0 \times 10^3/\mu L$ |
| Fibrinogen | 250 mg/dL |

The most likely cause of bleeding would be:

a. dilution of coagulation factors due to massive transfusion
b. intravascular coagulation secondary to microaggregates
c. hypofibrinogenemia
d. dilutional thrombocytopenia

165. The prothrombin time test requires that the patient's citrated plasma be combined with:

   a. platelet lipids
   b. thromboplastin
   c. $Ca^{++}$ and platelet lipids
   d. $Ca^{++}$ and thromboplastin


166. A patient develops unexpected bleeding and the following test results were obtained:

   Prolonged PT and APTT
   Decreased fibrinogen
   Increased fibrin split products
   Decreased platelets

   What is the most probable cause of these results?

   a. familial afibrinogenemia
   b. primary fibrinolysis
   c. DIC
   d. liver disease


167. A patient develops severe unexpected bleeding following four transfusions. The following test results were obtained:

   | PT and APTT | Prolonged |
   |---|---|
   | Platelets | $50 \times 10^3/\mu L$ |
   | Fibrinogen | 30 mg/dL |
   | Fibrin split products | Increased |

   Given these results, which of the following blood products should be recommended to the physician for this patient?

   a. Platelets
   b. Factor VIII
   c. Cryoprecipitate
   d. Fresh Frozen Plasma


168. What is the MCV if the hematocrit is 20%, the RBC is $1.5 \times 10^6/\mu L$, and the hemoglobin is 6 g/dL?

   a. 68 fL
   b. 75 fL
   c. 115 fL
   d. 133 fL

169. What is the MCV if the hematocrit is 20%, the RBC is 2.4 x 10⁶/μL, and the hemoglobin is 5 g/dL?

    a. 68 fL
    b. 83 fL
    c. 100 fL
    d. 120 fL

170. What is the MCH if the hematocrit is 20%, the RBC is 1.5 x 10⁶/μL, and the hemoglobin is 6 g/dL?

    a. 28 $\mu m^3$
    b. 30 $\mu m^3$
    c. 40 $\mu m^3$
    d. 75 $\mu m^3$

171. What is the MCH if the hematocrit is 20%, the RBC is 2.4 x 10⁶/μL, and the hemoglobin is 5 g/dL?

    a. 21 $\mu m^3$
    b. 23 $\mu m^3$
    c. 25 $\mu m^3$
    d. 84 $\mu m^3$

172. What is the MCHC if the hematocrit is 20%, the RBC is 1.5 x 10⁶/μL, and the hemoglobin is 6 g/dL?

    a. 28%
    b. 30%
    c. 40%
    d. 75%

173. What is the MCHC if the hematocrit is 20%, the RBC is 2.4 x 10⁶/μL, and the hemoglobin is 5 g/dL?

    a. 21%
    b. 25%
    c. 30%
    d. 34%

174. Given the following data:

| WBC | $8.5 \times 10^3/\mu L$ | Differential | |
|---|---|---|---|
| | | Segs | 56% |
| | | Bands | 2% |
| | | Lymphs | 30% |
| | | Monos | 6% |
| | | Eos | 6% |

What is the absolute lymphocyte count?

a. 170
b. 510
c. 2550
d. 4760

175. Given the following data:

| WBC | $8.5 \times 10^3/\mu L$ | Differential | |
|---|---|---|---|
| | | Segs | 56% |
| | | Bands | 2% |
| | | Lymphs | 30% |
| | | Monos | 6% |
| | | Eos | 6% |

What is the absolute eosinophil count?

a. 170
b. 510
c. 2550
d. 4760

176. A total leukocyte count is $10.0 \times 10^3/\mu L$ and 25 NRBCs are seen per 100 leukocytes on the differential. What is the corrected leukocyte count?

a. 2000/$\mu$L
b. 8000/$\mu$L
c. 10,000/$\mu$L
d. 12,000/$\mu$L

177. If the total leukocyte count is $20.0 \times 10^3/\mu L$ and 50 NRBCs are seen per 100 leukocytes on the differential, what is the corrected leukocyte count?

a. 6666/$\mu$L
b. 10,000/$\mu$L
c. 13,333/$\mu$L
d. 26,666/$\mu$L

178. The mean for hemoglobin is 14.0 and the standard deviation is 0.20. The acceptable control range is ± 2 standard deviations. What are the allowable limits for the control?

   a. 13.8-14.2
   b. 13.6-14.4
   c. 13.4-14.6
   d. 13.0-14.0

179. The mean for hemoglobin is 13.0 and the standard deviation is 0.15. The acceptable control range is ± 2 standard deviations. What are the allowable limits for the control?

   a. 13.0-14.0
   b. 12.9-13.1
   c. 12.7-13.3
   d. 12.5-13.5

180. Which of the following is the formula for manual white cell count?

   a. (number of cells counted x dilution x 10)/number of squares counted
   b. (number of cells counted x dilution)/10 x number of squares counted
   c. number of cells counted x dilution
   d. number of cells counted x number of squares counted

181. Which of the following is the formula for absolute cell count?

   a. number of cells counted/total count
   b. total count/number of cells counted
   c. 10 x total count
   d. % of cells counted x total count

182. Which of the following is the formula for mean corpuscular volume (MCV)?

   a. (Hgb x 10)/RBC
   b. Hgb/Hct
   c. (Hct x 10)/RBC
   d. RBC/Hct

183. Which of the following is the formula for mean corpuscular hemoglobin (MCH)?

   a. Hct/(RBC x 1000)
   b. Hgb/Hct
   c. RBC/Hct
   d. (Hgb x 10)/RBC

184. Which of the following is the formula for MCHC?

    a. (Hgb x 100)/Hct
    b. Hgb/RBC
    c. RBC/Hct
    d. (Hct x 1000)/RBC


185. If an RBC count is performed on a 1:100 dilution and the number of cells in one fifth of a square mm is 600, the total RBC count is:

    a. $1.5 \times 10^6/\mu L$
    b. $2.0 \times 10^6/\mu L$
    c. $3.0 \times 10^6/\mu L$
    d. $3.5 \times 10^6/\mu L$


186. If an RBC count is performed on a 1:200 dilution and the number of cells in one fifth of a square mm is 150, the total RBC count is:

    a. $1.5 \times 10^6/\mu L$
    b. $2.0 \times 10^6/\mu L$
    c. $3.0 \times 10^6/\mu L$
    d. $3.5 \times 10^6/\mu L$


187. If a WBC count is performed on a 1:10 dilution and the number of cells counted in 8 squares is 120, the total WBC count is:

    a. $1200/\mu L$
    b. $1500/\mu L$
    c. $12,000/\mu L$
    d. $15,000/\mu L$


188. If a WBC count is performed on a 1:100 dilution and the number of cells counted in 8 squares is 50, the total WBC count is:

    a. $5000/\mu L$
    b. $6250/\mu L$
    c. $50,000/\mu L$
    d. $62,500/\mu L$


189. In manual or visual endpoint coagulation tests, duplicates are needed because:

    a. reagents and samples must be paired
    b. coagulation controls are expensive
    c. high precision is less attainable in manual methodology
    d. the CAP requires duplicate testing

190. Using automated coagulation instruments, duplication of normal tests is no longer appropriate because:

   a. the laboratory can document precision by collecting data to reflect precision performance
   b. all technologists on all shifts can be taught quality control
   c. it is difficult to have duplicates done in a blind fashion
   d. one technologist can monitor quality control


191. The type of leukemia seen most commonly as a terminal event in plasma cell myeloma is:

   a. acute lymphoblastic leukemia
   b. acute monocytic leukemia
   c. acute myelomonocytic leukemia
   d. acute myelogenous leukemia


192. The most potent plasminogen activator in the contact phase of coagulation is:

   a. kallikrein
   b. streptokinase
   c. Factor XIIa
   d. fibrinogen


193. A test used to monitor streptokinase therapy is:

   a. reptilase time
   b. fibrin split products
   c. staphylococcal clumping test
   d. thrombin generation time


194. A bedside test that can be used to monitor heparin activity is the:

   a. activated clotting time
   b. Stypven time
   c. reptilase time
   d. partial thromboplastin time


195. After the removal of red blood cells from the circulation, hemoglobin is broken down into:

   a. iron, porphyrin, and amino acids
   b. iron, protoporphyrin, and globin
   c. heme, protoporphyrin, and amino acids
   d. heme, hemosiderin, and globin

196. Increased numbers of basophils are often seen in:

   a. acute infections
   b. chronic granulocytic leukemia
   c. chronic lymphocytic leukemia
   d. erythroblastosis fetalis (hemolytic disease of the newborn)


197. Normal platelets have a circulating life span of approximately:

   a. 5 days
   b. 10 days
   c. 20 days
   d. 30 days


198. Blood is diluted 1:200 and a platelet count is performed. 180 platelets were counted in the red cell counting area on one side of the hemocytometer and 186 on the other side. The total platelet count is:

   a. 146 x 10³/μL
   b. 183 x 10³/μL
   c. 366 x 10³/μL
   d. 732 x 10³/μL


199. The following coagulation results were obtained on a newborn:

|               |            | Reference Ranges |
| ------------- | ---------- | ---------------- |
| PT            | 12.8 sec   | 9.5-14.5 sec     |
| APTT          | 34.5 sec   | 20-35 sec        |
| Thrombin time | 14.0 sec   | 9-13 sec         |
| Fibrinogen    | 380 mg/dL  | 200-400 mg/dL    |

The results are most suggestive of:

   a. Factor VII deficiency
   b. normal newborn results
   c. hyperfibrinogenemia
   d. vitamin K deficiency


200. Which of the following technical factors will cause a decreased erythrocyte sedimentation rate?

   a. gross hemolysis
   b. small fibrin clots in the sample
   c. increased room temperature
   d. tilting of the tube

201. On a smear made directly from a finger stick, no platelets were found in the counting area. The first thing to do is:

 a. examine the slide for clumping
 b. obtain another smear
 c. perform a total platelet count
 d. request another finger stick

202. Of the following containers, the one best suited for collection of a cell count on peritoneal fluid is a:

 a. sterile plastic container
 b. test tube containing NaF
 c. capped syringe on ice
 d. tube containing EDTA

203. The calculated erythrocyte indices on an adult man are:

| MCV | 89 fL |
| MCH | 29 pg |
| MCHC | 38% |

The calculations have been rechecked; erythrocytes on the peripheral blood smear appear normocytic and normochromic with no abnormal forms. The next step is to:

 a. report the results
 b. examine another smear
 c. repeat the hemoglobin and hematocrit
 d. repeat the erythrocyte count and hematocrit

204. Thrombocytosis would be indicated by a platelet count of:

 a. $100 \times 10^3/\mu L$
 b. $200 \times 10^3/\mu L$
 c. $300 \times 10^3/\mu L$
 d. $600 \times 10^3/\mu L$

205. Which of the following is used for staining reticulocytes?

 a. Giemsa stain
 b. Wright's stain
 c. new methylene blue
 d. Prussian blue

206. The electrical resistance method of cell counting requires:

    a. equal sized particles
    b. a conductive liquid
    c. two internal electrodes for current
    d. three apertures for counting

207. What cell shape is MOST commonly associated with an increased MCHC?

    a. teardrop cells
    b. target cells
    c. spherocytes
    d. sickle cells

208. Given the following data:

| | |
|---|---|
| Hgb | 8 g/dL |
| Hct | 28% |
| RBC | $3.6 \times 10^6/\mu L$ |

The MCV is:

    a. 28 fL
    b. 35 fL
    c. 40 fL
    d. 77 fL

209. Which of the following factors is used only in the extrinsic coagulation pathway?

    a. II
    b. V
    c. VII
    d. VIII

210. A platelet count done by phase microscopy is $200 \times 10^3/\mu L$ (normal, 150-450 $\times 10^3/\mu L$). A standardized template bleeding time on the same person is 15 minutes (normal, 4.5 ± 1.5 minutes). This indicates that:

    a. the Duke method should have been used for the bleeding time
    b. the manual platelet count is in error
    c. abnormal platelet function should be suspected
    d. the results are as expected

211. If a blood smear is dried too slowly, the red blood cells are often:

    a. clumped
    b. crenated
    c. lysed
    d. destroyed

212. In performing a leukocyte count, blood is drawn to the 1.0 mark in the capillary of the pipet and then diluted to the 11 mark. The total number of cells counted in the 4 large corner squares of the Neubauer counting chamber is 200. The total leukocyte count per µL is:

   a. 1250
   b. 5000
   c. 8000
   d. 10,000

213. The presence of excessive rouleaux formation on a blood smear is often accompanied by an increased:

   a. reticulocyte count
   b. sedimentation rate
   c. hematocrit
   d. erythrocyte count

214. Five preoperative and control samples for APTT had prolonged times when run on an optical density coagulation instrument. The results for patients and controls were confirmed by using an alternate method of mechanical detection. Which of the following would best explain these results?

   a. incorrect anticoagulant used
   b. sample carryover
   c. reagent contamination
   d. improperly reconstituted controls

215. The following results are obtained:

| PT | Normal |
| APTT | Prolonged |
| APTT with absorbed plasma | Not corrected |

What is the deficient factor?

   a. antihemophilic factor (VIII)
   b. plasma thromboplastin component (IX)
   c. Stuart-Prower factor (X)
   d. Hageman factor (XII)

216. Which of the following factor deficiencies is associated with either no bleeding or only a minor bleeding tendency, even after trauma or surgery?

   a. Factor X
   b. Factor XII
   c. Factor XIII
   d. Factor V

217. An anemic patient has an RBC of 2.70 x 10⁶/µL and a hemoglobin of 13.5 g/dL, as determined by an electronic particle counter. Which of the following is the best explanation for these results?

    a. electrical interference
    b. lipemia
    c. high anticoagulant to blood ratio
    d. a high coincidence rate

218. The following results are obtained:

| | |
|---|---|
| PT | Normal |
| APTT | Prolonged |
| Absorbed plasma | Corrects APTT |

The factor deficiency is:

    a. VIII
    b. IX
    c. X
    d. V

219. Hemoglobins are read on a photoelectric colorimeter in the laboratory. While reading the hemoglobins, a problem of drifting is encountered. To assess the problem, the FIRST thing to do is:

    a. recalibrate the instrument
    b. check the filter
    c. set up new hemoglobin samples
    d. check the light source

220. A citrated blood specimen for coagulation studies is to be collected from a polycythemic patient. The anticoagulant should be:

    a. the standard volume
    b. reduced in volume
    c. changed to EDTA
    d. changed to oxalate

221. A person has a leukocyte count of 9.4 x 10³/µL on Saturday. On Monday he runs a marathon and his leukocyte count after the race is 14.8 x 10³/µL. The difference of the two leukocyte counts is due to:

    a. fluid increase
    b. pathologic variation
    c. analytic difference
    d. physiologic variation

222. The following CBC results were obtained from an automated cell counter on a patient sample with lipemic plasma:

| WBC | $7.2 \times 10^3/\mu L$ |
|---|---|
| RBC | $3.50 \times 10^6/\mu L$ |
| Hgb | 13.8 g/dL |
| Hct | 33.5% |
| MCV | 92 fL |
| MCH | 39.4 pg |
| MCHC | 41.0% |

Which of the following groups of tests would probably be in error?

a. WBC, RBC, MCV
b. RBC, Hct, MCV
c. RBC, Hgb, Hct
d. Hgb, MCH, MCHC

223. A patient's thrombin time is 25.5 seconds, and the control is 11.5 seconds. The patient's plasma is mixed with an equal part of normal plasma. The thrombin time is rerun and is 28.0 seconds with a control of 11.5 seconds. These results indicate:

a. fibrinogen deficiency
b. thrombocyte antibodies present
c. Factor VII deficiency
d. circulating anticoagulant

224. A patient's blood sample mixed with sucrose solution and incubated at 37°C shows moderate hemolysis. The direct antiglobulin test was negative. These results are suggestive of:

a. lupus erythematosus
b. polycythemia vera
c. acquired autoimmune hemolytic anemia
d. paroxysmal nocturnal hemoglobinuria

225. What completes the circuit between the stationary and the moving electrodes in the fibrometer?

a. fibrin strand
b. cam sensing device
c. third electrode
d. turbidity of reaction

226. The following laboratory results were obtained for a patient with an inherited autosomal dominant trait:

| Bleeding time | Prolonged |
| Platelet adhesiveness | Abnormal |
| PT | Normal |
| APTT | Normal |

These findings are most consistent with:

a. hemorrhagic disease of the newborn
b. Factor X deficiency
c. Factor XI deficiency
d. von Willebrand's disease

227. An enzyme deficiency associated with a moderate to severe hemolytic anemia after the patient is exposed to certain drugs and that is characterized by red cell inclusions formed by denatured hemoglobin is:

a. lactate dehydrogenase deficiency
b. G-6-PD deficiency
c. pyruvate kinase deficiency
d. hexokinase deficiency

228. The following results were obtained from a postsurgical patient receiving total parenteral nutrition:

| Hospital day | 17 | 18 | 19 |
|---|---|---|---|
| Hgb (g/dL) | 12.1 | 11.6 | 9.4 |
| Hct (%) | 29.2 | 29.4 | 28.8 |

The most consistent explanation for the above data is:

a. acute surgical bleeder
b. specimen on day 19 from wrong patient
c. improperly mixed specimen on day 19
d. lipid interference on days 17 and 18

229. Aliquots of plasma with a prolonged PT and prolonged APTT are mixed using various ratios of patient plasma and normal plasma. All samples are incubated at 37°C and tested at 10-, 30-, and 60-minute intervals. The PT and APTT results on all of the mixtures are corrected. The results would indicate the presence of:

a. circulating anticoagulant
b. factor deficiency
c. contaminated reagent
d. antibodies

230. To prepare 25 mL of 3% acetic acid, how much glacial acetic acid is needed?

    a. 7.5 mL
    b. 3.0 mL
    c. 1.5 mL
    d. 0.75 mL

231. An automated platelet count is 15 x $10^3/\mu L$. The technologist should:

    a. phone result to physician immediately
    b. review peripheral smear
    c. report count
    d. repeat collection

232. A red blood cell about 5 μm in diameter that stains bright red and shows no central pallor is a:

    a. spherocyte
    b. leptocyte
    c. microcyte
    d. macrocyte

233. The laboratory tests performed on a patient indicate macrocytosis, anemia, leukopenia, and thrombocytopenia. Which of the following disorders is the patient most likely to have?

    a. iron deficiency
    b. hereditary spherocytosis
    c. vitamin $B_{12}$ deficiency
    d. acute hemorrhage

234. Peripheral blood smears from patients with untreated pernicious anemia are characterized by:

    a. pancytopenia and macrocytosis
    b. pancytopenia and leukocytosis
    c. leukocytosis and ovalocytosis
    d. pancytopenia and microcytosis

235. The characteristic erythrocyte found in pernicious anemia is:

    a. microcytic
    b. spherocytic
    c. hypochromic
    d. macrocytic

236. The white cell feature most characteristic of pernicious anemia is:

    a. eosinophilia
    b. toxic granulation
    c. hypersegmentation
    d. atypical lymphocytes


237. Platelet activity is affected by:

    a. anticoagulant therapy
    b. aspirin
    c. hyperglycemia
    d. hypoglycemia


238. A coagulation factor synthesized in the liver and vitamin K dependent is:

    a. fibrinogen
    b. prothrombin
    c. Factor VIII
    d. Factor XIII


239. Which of the following coagulation factors is considered to be labile?

    a. II
    b. V
    c. VII
    d. X


240. If a clot incubated at 37°C dissolves within 24 hours, which of the following should be suspected?

    a. fibrinolysins
    b. low fibrinogen level
    c. Factor VIII deficiency
    d. thrombocytopenia


241. In infectious mononucleosis, lymphocytes tend to be:

    a. small with little cytoplasm
    b. normal
    c. decreased in number
    d. enlarged and indented by surrounding structures

242. Prothrombin is:

   a. a protein formed by the liver in the presence of vitamin K
   b. an enzyme that converts fibrinogen into fibrin threads
   c. the end product of the reaction between fibrinogen and thrombin
   d. a protein released by platelets during coagulation

243. Using a WBC pipet, blood is drawn to the 1.0 mark and diluted to the 11.0 mark. 182 cells are counted in 4 square millimeters. The count is:

   a. 4500/μL
   b. 9100/μL
   c. 45,500/μL
   d. 91,000/μL

244. The direct antiglobulin test is often positive in:

   a. congenital hemolytic spherocytosis
   b. march hemoglobinuria
   c. acquired hemolytic anemia
   d. thalassemia major

245. The laboratory findings on a patient are as follows:

| MCV | 55 fL |
| MCHC | 25% |
| MCH | 17 pg |

A stained blood film of this patient would most likely reveal a red cell picture that is:

   a. microcytic, hypochromic
   b. macrocytic, hypochromic
   c. normocytic, normochromic
   d. microcytic, normochromic

246. A bleeding time is used to evaluate the activity of:

   a. platelets
   b. prothrombin
   c. labile factor
   d. Factor XIII

247. Most childhood leukemias are:

    a. acute lymphocytic
    b. acute monocytic
    c. chronic myelocytic
    d. chronic lymphocytic


248. A sedimentation rate is set up 2 hours after the specimen is received by the laboratory. Ten minutes before the sedimentation rate is to be read, the technician notices that the tube was tilted. The technician should then:

    a. remix the blood and set up the procedure again
    b. report the result, after waiting 10 minutes
    c. obtain a new specimen and set up the sedimentation rate again
    d. correct the sedimentation rate for the degree of the angle


249. An increased amount of cytoplasmic basophilia in a blood cell indicates:

    a. increased cytoplasmic maturation
    b. decreased cytoplasmic maturation
    c. reduction in size of the cell
    d. decreased nuclear maturation


250. A patient has the following laboratory results:

| RBC | $2.00 \times 10^6/\mu L$ |
| Hct | 24% |
| Hgb | 6.8 g/dL |
| Reticulocytes | 0.8% |

The mean corpuscular volume (MCV) of the patient is:

    a. 35 fL
    b. 83 fL
    c. 120 fL
    d. 150 fL


251. All of the findings listed below may be seen in acquired hemolytic anemias of the auto-immune variety. The one considered to be the MOST characteristic is:

    a. increased osmotic fragility
    b. leukopenia and thrombocytopenia
    c. peripheral spherocytosis
    d. positive direct antiglobulin test

252. Cell description:

| | |
|---|---|
| Size | 12-16 μm |
| Nucleus | Oval, notched, folded over to horseshoe shape |
| Chromatin | Fine lacy, stains light purple-pink |
| Nucleoli | None present |
| Cytoplasm | Abundant, slate gray, with many fine lilac-colored granules |

This cell is a:

a. promyelocyte
b. lymphocyte
c. neutrophil
d. monocyte

253. While running prothrombin times at a temperature of 37°C and with proper concentration of reagents, the control is 16 seconds instead of the expected 12 seconds. The next step should be to:

a. run another control
b. change the reagent lines
c. readjust the timer to compensate for the variation
d. calculate a correction factor to be used on the results

254. The ideal capillary blood collection site on a newborn is:

a. tip of the thumb
b. ear lobe
c. plantar surface of the heel
d. the great toe

255. The following results were obtained on a patient's blood:

| | |
|---|---|
| Hgb | 11.5 g/dL |
| Hct | 40% |
| MCV | 89 fL |
| MCH | 26 pg |
| MCHC | 29% |

Examination of a Wright's stained smear of the same sample would most likely show:

a. macrocytic, normochromic erythrocytes
b. microcytic, hypochromic erythrocytes
c. normocytic, hypochromic erythrocytes
d. normocytic, normochromic erythrocytes

256. In the normal adult, the spleen acts as a site for:

   a. storage of red blood cells
   b. production of red blood cells
   c. synthesis of erythropoietin
   d. removal of imperfect and aging cells


257. Supravital staining is important for reticulocytes since the cells must be living in order to stain the:

   a. remaining RNA in the cell
   b. iron before it precipitates
   c. cell membrane before it dries out
   d. denatured hemoglobin in the cell


258. Heparin acts by:

   a. precipitating calcium
   b. binding calcium
   c. activating plasmin
   d. inhibiting thrombin


259. A patient has been taking aspirin regularly for arthritic pain. Which one of the following tests is most likely to be abnormal in this patient?

   a. platelet count
   b. template bleeding time
   c. prothrombin time
   d. activated partial thromboplastin time


260. In an automated cell counter with a three-digit readout capacity, the WBC printed result is 99.9. The next step is to:

   a. repeat after warming the sample to 37°C
   b. make an appropriate dilution of the sample
   c. recalibrate the machine from pooled samples
   d. request a new sample immediately


261. Evidence of active red cell regeneration may be indicated on a blood smear by:

   a. basophilic stippling, nucleated red blood cells, and polychromasia
   b. hypochromia, macrocytes, and nucleated red blood cells
   c. hypochromia, basophilic stippling, and nucleated red blood cells
   d. Howell-Jolly bodies, Cabot rings, and basophilic stippling

262. When evaluating a smear for a reticulocyte count, the technician observes that the red blood cells are overlapping throughout the entire slide. The most likely explanation is:

    a. grease on the slide prevented even spreading
    b. improper proportions of blood and stain were used
    c. the slide was dried too quickly
    d. the drop used for the slide preparation was too large


263. A specimen run on an automatic cell counter has a platelet count of 19 x 10³/µL. The first thing the technician should do is:

    a. report the count after the batch run is completed
    b. request a new specimen
    c. review the stained blood smear
    d. notify the laboratory manager


264. An automated platelet count indicates platelet clumping, which is confirmed by examining the smear. The technician should:

    a. repeat the count on the same sample
    b. report the automated count
    c. perform a manual count
    d. re-collect in sodium citrate


265. A common source of interference in the cyanmethemoglobin method is:

    a. hemolysis
    b. very high WBC count
    c. cold agglutinins
    d. clumped platelets


266. In the APTT test, the patient's plasma is mixed with:

    a. ADP and calcium
    b. tissue thromboplastin and collagen
    c. phospholipid and calcium
    d. tissue thromboplastin and calcium


267. The APTT:

    a. tests the extrinsic coagulation pathway
    b. monitors Coumadin therapy
    c. requires tissue thromboplastin
    d. monitors heparin therapy

268. The light-colored zone adjacent to the nucleus in a plasmacyte is the:

    a. ribosome
    b. chromatin
    c. mitochondria
    d. Golgi area

269. The following hemoglobin results were obtained for a patient:

    | Monday morning | 11.8 g/dL |
    |---|---|
    | Monday afternoon | 11.3 g/dL |
    | Tuesday morning | 11.7 g/dL |

    What can be concluded about the results?

    a. One value probably resulted from laboratory error.
    b. There is poor precision; daily QA charts should be checked.
    c. The patient was probably bleeding temporarily.
    d. There is no significant change in the patient's hemoglobin.

270. A 15-year-old girl is taking primaquine for a parasitic infection and notices her urine is a brownish color. A CBC shows mild anemia. The laboratorian performing the reticulocyte count notices numerous irregular shaped granules near the periphery of the RBC. These cellular inclusions are most likely:

    a. Howell-Jolly bodies
    b. basophilic stippling
    c. Heinz bodies
    d. Pappenheimer bodies

271. Polychromatic red cells when stained with a supravital stain are called:

    a. siderocytes
    b. reticulocytes
    c. schistocytes
    d. spherocytes

272. The term "shift to the left" refers to:

    a. a microscope adjustment
    b. immature cell forms in the peripheral blood
    c. a trend on a Levy-Jennings chart
    d. a calibration adjustment on an instrument

*The remaining questions (\*) have been identified as more appropriate for the entry level medical technologist.*

*273. The greatest activity of serum muramidase occurs with:

    a. cancer of the prostate
    b. chronic myeloproliferative disease
    c. acute monocytic leukemia
    d. Gaucher's disease

*274. A Wright's stained peripheral smear reveals the following:

Erythrocytes enlarged 1.5 to 2 times normal size
Schüffner's dots
Parasites with irregular "spread-out" trophozoites, golden-brown pigment
12-24 merozoites
Wide range of stages

This is consistent with *Plasmodium*:

    a. *falciparum*
    b. *malariae*
    c. *ovale*
    d. *vivax*

*275. In an uncomplicated case of severe iron deficiency anemia, which of the following sets represents the typical pattern of results?

| | Serum Iron | Serum TIBC | % Saturation | Marrow % Sideroblasts | Marrow Iron Stores | Serum Ferritin | Hgb A$_2$ |
|---|---|---|---|---|---|---|---|
| a. | decreased | increased | decreased | decreased | increased | increased | increased |
| b. | decreased | decreased | decreased | decreased | decreased | decreased | decreased |
| c. | decreased | increased | decreased | decreased | decreased | decreased | decreased |
| d. | decreased | decreased | increased | increased | increased | increased | increased |

*276. On an electronic particle counter, if the RBC count is erroneously increased, how will other parameters be affected?

    a. increased MCHC
    b. increased hemoglobin
    c. decreased MCH
    d. increased MCV

*277. Refer to the following diagram:

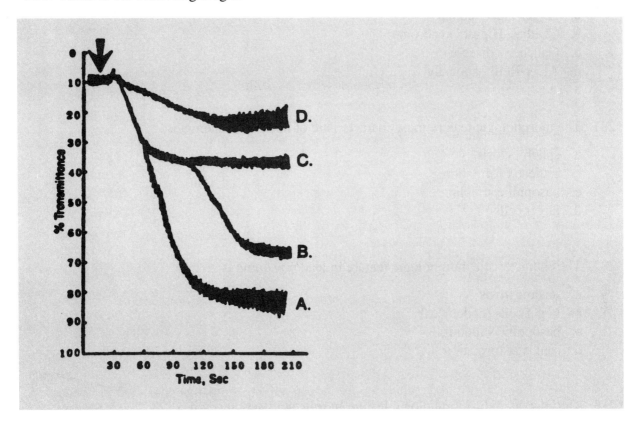

In the platelet aggregation curves shown above, the aggregating agent was added at the point indicated by the arrow. Select the appropriate aggregation curve for recent aspirin ingestion. (Aggregating agent is ADP or epinephrine).

a. A
b. B
c. C
d. D

*278. Of the following, the disease most closely associated with glucocerebrosidase deficiency is:

a. Gaucher's disease
b. Chédiak-Higashi syndrome
c. Pelger-Huët anomaly
d. May-Hegglin anomaly

*279. Of the following, the disease most closely associated with cytoplasmic granule fusion is:

a. Chédiak-Higashi syndrome
b. Pelger-Huët anomaly
c. May-Hegglin anomaly
d. Alder-Reilly anomaly

*280. Of the following, the disease most closely associated with mucopolysaccharidosis is:

   a. Pelger-Huët anomaly
   b. Chédiak-Higashi syndrome
   c. Gaucher's disease
   d. Alder-Reilly anomaly


*281. The morphologic feature most characteristic of hemolytic anemia is:

   a. spherocytosis
   b. rouleaux formation
   c. basophilic stippling
   d. target cells


*282. The characteristic morphologic feature in lead poisoning is:

   a. macrocytosis
   b. target cells (codocytes)
   c. basophilic stippling
   d. rouleaux formation


*283. The characteristic morphologic feature in folic acid deficiency is:

   a. macrocytosis
   b. target cells
   c. basophilic stippling
   d. rouleaux formation


*284. A platelet determination was performed on an automated instrument and a very low value was obtained. The platelets appeared adequate when estimated from the stained blood film. The best explanation for this discrepancy is:

   a. many platelets are abnormally large
   b. blood sample is hemolyzed
   c. white cell fragments are present in the blood
   d. red cell fragments are present in the blood


*285. Which of the following tests can be useful in differentiating leukemoid reactions from chronic granulocytic leukemias?

   a. peroxidase stain
   b. Sudan black B stain
   c. surface membrane markers
   d. leukocyte alkaline phosphatase

*286. Which of the following characteristics are common to hereditary spherocytosis, hereditary elliptocytosis, hereditary stomatocytosis, and paroxysmal nocturnal hemoglobinuria?

a. autosomal dominant inheritance
b. red cell membrane defects
c. positive direct antiglobulin test
d. measured platelet count


*287. In synovial fluid, the most characteristic microscopic finding in gout is:

a. calcium pyrophosphate crystals
b. cartilage debris
c. monosodium urate crystals
d. hemosiderin-laden macrophages


*288. In synovial fluid, the most characteristic microscopic finding in osteoarthritis is:

a. neutrophils with 0.5- to 1.5-μm inclusions
b. cartilage debris
c. monosodium urate crystals
d. hemosiderin-laden macrophages


*289. In synovial fluid, the most characteristic finding in rheumatoid arthritis is:

a. cartilage debris
b. monosodium urate crystals
c. hemosiderin-laden macrophages
d. neutrophils with 0.5- to 1.5-μm inclusions


*290. In synovial fluid, the most characteristic finding in pseudogout is:

a. calcium pyrophosphate dihydrate crystals
b. cartilage debris
c. monosodium urate crystals
d. hemosiderin-laden macrophages


*291. In synovial fluid, the most characteristic finding in traumatic arthritis is:

a. monosodium urate crystals
b. cartilage debris
c. calcium pyrophosphate dihydrate crystals
d. hemosiderin-laden macrophages

*292. T-cell acute lymphocytic leukemia (ALL) is closely related to:

a. chronic lymphocytic leukemia (CLL)
b. autoimmune disease
c. lymphoblastic lymphoma
d. acute granulocytic leukemia (AGL)

*293. A patient diagnosed with polycythemia vera 5 years ago now has a normal hematocrit, decreased hemoglobin, and microcytic, hypochromic red cells. What is the most probable cause for the current blood situation?

a. phlebotomy
b. myelofibrosis
c. preleukemia
d. aplastic anemia

*294. The stain that identifies intracellular carbohydrate, glycogen, mucopolysaccharide, muco-protein, glycoprotein, and glycolipid is:

a. Sudan black B
b. leukocyte alkaline phosphatase (LAP)
c. periodic acid–Schiff (PAS)
d. peroxidase

*295. The stain that selectively identifies phospholipid in the membranes of primary and secondary granules within myeloid cells is:

a. Sudan black B
b. leukocyte alkaline phosphatase (LAP)
c. periodic acid–Schiff (PAS)
d. peroxidase

*296. A patient has been treated for polycythemia vera for several years. His blood smear now shows:

Oval macrocytes
Howell-Jolly bodies
Hypersegmented neutrophils
Large, agranular platelets

The most probable cause of this blood picture is:

a. iron deficiency
b. alcoholism
c. dietary $B_{12}$ deficiency
d. chemotherapy

*297. In polycythemia vera, the leukocyte alkaline phosphatase activity is:

a. elevated
b. normal
c. decreased

*298. Terminal deoxynucleotidyl transferase (TdT) is a marker found on:

a. hairy cells
b. myeloblasts
c. monoblasts
d. lymphoblasts

*299. The M:E ratio in chronic granulocytic leukemia is usually:

a. normal
b. high
c. low
d. variable

*300. The M:E ratio in erythroleukemia is usually:

a. normal
b. high
c. low
d. variable

*301. The M:E ratio in acute granulocytic leukemia is usually:

a. normal
b. high
c. low
d. variable

*302. The M:E ratio in polycythemia vera is usually:

a. normal
b. high
c. low
d. variable

*303. Giant, bizarre-shaped, multinucleated erythroid precursors are present in which of the following?

a. chronic granulocytic leukemia
b. myelofibrosis with myeloid metaplasia
c. erythroleukemia
d. acute granulocytic leukemia


*304. In acute granulocytic leukemia, the myeloblasts stain positive with all of the following EXCEPT:

a. specific esterase
b. Sudan black B
c. peroxidase
d. PAS


*305. The leukocyte alkaline phosphatase activity is increased in:

a. erythroleukemia
b. leukemoid reaction
c. chronic granulocytic leukemia
d. acute granulocytic leukemia


*306. In the immunologic classification of acute lymphocytic leukemia (ALL), the acid phosphatase stain is usually positive for:

a. null cell ALL
b. T cell ALL
c. common ALL
d. B cell ALL


*307. The peripheral blood monocyte is an intermediate stage in the formation of the:

a. plasmacyte
b. Türk irritation cell
c. histiocyte
d. hairy cell


*308. Which of the following has a B cell origin?

a. Sézary syndrome
b. malignant lymphoma, lymphoblastic type
c. Sternberg sarcoma
d. Waldenström's macroglobulinemia

*309. Which of the following is NOT a characteristic of hemoglobin H?

    a. it is a tetramer of beta chains
    b. it is relatively unstable and thermolabile
    c. electrophoretically, it represents a "fast" hemoglobin
    d. its oxygen affinity is lower than that of Hgb A


*310. Which of the following are found in association with megaloblastic anemia?

    a. neutropenia and thrombocytopenia
    b. decreased LD activity
    c. increased erythrocyte folate levels
    d. decreased plasma bilirubin levels


*311. Which of the following are characteristic of Auer rods?

    a. They contain lactoferrin.
    b. They are lysosome and acid phosphatase–positive.
    c. They are found in the leukemic phase of lymphoma.
    d. They are found in acute lymphocytic leukemia.


*312. Mechanism of cortisol-induced neutrophilia includes:

    a. an acute shift in granulocytes from the marginating pool to the circulating pool
    b. an increased exit of granulocytes from the circulation
    c. a decreased exit of granulocytes from the bone marrow
    d. granulocyte return from the tissues to the circulating pool


*313. A characteristic of cyclic neutropenia is:

    a. episodes of neutropenia beginning in infancy and recurring at 3-week intervals
    b. presence of leukoagglutinins in the serum
    c. presence of serum neutropenic factors
    d. production of neutropenia in persons transfused with plasma from an affected patient


*314. Precursors of tissue macrophages of the reticuloendothelial system most likely are:

    a. T lymphocytes
    b. B lymphocytes
    c. monocytes
    d. mast cells

*315. Which of the following cells are most likely identified in lesions of mycosis fungoides?

    a. T lymphocytes
    b. B lymphocytes
    c. monocytes
    d. mast cells

*316. The atypical lymphocyte seen in the peripheral smear of patients with infectious mono-
nucleosis is reacting to which of the following?

    a. T lymphocytes
    b. B lymphocytes
    c. monocytes
    d. mast cells

*317. Which of the following cells are the atypical lymphocytes seen on the peripheral blood
smear of patients with infectious mononucleosis?

    a. T lymphocytes
    b. B lymphocytes
    c. monocytes
    d. mast cells

*318. Which of the following platelet responses is most likely associated with Glanzmann's
thrombasthenia?

    a. decreased platelet aggregation to ristocetin
    b. defective ADP release; normal response to ADP
    c. decreased amount of ADP in platelets
    d. markedly decreased aggregation to epinephrine, ADP, and collagen

*319. Which of the following platelet responses is most likely associated with hemophilia A
(Factor VIII deficiency)?

    a. defective ADP release; normal response to ADP
    b. decreased amount of ADP in platelets
    c. absent aggregation to epinephrine, ADP, and collagen
    d. normal platelet aggregation

*320. A 20-year-old black man has peripheral blood changes suggesting thalassemia minor. The
quantitative hemoglobin $A_2$ level is normal, but the hemoglobin F level is 5% (normal =
less than 2%). This is most consistent with:

    a. alpha thalassemia minor
    b. beta thalassemia minor
    c. delta-beta thalassemia minor
    d. hereditary persistence of fetal hemoglobin

*321. A native of Thailand has a normal hemoglobin level. Hemoglobin electrophoresis on cellulose acetate shows 45% Hgb A and approximately 40% of a hemoglobin with the mobility of Hgb $A_2$. This is most consistent with:

a. Hgb C trait
b. Hgb E trait
c. Hgb O trait
d. Hgb D trait

*322. A 20-year-old woman with sickle cell anemia whose usual hemoglobin concentration is 8 g/dL develops fever, increased weakness, and malaise. The hemoglobin concentration is 4 g/dL and the reticulocyte count is 0.1%. The most likely explanation for this clinical picture is:

a. increased hemolysis due to hypersplenism
b. aplastic crisis
c. thrombotic crisis
d. occult blood loss

*323. Megaloblastic asynchronous development in the bone marrow indicates which one of the following?

a. proliferation of erythrocyte precursors
b. impaired synthesis of DNA
c. inadequate production of erythropoietin
d. deficiency of G-6-PD

*324. The type of leukemia seen most commonly as a terminal event in multiple myeloma is:

a. acute lymphoblastic leukemia
b. acute monocytic leukemia
c. acute myelogenous (myelocytic) leukemia
d. chronic myelogenous leukemia

*325. A prolonged thrombin time and a normal reptilase-R time are characteristic of:

a. dysfibrinogenemia
b. increased fibrin split products
c. fibrin monomer-split product complexes
d. therapeutic heparinization

*326. The preferred blood product for a bleeding patient with von Willebrand's disease is transfusion with:

a. Factor II, VII, IX, X concentrates
b. Platelet Concentrates
c. Fresh Frozen Plasma and Platelets
d. Cryoprecipitated AHF

*327. Hageman factor (XII) is involved in each of the following reactions EXCEPT:

    a. activation of C1 to C1 esterase
    b. activation of plasminogen
    c. activation of Factor XI
    d. transformation of fibrinogen to fibrin

*328. Cytochemical stains were performed on bone marrow smears from an acute leukemia patient. All blasts were periodic acid–Schiff (PAS) negative. The majority of the blasts showed varying amounts of Sudan black B positivity. Some of the blasts stained positive for naphthol AS-D acetate esterase, some were positive for naphthol AS-D chloroacetate esterase, and some blasts stained positive for both esterases. What type of leukemia is indicated?

    a. lymphocytic
    b. myelogenous
    c. myelomonocytic
    d. erythroleukemia

*329. Which substrate is used for the detection of specific esterase?

    a. acetate
    b. chloroacetate
    c. pararosanilin acetate
    d. phenylene diacetate

*330. Neutropenia is NOT usually associated with:

    a. viral infections
    b. Hodgkin's disease
    c. select antibiotics
    d. chemotherapy

*331. Long-term exposure to certain antibiotics such as penicillin has been found to result in:

    a. leukopenia
    b. thrombocytosis
    c. lymphocytosis
    d. polycythemia

*332. Platelet aggregation will occur with the end production of:

    a. cyclooxygenase
    b. arachidonic acid
    c. prostacyclin
    d. thromboxane $A_2$

*333. Which cell type shows the most intense staining with peroxidase?

   a. segmented neutrophil
   b. basophil
   c. band
   d. monocyte

*334. The mean value of a reticulocyte count on specimens of cord blood from healthy, full-term newborns is about:

   a. 0.5%
   b. 2.0%
   c. 5.0%
   d. 8.0%

*335. In normal adult bone marrow, the most common granulocyte is the:

   a. basophil
   b. myeloblast
   c. eosinophil
   d. metamyelocyte

*336. Which one of the following is a true statement about megakaryocytes in a bone marrow aspirate?

   a. An average of 1 to 3 should be found in each low-power field (10x).
   b. The majority of forms are the MK$_1$ stage.
   c. Morphology must be determined from the biopsy section.
   d. Quantitative estimation is done using the 100x oil immersion lens.

*337. In addition to a Romanowsky stain, routine evaluation of a bone marrow should include which of the following stains?

   a. chloroacetate esterase
   b. periodic acid–Schiff (PAS)
   c. Prussian blue
   d. Sudan black B

*338. A hypercellular marrow with an M:E ratio of 6:1 is most commonly due to:

   a. lymphoid hyperplasia
   b. granulocytic hyperplasia
   c. normoblastic hyperplasia
   d. myeloid hypoplasia

*339. The most likely cause of the macrocytosis that often accompanies anemia of myelofibrosis is:

    a. folic acid deficiency
    b. increased reticulocyte count
    c. inadequate $B_{12}$ absorption
    d. pyridoxine deficiency


*340. The Philadelphia chromosome is formed by a translocation between the:

    a. long arm of chromosome 22 and long arm of chromosome 9
    b. long arm of chromosome 21 and long arm of chromosome 9
    c. long arm of chromosome 21 and short arm of chromosome 6
    d. long arm of chromosome 22 and short arm of chromosome 6


*341. A 30-year-old man who had been diagnosed as having leukemia 2 years previously was readmitted because of cervical lymphadenopathy. Laboratory findings included the following:

| WBC | $39.6 \times 10^3/\mu L$ | Differential | |
|---|---|---|---|
| RBC | $3.25 \times 10^6/\mu L$ | Polys | 7% |
| Hgb | 9.4 g/dL | Lymphs | 4% |
| Hct | 28.2% | Monos | 2% |
| MCV | 86.7 fL | Eos | 3% |
| MCH | 29.0 pg | Basos | 48% |
| MCHC | 33.4% | Myelos | 13% |
| Platelets | $53 \times 10^3/\mu L$ | Promyelos | 2% |
| | | Metamyelos | 8% |
| | | Blasts | 13% |
| | | NRBCs | 11% |
| | | Megakaryoblasts | 3% |

Bone marrow: 95% cellularity, 50% blast cells (some with peroxidase and Sudan black B positivity)

| | |
|---|---|
| LAP | 11 |
| Philadelphia chromosome | Positive |

These results are most consistent with:

a. acute myeloid leukemia
b. erythroleukemia
c. chronic myelogenous leukemia (CML)
d. CML in blast transformation

*342. A 30-year-old woman was admitted to the hospital for easy bruising and menorrhagia. Laboratory findings included the following:

| WBC | 3.5 x 10³/µL | Differential | |
|---|---|---|---|
| RBC | 2.48 x 10⁶/µL | Polys | 3% |
| Platelets | 30 x 10³/µL | Lymphs | 2% |
| Hgb | 8.6 g/dL | Monos | 2% |
| Hct | 25.0% | Myelos | 4% |
| MCV | 100.7 fL | Abnormal immature | 58% |
| MCH | 34.7 pg | Blasts | 31% |
| MCHC | 34.3% | NRBCs | 1% |

Auer rods, 1+ macrocytes, 1+ polychromasia

| PT | 34.0 sec |
|---|---|
| APTT | 62.5 sec |
| Thrombin time | 15.0 sec |
| FSP | > 40 µg/mL |
| Fibrinogen | 315 mg/dL (control, 200-400) |

The cells identified as "abnormal immature" were described as having lobulated nuclei with prominent nucleoli; the cytoplasm had intense azurophilic granulation over the nucleus, with some cells containing 1 to 20 Auer rods frequently grouped in bundles. A 15-17 chromosomal translocation was noted. Cells were SBB, peroxidase, and NAS-D-chloroacetate positive, PAS negative. Which of the following types of acute leukemia is most likely?

a. myeloblastic
b. promyelocytic
c. myelomonocytic
d. monocytic


*343. The absence of intermediate maturing cells between the blast and mature neutrophil commonly seen in acute myelocytic leukemia and myelodysplastic syndromes is called:

a. subleukemia
b. aleukemic leukemia
c. leukemic hiatus
d. leukemoid reaction

*344. Which of the following leukemias is characterized by immature cells that are Sudan black B positive with discrete fine granules, peroxidase negative, PAS variable, strongly alpha naphthyl acetate esterase positive, and muramidase positive?

a. acute lymphocytic
b. chronic lymphocytic
c. acute myelocytic
d. acute myelomonocytic

*345. Which of the following will distinguish early myeloid metaplasia from chronic myelogenous leukemia?

a. bone marrow hyperplasia
b. bone marrow fibrosis
c. increased leukocytic alkaline phosphatase (LAP)
d. megaloblastosis

*346. A 50-year-old man was admitted into the hospital with acute leukemia. Laboratory findings included the following:

| | |
|---|---|
| Myeloperoxidase stain | Blast cells negative |
| PAS stain | Blast cells demonstrate a blocking pattern |
| TdT | Blast cells positive |
| Surface immunoglobulin | Blast cells negative |
| CD2 | Blast cells negative |
| Philadelphia chromosome | Positive |

These results are most consistent with:

a. acute myelogenous leukemia
b. chronic lymphocytic leukemia in lymphoblastic transformation
c. T-cell acute lymphocytic leukemia
d. chronic myelogenous leukemia in lymphoblastic transformation

*347. A bone marrow report described cells containing 1-2 nucleoli, moderately coarse nuclear chromatin, a high N/C ratio, and a coarse staining pattern with PAS. These cells are most likely:

a. myeloblasts
b. lymphocytes
c. monoblasts
d. lymphoblasts

*348. In an adult with rare homozygous delta-beta thalassemia, the hemoglobin produced is:

    a. A
    b. Bart's
    c. F
    d. H

*349. Which of the following cells contains hemosiderin?

    a. megakaryocyte
    b. osteoclast
    c. histiocyte
    d. mast cell

*350. Which of the following cells is the largest cell in the bone marrow:

    a. megakaryocyte
    b. histiocyte
    c. osteoblast
    d. mast cell

*351. Which of the following stains is closely associated with the lysosomal enzyme in primary (azurophilic) granules?

    a. peroxidase
    b. Sudan black B
    c. periodic acid–Schiff (PAS)
    d. Prussian blue

*352. Which of the following may be used to stain glycogen, polysaccharides, and glycoproteins?

    a. peroxidase
    b. Sudan black B
    c. periodic acid–Schiff (PAS)
    d. nitroblue tetrazolium (NBT)

*353. Which of the following stains is used to demonstrate iron, ferritin, and hemosiderin?

    a. peroxidase
    b. Sudan black B
    c. periodic acid–Schiff (PAS)
    d. Prussian blue

*354. Which of the following is NOT useful in distinguishing thalassemia minor from iron deficiency anemia?

    a. free erythrocyte protoporphyrins (FEP)
    b. serum ferritin
    c. hemoglobin electrophoresis
    d. osmotic fragility

*355. Which of the following is increased in erythrocytosis secondary to a congenital heart defect?

    a. arterial oxygen saturation
    b. serum vitamin $B_{12}$
    c. leukocyte alkaline phosphatase activity
    d. erythropoietin

*356. Biochemical abnormalities characteristic of polycythemia vera include:

    a. increased serum $B_{12}$ binding capacity
    b. hypouricemia
    c. hypohistaminemia
    d. decreased leukocyte alkaline phosphatase activity

*357. A 10-year-old patient's bone marrow is classified morphologically by the French-American-British (FAB) system as an L3 ALL. Which of the following results supports this diagnosis?

    a. terminal deoxynucleotidyl transferase (TdT) positive
    b. Pelger-Huët–like neutrophils are found
    c. surface immunoglobulin positive
    d. E-rosette positive

*358. Abnormalities found in erythroleukemia include:

    a. rapid DNA synthesis
    b. marrow fibrosis
    c. megaloblastoid development
    d. increased erythrocyte survival

*359. Which of the following bone marrow findings favors the diagnosis of multiple myeloma?

    a. presence of Reed-Sternberg cells
    b. sheaths of immature plasma cells
    c. presence of flame cells and Russell bodies
    d. presence of plasmacytic satellitosis

*360. Leukocyte alkaline phosphatase activity is decreased in:

a. acute infections
b. pregnant women
c. polycythemia vera
d. paroxysmal nocturnal hemoglobinuria

*361. Bone marrow examination reveals a hypercellular marrow consisting of probable lympho-blasts with receptors for sheep rosettes and TdT; however, the lymphoblasts are negative for SIgs, Ia antigen, CALLA, Fc, and complement receptors. The most likely diagnosis is:

a. null-cell acute lymphocytic leukemia (non-B, non-T cell ALL)
b. chronic lymphocytic leukemia (CLL)
c. T-cell leukemia (T-ALL)
d. hairy-cell leukemia

*362. Which one of the following hypochromic anemias is usually associated with a normal free erythrocyte protoporphyrin level?

a. anemia of chronic disease
b. iron deficiency
c. lead poisoning
d. thalassemia minor

*363. A useful chemical test for the diagnosis of hairy-cell leukemia is the:

a. peroxidase test
b. Sudan black B test
c. periodic acid–Schiff test
d. tartrate-resistant acid phosphatase test

*364. What feature would NOT be expected in pseudo–Pelger-Huët cells?

a. hyperclumped chromatin
b. decreased granulation
c. normal peroxidase activity
d. normal neutrophils

*365. The hypoproliferative red cell population in the bone marrow of uremic patients is caused by:

a. infiltration of bone marrow by toxic waste products
b. decreased levels of circulating erythropoietin
c. defective globin synthesis
d. overcrowding of bone marrow space by increased myeloid precursors

*366. The granules of Alder-Reilly anomaly will stain positively with:

    a. Sudan black B
    b. periodic acid–Schiff
    c. myeloperoxidase
    d. naphthol-AS-D chloroacetate esterase

Questions 367-368 refer to the following illustration:

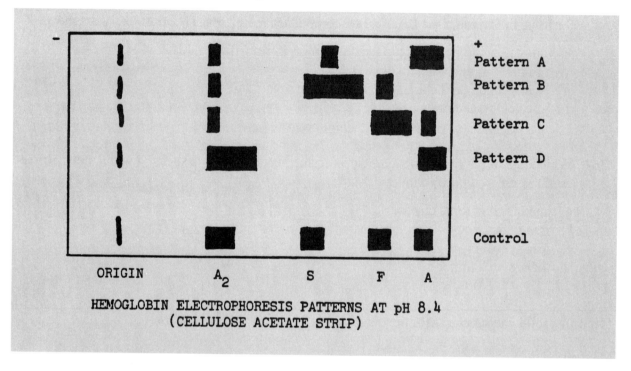

*367. Which electrophoresis pattern is consistent with sickle cell trait?

    a. pattern A
    b. pattern B
    c. pattern C
    d. pattern D

*368. Which pattern is consistent with thalassemia major?

    a. pattern A
    b. pattern B
    c. pattern C
    d. pattern D

*369. A 40-year-old white male was admitted to the hospital for treatment of anemia, weariness, weight loss, and loss of libido. The patient presented with the following laboratory data:

| | |
|---|---|
| WBC | $5.8 \times 10^3/\mu L$ |
| RBC | $3.7 \times 10^6/\mu L$ |
| Hgb | 10.0 g/dL |
| Hct | 32% |
| MCV | 86 fL |
| MCH | 26 pg |
| MCHC | 32% |
| Serum iron | 220 µg/dL |
| TIBC | 300 µg/dL |
| Serum ferritin | 2800 ng/mL |

Examination of the bone marrow revealed erythroid hyperplasia with a shift to the left of erythroid precursors. Prussian blue staining revealed markedly elevated iron stores noted with occasional sideroblasts seen. These data are most consistent with which of the following conditions?

a. iron deficiency anemia
b. anemia of chronic disease
c. hemochromatosis
d. acute blood loss

*370. A 56-year-old man was admitted to the hospital for treatment of a bleeding ulcer. The following laboratory data were obtained:

| | |
|---|---|
| RBC | $4.2 \times 10^6/\mu L$ |
| WBC | $5.0 \times 10^3/\mu L$ |
| Hct | 30% |
| Hgb | 8.5 g/dL |
| Serum iron | 40 µg/dL |
| TIBC | 460 µg/dL |
| Serum ferritin | 12 ng/mL |

Examination of the bone marrow revealed the absence of iron stores. These data are most consistent with which of the following conditions?

a. iron deficiency anemia
b. anemia of chronic disease
c. hemochromatosis
d. acute blood loss

*371. A 89-year-old white female was transferred to the hospital from a nursing facility for treatment of chronic urinary tract infection with proteinuria. The patient presented with the following laboratory data:

| | |
|---|---|
| WBC | $10.0 \times 10^3/\mu L$ |
| RBC | $3.1 \times 10^6/\mu L$ |
| Hgb | 7.2 g/dL |
| Hct | 24% |
| MCV | 78 fL |
| MCH | 23 pg |
| MCHC | 31% |
| Serum iron | 29 µg/dL |
| TIBC | 160 µg/dL |
| Serum ferritin | 100 ng/mL |

Examination of the bone marrow revealed a slightly fatty marrow with increased storage iron as detected by the Prussian blue technique. These data are most consistent with which of the following conditions?

a. iron deficiency anemia
b. anemia of chronic disease
c. hemochromatosis
d. acute blood loss


*372. The following are compounds formed in the synthesis of heme:

| | |
|---|---|
| 1. coproporphyrinogen | 2. porphobilinogen |
| 3. uroporphyrinogen | 4. protoporphyrinogen |

Which of the following responses lists these compounds in the order in which they are formed?

a. 4, 3, 1, 2
b. 2, 3, 1, 4
c. 2, 4, 3, 1
d. 2, 1, 3, 4


*373. Which of the following is a congenital nonspherocytic hemolytic anemia in which there are red cell inclusions when blood smears are stained with Prussian blue?

a. paroxysmal nocturnal hemoglobinuria
b. pyruvate kinase deficiency
c. thalassemia
d. G-6-PD deficiency

*374. An EDTA blood sample has a white count of 7.0 x 10³/μL. The specimen is selected as a patient precision control. It is refrigerated and run seven times within a 24-hour period, being inverted by hand 10 times before each run. The following results are obtained (commercial control in range):

| Time From Collection (hr) | WBC Count |
|---|---|
| 0 | 7200 |
| 2 | 9600 |
| 6 | 5400 |
| 8 | 8300 |
| 12 | 9200 |
| 15 | 6400 |
| 20 | 5900 |
| 23 | 7400 |

The best explanation for the results is:

a. the patient specimen was inadequately mixed
b. the white cells have deteriorated due to prolonged exposure to EDTA
c. the above represents normal random variation within the sample
d. the white blood cell values are valid only for a 12-hour period

*375. The following results were obtained on a leukocyte alkaline phosphatase stain:

| Score | 4+ | 3+ | 2+ | 1+ | 0 |
|---|---|---|---|---|---|
| No. of cells counted | 35 | 33 | 28 | 2 | 4 |

These reactions are most consistent with:

a. leukemoid reaction
b. nephrotic syndrome
c. chronic granulocytic leukemia
d. progressive muscular dystrophy

*376. A patient has a white blood count of 50 x 10³/μL. To distinguish between bacterial infection and chronic granulocytic leukemia the most useful test is:

a. Wright's stain
b. peroxidase
c. periodic acid–Schiff (PAS)
d. leukocyte alkaline phosphatase (LAP)

*377. The following laboratory data were obtained from a 40-year-old woman with a long history of abnormal bleeding:

| | |
|---|---|
| Prothrombin time | Normal |
| APTT | Prolonged |
| Factor VIII coagulant activity | Decreased |
| Factor VIII–related antigen | Markedly decreased |
| Platelet count | Normal |
| Template bleeding time | Prolonged |

Which of the following disorders does this woman most likely have?

a. classic hemophilia
b. von Willebrand's disease
c. Christmas disease
d. disseminated intravascular coagulation (DIC)

*378. The following laboratory data were obtained from a 27-year-old man with a long history of abnormal bleeding:

| | |
|---|---|
| Prothrombin time | Normal |
| APTT | Markedly prolonged |
| Factor VIII coagulant activity | Markedly decreased |
| Factor VIII–related antigen | Normal |
| Platelet count | Normal |
| Template bleeding time | Normal |

Which of the following disorders does this man most likely have?

a. classic hemophilia
b. von Willebrand's disease
c. Christmas disease
d. disseminated intravascular coagulation (DIC)

*379. In von Willebrand's disease, platelets give an abnormal aggregation result in the presence of:

a. adenosine diphosphate
b. epinephrine
c. collagen
d. ristocetin

*380. A heparinized blood sample is collected from a patient during open-heart surgery. The surgeon requests a complete blood count on the specimen. The most appropriate course of action is:

a. perform the complete blood count as requested
b. report only the hemoglobin and hematocrit on heparinized blood
c. report only the white cell and platelet counts on heparinized blood
d. report the white cell and red cell counts on heparinized blood

*381. Which of the following stains can be used to differentiate siderotic granules (Pappenheimer bodies) from basophilic stippling?

    a. Wright's
    b. Prussian blue
    c. crystal violet
    d. periodic acid–Schiff


*382. The main function of the hexose monophosphate shunt in the erythrocyte is to:

    a. regulate the level of 2,3-DPG
    b. provide reduced glutathione to prevent oxidation of hemoglobin
    c. prevent the reduction of heme iron
    d. provide energy for membrane maintenance


*383. A patient has a congenital nonspherocytic hemolytic anemia. After exposure to antimalarial drugs, the patient experiences a severe hemolytic episode. This episode is characterized by red cell inclusions caused by hemoglobin denaturation. Which of the following conditions is most consistent with these findings?

    a. G-6-PD deficiency
    b. thalassemia major
    c. pyruvate kinase deficiency
    d. paroxysmal nocturnal hemoglobinuria


*384. A patient is admitted with a history of chronic bleeding secondary to peptic ulcer. Hematology workup reveals a severe microcytic, hypochromic anemia. Iron studies were requested. Which of the following would be expected in this case?

    a. decreased serum iron, increased TIBC, increased storage iron
    b. increased serum iron, decreased TIBC, increased storage iron
    c. decreased serum iron, increased TIBC, decreased storage iron
    d. increased serum iron, normal TIBC, decreased storage iron


*385. When using the turbidity (solubility) method for detecting the presence of hemoglobin S, an incorrect interpretation may be made when there is a(n):

    a. unusually high concentration of hemoglobin
    b. glucose concentration greater than 150 mg/dL
    c. blood specimen greater than 2 hours old
    d. increased total serum protein

*386. A 50-year-old patient was found to have the following lab results:

Hgb    7.0 g/dL
Hct    20%
RBC    $2.0 \times 10^6/\mu L$

It was determined that the patient was suffering from pernicious anemia. Which of the following sets of data most likely was obtained on the patient?

|  | WBCs | Platelets | Reticulocytes |
|---|---|---|---|
| a. | 17,500 | 350,000 | 5.2% |
| b. | 7500 | 80,000 | 4.1% |
| c. | 5000 | 425,000 | 2.9% |
| d. | 3500 | 80,000 | 0.8% |

*387. The automated platelet count on an EDTA specimen is $58 \times 10^3/\mu L$. The platelet estimate on the blood smear appears normal, but it was noted that the platelets were surrounding the neutrophils. The next step should be to:

a. report the automated platelet count since it is more accurate than a platelet estimate
b. warm the EDTA tube and repeat the automated platelet count
c. rerun the original specimen since the platelet count and blood smear estimate do not match
d. re-collect a specimen for a platelet count using a different anticoagulant

*388. A phase-platelet count was performed and the total platelet count was 356,000/$\mu L$. Ten fields on the stained blood smear were examined for platelets and the results per field were:

16, 18, 15, 20, 19, 17, 19, 18, 20, 16

The next step would be to:

a. report the phase-platelet count since it correlated well with the slide
b. repeat the phase-platelet count on a re-collected specimen and check for clumping
c. check 10 additional fields on the blood smear
d. repeat the platelet count using a different method

*389. Aspirin affects platelet function by interfering with platelets' metabolism of:

a. prostaglandins
b. lipids
c. carbohydrates
d. nucleic acids

*390. A yellow peritoneal fluid specimen produced the following cell counts:

| | |
|---|---|
| Total WBC | 1600/μL |
| Total RBC | 200/μL |
| Segs | 2% |
| Lymphs | 5% |
| Large mononuclear cells | 93% |

Subsequent testing procedures should include:

a. blood cultures
b. serological studies
c. cytology examination
d. tissue culture

*391. Of the following, the disease most closely associated with pale blue inclusions in granulo-cytes and giant platelets is:

a. Gaucher's disease
b. Alder-Reilly anomaly
c. May-Hegglin anomaly
d. Pelger-Huët anomaly

*392. A 54-year-old man was admitted with pulmonary embolism and given streptokinase. Which of the following would be most useful in monitoring this therapy?

a. activated partial thromboplastin time
b. bleeding time
c. prothrombin time
d. thrombin time

*393. The combination of increased capillary fragility and prolonged bleeding time suggests a deficiency in:

a. thromboplastin
b. prothrombin
c. platelets
d. fibrinogen

*394. Which of the following stains is helpful in the diagnosis of suspected erythroleukemia?

a. peroxidase
b. nonspecific esterase
c. periodic acid–Schiff (PAS)
d. acid phosphatase

*395. A 14-year-old boy is seen in the ER, complaining of a sore throat, swollen glands, and fatigue. The CBC results are:

| WBC | 16.0 x 10³/μL | Differential | |
|---|---|---|---|
| RBC | 4.37 x 10⁶/μL | Segs | 30% |
| Hgb | 12.8 g/dL | Bands | 2% |
| Hct | 38.4% | Lymphs | 50% |
| Platelets | 390 x 10³/μL | Monos | 3% |
| | | Atypical lymphs | 15% |

What is the most likely diagnosis?

a. acute lymphocytic leukemia
b. chronic lymphocytic leukemia
c. viral hepatitis
d. infectious mononucleosis

*396. A patient has the following laboratory data:

| RBC | 2.35 x 10⁶/μL |
|---|---|
| WBC | 3.0 x 10³/μL |
| Platelets | 95.0 x 10³/μL |
| Hgb | 9.5 g/dL |
| Hct | 27% |
| MCV | 115 fL |
| MCHC | 35% |
| MCH | 40 pg |

Which of the following tests would contribute toward a diagnosis?

a. reticulocyte count
b. platelet factor 3
c. serum $B_{12}$ and folate
d. leukocyte alkaline phosphatase

*397. Laboratory tests performed on a patient indicate macrocytosis, anemia, leukopenia, and thrombocytopenia. Which of the following disorders is the patient most likely to have?

a. anemia of chronic disorder
b. vitamin $B_{12}$ deficiency
c. iron deficiency
d. acute hemorrhage

*398. Which of the following stains is most frequently used to differentiate acute myelocytic from acute lymphocytic leukemia?

a. alkaline phosphatase
b. nonspecific esterase
c. acid phosphatase
d. peroxidase


*399. Which of the following test systems has the SMALLEST standard deviation?

a. manual white cell count
b. reticulocyte count
c. leukocyte alkaline phosphatase score
d. hemoglobin by cyanmethemoglobin


*400. The cell series most readily identified by a positive Sudan black B is:

a. erythrocytic
b. myelocytic
c. plasmocytic
d. lymphocytic


*401. Higher levels of employee motivation occur when the supervisor:

a. sets goals to be accomplished
b. provides all the details of the task
c. constantly monitors progress
d. immediately corrects every error


*402. The following coagulation studies were obtained:

| | |
|---|---|
| Bleeding time | 3 min |
| Platelets | 350 x 10³/µL |
| Platelet adhesiveness | Normal |
| APTT | 45.0 sec |
| APTT control | 32.0 sec |
| Factor VIII | 5% |

These results would most likely indicate:

a. classic hemophilia
b. Christmas disease
c. Hageman factor deficiency
d. immune thrombocytopenic purpura

*403. A phase-platelet count is performed using a red cell pipet. 155 platelets are counted on one side of the hemacytometer in the red cell counting area, and 145 are counted on the other side in the same area. After making the appropriate calculations, the next step would be to:

a. repeat the procedure, using a 1:20 dilution in a white cell pipet
b. report the calculated value
c. collect a new specimen
d. repeat the procedure, using a 1:200 dilution in the red cell pipet

*404. A patient is diagnosed as having bacterial septicemia. Which of the following would best describe the expected change in his peripheral blood?

a. granulocytic leukemoid reaction
b. lymphocytic leukemoid reaction
c. neutropenia
d. eosinophilia

*405. A deficiency of protein C is associated with which of the following?

a. prolonged activated partial thromboplastin time (APTT)
b. decreased fibrinogen level (less than 100 mg/dL)
c. increased risk of thrombosis
d. spontaneous hemorrhage

*406. Dwarf or micromegakaryocytes may be found in the peripheral blood of patients with:

a. pernicious anemia
b. DIC
c. myelofibrosis with myeloid metaplasia
d. chronic lymphocytic leukemia

*407. In laser flow cytometry, histograms combining the data from forward-angle light scatter with the data from right-angle light scatter permit the operator to:

a. quantitate cell surface protein
b. determine absolute cell size
c. distinguish internal cell structures
d. differentiate cell populations from one another

*408. Which of the following is characteristic of cellular changes as megakaryoblasts mature into megakaryocytes within the bone marrow?

a. progressive decrease in overall cell size
b. increasing basophilia of cytoplasm
c. nuclear division without cytoplasmic division
d. fusion of the nuclear lobes

*409. The first step in the determination of functional antithrombin III (AT III) is to:

a. neutralize plasma antithrombin
b. neutralize thrombin with test plasma
c. incubate plasma with anti-AT III
d. precipitate AT III with plasma


*410. Biological assays for antithrombin III (AT III) are based on the inhibition of:

a. Factor VIII
b. heparin
c. serine proteases
d. anti-AT III globulin


*411. A patient has pancytopenia, decreased total serum iron, and decreased serum iron-binding capacity, and shows a homogeneous fluorescence pattern with a high titer on a fluorescent antinuclear antibody test. This is suggestive of:

a. polycythemia vera
b. lupus erythematosus
c. iron deficiency anemia
d. hemoglobin SC disease


*412. In immunophenotyping by flow cytometry the emitting fluorescence intensity is proportional to the:

a. DNA content in the cell
b. amount of cell surface antigen
c. RNA content in the cell
d. size of the cell nucleus


*413. vWF antigen can be found in which of the following?

a. myeloblast
b. monoblast
c. lymphoblast
d. megakaryoblast


*414. Plasma from a patient with lupus coagulation inhibitor can show:

a. a prolonged APTT and normal PT
b. may exhibit bleeding tendencies
c. no change with platelet neutralization
d. complete correction when incubated with normal plasma

*415. The Prussian blue staining of peripheral blood identifies:

    a. Howell-Jolly bodies
    b. siderotic granules
    c. reticulocytes
    d. basophilic stippling


*416. A patient with thalassemia minor characteristically has a(n):

    a. elevated $A_2$ hemoglobin
    b. low fetal hemoglobin
    c. high serum iron
    d. normal red cell fragility


*417. Which cells are involved in immediate hypersensitivity reactions?

    a. eosinophils
    b. basophils
    c. plasma cells
    d. reactive lymphocytes


*418. An oncology patient has the following results:

|  | Day 1 | Day 3 |
|---|---|---|
| WBC | $8.0 \times 10^3/\mu L$ | $2.0 \times 10^3/\mu L$ |
| RBC | $3.50 \times 10^6/\mu L$ | $3.45 \times 10^6/\mu L$ |
| Hgb | 10.0 g/dL | 9.9 g/dL |
| Hct | 29.8% | 29.5% |
| Platelets | $180 \times 10^3/\mu L$ | $150 \times 10^3/\mu L$ |

The most probable explanation is:

    a. chemotherapy
    b. cold antibody
    c. clotted specimen
    d. inadequate mixing

| | | | | |
|---|---|---|---|---|
| 1. d | | | 124. b | 165. d |
| 2. a | | | 125. d | 166. c |
| 3. a | | | 126. d | 167. c |
| 4. c | | | 127. b | 168. d |
| 5. c | | | 128. a | 169. b |
| 6. d | | | 129. d | 170. c |
| 7. b | | | 130. c | 171. a |
| 8. c | | | 131. d | 172. b |
| 9. d | | | 132. d | 173. b |
| 10. b | 51. d | 92. d | 133. a | 174. c |
| 11. a | 52. a | 93. c | 134. d | 175. b |
| 12. b | 53. d | 94. a | 135. d | 176. b |
| 13. b | 54. a | 95. a | 136. d | 177. c |
| 14. d | 55. c | 96. a | 137. b | 178. b |
| 15. d | 56. a | 97. a | 138. a | 179. c |
| 16. b | 57. c | 98. a | 139. d | 180. a |
| 17. d | 58. c | 99. d | 140. d | 181. d |
| 18. a | 59. c | 100. d | 141. a | 182. c |
| 19. b | 60. b | 101. a | 142. a | 183. d |
| 20. d | 61. a | 102. a | 143. a | 184. a |
| 21. b | 62. d | 103. b | 144. d | 185. c |
| 22. d | 63. d | 104. b | 145. d | 186. a |
| 23. a | 64. b | 105. d | 146. b | 187. b |
| 24. c | 65. b | 106. c | 147. c | 188. b |
| 25. a | 66. b | 107. d | 148. c | 189. c |
| 26. a | 67. a | 108. a | 149. c | 190. a |
| 27. d | 68. c | 109. a | 150. b | 191. d |
| 28. d | 69. d | 110. d | 151. d | 192. a |
| 29. a | 70. d | 111. c | 152. b | 193. b |
| 30. b | 71. c | 112. b | 153. c | 194. a |
| 31. d | 72. d | 113. a | 154. a | 195. b |
| 32. a | 73. d | 114. d | 155. d | 196. b |
| 33. d | 74. d | 115. b | 156. b | 197. b |
| 34. a | 75. b | 116. c | 157. b | 198. c |
| 35. a | 76. b | 117. d | 158. c | 199. b |
| 36. c | 77. a | 118. d | 159. d | 200. b |
| 37. a | 78. d | 119. a | 160. b | 201. a |
| 38. d | 79. a | 120. b | 161. c | 202. d |
| 39. c | 80. d | 121. b | 162. b | 203. c |
| 40. a | 81. c | 122. d | 163. c | 204. d |
| 41. a | 82. d | 123. b | 164. d | 205. c |

| | | | | |
|---|---|---|---|---|
| 206. b | 249. b | 292. c | 335. d | 378. a |
| 207. c | 250. c | 293. a | 336. a | 379. d |
| 208. d | 251. d | 294. c | 337. c | 380. b |
| 209. c | 252. d | 295. a | 338. b | 381. b |
| 210. c | 253. a | 296. d | 339. a | 382. b |
| 211. b | 254. c | 297. a | 340. a | 383. a |
| 212. b | 255. c | 298. d | 341. d | 384. c |
| 213. b | 256. d | 299. b | 342. b | 385. d |
| 214. c | 257. a | 300. c | 343. c | 386. d |
| 215. b | 258. d | 301. b | 344. d | 387. d |
| 216. b | 259. b | 302. a | 345. c | 388. a |
| 217. b | 260. b | 303. c | 346. d | 389. a |
| 218. a | 261. a | 304. d | 347. d | 390. c |
| 219. d | 262. d | 305. b | 348. c | 391. c |
| 220. b | 263. c | 306. b | 349. c | 392. d |
| 221. d | 264. d | 307. c | 350. a | 393. c |
| 222. d | 265. b | 308. d | 351. a | 394. c |
| 223. d | 266. c | 309. d | 352. c | 395. d |
| 224. d | 267. d | 310. a | 353. d | 396. c |
| 225. a | 268. d | 311. b | 354. d | 397. b |
| 226. d | 269. d | 312. a | 355. d | 398. d |
| 227. b | 270. c | 313. a | 356. a | 399. d |
| 228. d | 271. b | 314. c | 357. c | 400. b |
| 229. b | 272. b | 315. a | 358. c | 401. a |
| 230. d | 273. c | 316. b | 359. b | 402. a |
| 231. b | 274. d | 317. a | 360. d | 403. b |
| 232. a | 275. c | 318. d | 361. c | 404. a |
| 233. c | 276. c | 319. d | 362. d | 405. c |
| 234. a | 277. c | 320. c | 363. d | 406. c |
| 235. d | 278. a | 321. b | 364. c | 407. d |
| 236. c | 279. a | 322. b | 365. b | 408. c |
| 237. b | 280. d | 323. b | 366. b | 409. b |
| 238. b | 281. a | 324. c | 367. a | 410. c |
| 239. b | 282. c | 325. d | 368. c | 411. b |
| 240. a | 283. a | 326. d | 369. c | 412. b |
| 241. d | 284. a | 327. d | 370. a | 413. d |
| 242. a | 285. d | 328. c | 371. b | 414. a |
| 243. a | 286. b | 329. b | 372. b | 415. b |
| 244. c | 287. c | 330. b | 373. c | 416. a |
| 245. a | 288. b | 331. a | 374. a | 417. b |
| 246. a | 289. d | 332. d | 375. a | 418. a |
| 247. a | 290. a | 333. a | 376. d | |
| 248. c | 291. b | 334. c | 377. b | |

# CHAPTER 12

## *Immunology*

*The following items have been identified as appropriate for both entry level medical technologists and medical laboratory technicians.*

1. Which of the following statements about immunoglobulins is true?

   a. Immunoglobulins are produced by T lymphocytes.
   b. The IgA class is determined by the gamma heavy chain.
   c. The IgA class exists as serum and secretory molecules.
   d. There are two subclasses of IgG.

2. The classic antibody response pattern following infection with hepatitis A is:

   a. increase in IgM antibody; decrease in IgM antibody; increase in IgG antibody
   b. detectable presence of IgG antibody only
   c. detectable presence of IgM antibody only
   d. decrease in IgM antibody; increase in IgG antibody of the IgG3 subtype

3. Which of the following is the major residual split portion of C3?

   a. C3a
   b. C3b
   c. C4
   d. C1q

Questions 4-7 refer to the curve below, which was obtained by adding increasing amounts of a soluble antigen to fixed volumes of monospecific antiserum.

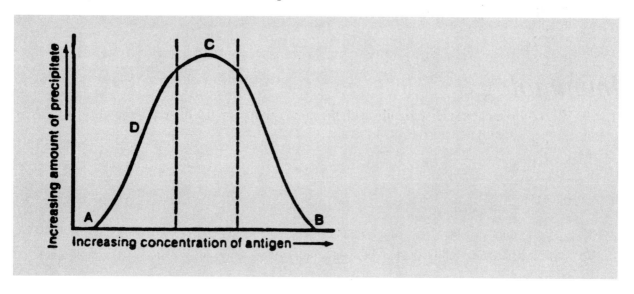

4. The area on the curve for equivalence precipitate is:

    a.  A
    b.  B
    c.  C
    d.  D

5. The area on the curve where no precipitate formed due to antigen excess is:

    a.  A
    b.  B
    c.  C
    d.  D

6. The area on the curve for prozone is:

    a.  A
    b.  B
    c.  C
    d.  D

7. The area on the curve where soluble antigen-antibody complexes have begun to form is:

    a.  A
    b.  B
    c.  C
    d.  D

8. Which of the following releases histamine and other mediators from basophils?

   a. C3a
   b. properdin factor B
   c. C1q
   d. C4

9. The component associated only with the alternative pathway of complement activation is:

   a. C4
   b. C1q
   c. properdin factor B
   d. C3a

10. Which of the following is cleaved as a result of activation of the classical complement pathway?

    a. properdin factor B
    b. C1q
    c. C4
    d. C3b

11. The enzyme-linked immunosorbent assay (ELISA) technique for the detection of HBsAg:

    a. requires radiolabeled C1q
    b. is quantitated by degree of fluorescence
    c. uses anti-HBs linked to horseradish peroxidase
    d. uses beads coated with HBsAg

12. Rheumatoid factor is:

    a. an antigen found in the serum of patients with rheumatoid arthritis
    b. identical to the rheumatoid arthritis precipitin
    c. IgG or IgM autoantibody
    d. capable of forming circulating immune complexes only when IgM-type autoantibody is present

13. The presence of immune complexes indicates:

    a. polyclonal hypergammaglobulinemia
    b. inflammatory tissue injury
    c. protection from complement-dependent neutrophil chemotaxis
    d. normal host response to antigenic exposure

Questions 14-17 refer to the following illustration of the hepatitis B virus:

14. Select the corresponding lettered component indicated on the diagram for surface antigen.

    a. A
    b. B
    c. C
    d. D


15. Select the corresponding lettered component indicated on the diagram for e antigen.

    a. A
    b. B
    c. C
    d. D


16. Select the corresponding lettered component indicated on the diagram for core antigen.

    a. A
    b. B
    c. C
    d. D


17. Select the corresponding lettered component indicated on the diagram for viral DNA.

    a. A
    b. B
    c. C
    d. D

18. The complement component C3:

   a. is increased (in plasma levels) when complement activation occurs
   b. can be measured by immunoprecipitin assays
   c. releases histamine from basophils or mast cells
   d. is NOT involved in the alternate complement pathway

19. Chronic carriers of HBV:

   a. have chronic symptoms of hepatitis
   b. continue to carry the HBV
   c. do not transmit infection
   d. carry the HBV but are not infectious

20. The antigen marker most closely associated with transmissibility of HBV infection is:

   a. HBs
   b. HBe
   c. HBc
   d. HBV

21. Hepatitis C (nonenteric form of non-A, non-B hepatitis) differs from hepatitis A and hepatitis B because it:

   a. has a highly stable incubation period
   b. is associated with a high incidence of icteric hepatitis
   c. is associated with a high incidence of the chronic carrier state
   d. is seldom implicated in cases of posttransfusion hepatitis

22. Which of the following mediators is released during T-cell activation?

   a. immunoglobulins
   b. thymosin
   c. serotonin
   d. lymphokines

23. The J-chain is associated with which of the following immunoglobulins?

   a. IgA
   b. IgG
   c. IgE
   d. IgD

24. Initiation of the activation mechanism of the alternative complement pathway differs from that of the classical pathway in that:

    a. antigen-antibody complexes containing IgM or IgG are required
    b. endotoxin alone cannot initiate activation
    c. C1 component of complement is involved
    d. antigen-antibody complexes containing IgA or IgE may initiate activation

25. The C3b component of complement:

    a. is undetectable in pathologic sera
    b. is a component of the C3 cleaving enzyme of the classical pathway
    c. is cleaved by C3 inactivator into C3c and C3d
    d. migrates farther toward the cathode than C3

26. The serum hemolytic complement level ($CH_{50}$):

    a. is a measure of total complement activity
    b. provides the same information as a serum factor B level
    c. is detectable when any component of the classical system is congenitally absent
    d. can be calculated from the serum concentrations of the individual components

27. A 26-year-old nurse developed fatigue, a low-grade fever, polyarthritis, and urticaria. Two months earlier she had cared for a patient with hepatitis. Which of the following findings are likely to be observed in this nurse?

    a. a negative hepatitis B surface antigen test
    b. elevated AST and ALT levels
    c. a positive rheumatoid factor
    d. a positive Monospot™ test

28. The FTA-ABS test for the serologic diagnosis of syphilis is:

    a. less sensitive and specific than the VDRL if properly performed
    b. likely to remain positive after adequate antibiotic therapy
    c. currently recommended for testing cerebrospinal fluid
    d. preferred over darkfield microscopy for diagnosing primary syphilis

29. The hyperviscosity syndrome is most likely to be seen in monoclonal disease of which of the following immunoglobulin classes?

    a. IgA
    b. IgM
    c. IgG
    d. IgD

30. The curve below was obtained by adding increasing amounts of a soluble antigen to fixed volumes of monospecific antiserum:

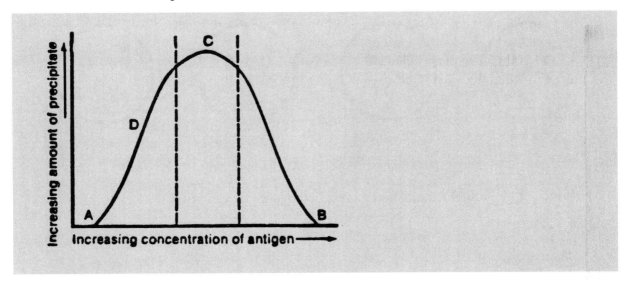

The area in which the addition of more antibody would result in the formation of additional precipitate is:

a. A
b. B
c. C
d. D

31. Antibody class and antibody subclass are determined by major physiochemical differences and antigenic variation found primarily in the:

a. constant region of heavy chain
b. constant region of light chain
c. variable regions of heavy and light chains
d. constant regions of heavy and light chains

32. Which of the following complement components is a strong chemotactic factor as well as a strong anaphylatoxin?

a. C3a
b. C3b
c. C5a
d. C4a

33. Which of the following complement components or pair of components is a viral neutralizer?

a. C1
b. C1, 4
c. C2b
d. C3a

Questions 34-37 refer to the following illustration:

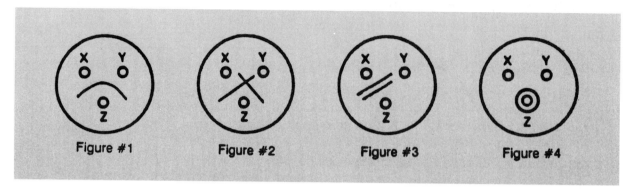

Figure #1    Figure #2    Figure #3    Figure #4

34. Which of the figures demonstrates a reaction pattern of identity?

   a. Figure #1
   b. Figure #2
   c. Figure #3
   d. Figure #4

35. Which of the figures demonstrates a reaction pattern of nonidentity?

   a. Figure #1
   b. Figure #2
   c. Figure #3
   d. Figure #4

36. Which of the figures demonstrates a reaction pattern showing two different antigenic molecular species?

   a. Figure #1
   b. Figure #2
   c. Figure #3
   d. Figure #4

37. A nonspecific precipitin reaction is demonstrated in:

   a. Figure #1
   b. Figure #2
   c. Figure #3
   d. Figure #4

38. Which of the following activities is associated with C3b?

    a. opsonization
    b. anaphylaxis
    c. vasoconstriction
    d. chemotaxis


39. Immediate hypersensitivity is most commonly associated with:

    a. transfusion reaction
    b. anaphylactic reaction
    c. contact dermatitis
    d. bacterial septicemia


40. A transfusion reaction to erythrocyte antigens will activate which of the following immunopathologic mechanisms?

    a. immediate hypersensitivity
    b. Arthus reaction
    c. delayed hypersensitivity
    d. immune cytolysis


41. Delayed hypersensitivity is related to:

    a. contact sensitivity to inorganic chemicals
    b. transfusion reaction
    c. anaphylactic reaction
    d. bacterial septicemia


42. High titers of antimicrosomal antibodies are most often found in:

    a. rheumatoid arthritis
    b. systemic lupus erythematosus
    c. chronic hepatitis
    d. thyroid disease


43. Systemic lupus erythematosus patients often have which of the following test results?

    a. high titers of DNA antibody
    b. decreased serum immunoglobulin levels
    c. high titers of anti–smooth muscle antibodies
    d. high titers of antimitochondrial antibody

44. Anti-RNA antibodies are often present in individuals having an antinuclear antibody immunofluorescent pattern that is:

    a. speckled
    b. rim
    c. diffuse
    d. nucleolar

45. Antibodies to which of the following immunoglobulins are known to have produced anaphylactic reactions following blood transfusion?

    a. IgA
    b. IgD
    c. IgE
    d. IgG

46. The latex agglutination titer commonly considered as the lower limit of positivity for diagnosis of rheumatoid arthritis is:

    a. 1:2
    b. 1:40
    c. 1:160
    d. 1:640

47. A 16-year-old boy with infectious mononucleosis has a cold agglutinin titer of 1:2000. An important consideration of this antibody's clinical relevance is the:

    a. thermal range
    b. titer at 4°C
    c. specificity
    d. light chain type

48. Which of the following is an important cellular mediator of immune complex tissue injury?

    a. monocyte
    b. neutrophil
    c. basophil
    d. eosinophil

49. A serologic test for syphilis that depends upon the detection of cardiolipin-lecithin-cholesterol antigen is:

    a. FTA-ABS
    b. RPR
    c. MHA-TP
    d. TPI

50. In the FTA-ABS test, the presence of a beaded pattern of fluorescence along the treponeme indicates:

    a. positive identification of *Treponema pallidum*
    b. presumptive diagnosis of active syphilis
    c. presence of nontreponemal antibody (NTA)
    d. false-positive reaction

51. The most important use of a nontreponemal antibody (NTA) test alone is in:

    a. establishing the diagnosis of acute active syphilis
    b. establishing the diagnosis of chronic syphilis
    c. evaluating the success of therapy
    d. determining the prevalence of disease in the general population

52. The serologic test for syphilis recommended for detecting antibody in cerebrospinal fluid is:

    a. nontreponemal antibody
    b. CSF-VDRL
    c. FTA-ABS
    d. MHA-TP

53. The initial immune response following fetal infection with rubella is the production of which class(es) of antibodies?

    a. IgG
    b. IgA
    c. IgM
    d. both IgG and IgA

54. Within one week after exposure to rash illness, a maternal serum rubella titer that is equal to or greater than 1:8 indicates:

    a. probable immunity to rubella
    b. evidence of acute rubella infection
    c. susceptibility to rubella infection
    d. absence of acute rubella

55. Which IgG subclass is most efficient at crossing the placenta?

    a. IgG1
    b. IgG2
    c. IgG3
    d. IgG4

56. The area of the immunoglobulin molecule referred to as the hinge region is located between which domains?

    a. VH and VL
    b. CH1 and CH2
    c. CH2 and CH3
    d. CH3 and VL

57. Which class of immunoglobulin is thought to function as an antigenic receptor site on the surface of immature B lymphocytes?

    a. IgD
    b. IgM
    c. IgA
    d. IgG

58. Which of the following terms describes a graft between genetically unidentical individuals belonging to the same species?

    a. autograft
    b. isograft
    c. allograft
    d. xenograft

59. Which of the following is the "recognition unit" in the classical complement pathway?

    a. C1q
    b. C3a
    c. C4
    d. C5

60. Which of the following is the "C3 activation unit" in the classical complement pathway?

    a. C1q
    b. C3
    c. C4b, C2a
    d. C5, C6, C7, C8, C9

61. Which of the following is the "membrane attack complex" of complement activation?

    a. C1
    b. C3
    c. C4, C2, C3
    d. C5b, C6, C7, C8, C9

62. A series of eight tubes are set up with 0.79 mL of diluent in each. A serial dilution is performed by adding 10 μL of serum to the first tube and then transferring 10 μL through each remaining tube. What is the serum dilution of tube 7?

   a. 1:2.431 x 10$^{11}$
   b. 1:2.621 x 10$^{11}$
   c. 1:1.920 x 10$^{13}$
   d. 1:2.097 x 10$^{13}$

63. Patients suffering from Waldenström's macroglobulinemia demonstrate excessively increased concentrations of which of the following?

   a. IgG
   b. IgA
   c. IgM
   d. IgD

64. The presence of HbsAg, anti-HBc and often HbeAg is characteristic of:

   a. early acute phase HBV hepatitis
   b. early convalescent phase HBV hepatitis
   c. recovery phase of acute HBV hepatitis
   d. carrier state of acute HBV hepatitis

65. The disappearance of HBsAg and HBeAg, the persistence of anti-HBc, the appearance of anti-HBs, and often of anti-HBe indicate:

   a. early acute HBV hepatitis
   b. early convalescent phase HBV hepatitis
   c. recovery phase of acute HBV hepatitis
   d. carrier state of acute HBV hepatitis

66. The immunoglobulin class typically found to be present in saliva, tears, and other secretions is:

   a. IgG
   b. IgA
   c. IgM
   d. IgD

67. The immunoglobulin class associated with immediate hypersensitivity or atopic reactions is:

   a. IgA
   b. IgM
   c. IgD
   d. IgE

68. Adenovirus infections primarily involve the:

    a. respiratory tract
    b. gastrointestinal tract
    c. genital tract
    d. urinary tract


69. In primary biliary cirrhosis, which of the following antibodies is seen in high titers?

    a. antimitochondrial
    b. anti–smooth muscle
    c. anti-DNA
    d. anti–parietal cell


70. In chronic active hepatitis, high titers of which of the following antibodies are seen?

    a. antimitochondrial
    b. anti–smooth muscle
    c. anti-DNA
    d. anti–parietal cell


71. In the indirect fluorescent antinuclear antibody test, a homogeneous pattern indicates the presence of antibody to:

    a. RNP
    b. Sm
    c. RNA
    d. DNA


72. In the indirect fluorescent antinuclear antibody test, a speckled pattern may indicate the presence of antibody to:

    a. histone
    b. Sm
    c. RNA
    d. DNA


73. Which of the following is used to detect allergen-specific IgE?

    a. RIST
    b. IEP
    c. RAST
    d. CRP

74. In skin tests, a wheal and flare development is indicative of:

    a. immediate hypersensitivity
    b. delayed hypersensitivity
    c. anergy
    d. Arthus reaction


75. Carcinoembryonic antigen (CEA) is most likely to be produced in a malignancy involving the:

    a. brain
    b. testes
    c. bone
    d. colon


76. In direct fluorescent antibody screening for the diagnosis of primary syphilis, which of the following labeled antibody reagents is used?

    a. antibody to spirochetes
    b. antibody to cardiolipin
    c. antibody to circulating antibodies
    d. antibody to antibodies in situ


77. Antiserum and a patient's serum specimen are added to opposing wells in an agar plate and an electrical current is then applied to this plate. This process is called:

    a. counterimmunoelectrophoresis
    b. radial immunodiffusion
    c. electroimmunodiffusion
    d. immunoelectrophoresis


78. A patient has the following test results:

| | |
|---|---|
| ANA | Positive, 1:320 |
| ASO | 50 Todd units |
| Complement | Decreased |
| RA | Positive |

The above results could be seen in patients with:

    a. rheumatic fever
    b. rheumatoid arthritis
    c. lupus erythematosus
    d. glomerulonephritis

79. The rheumatoid factor in rheumatoid arthritis usually belongs to which immunoglobulin class?

a. IgM
b. IgA
c. IgG
d. IgE

80. Refer to the following data:

|  | HBsAg | Anti-HBc IgM | Anti-HAV IgM |
|---|---|---|---|
| Patient 1 | – | – | + |
| Patient 2 | + | + | – |
| Patient 3 | – | + | – |

From the test results above, it can be concluded that patient 3 has:

a. recent acute hepatitis A
b. acute hepatitis B
c. acute hepatitis C (non-A/non-B hepatitis)
d. chronic hepatitis B

81. A single, reliable screening test for detecting neonatal infection in the absence of clinical signs is:

a. serum immunoelectrophoresis
b. differential leukocyte count
c. CD4 cell counts
d. quantitative serum IgM determination

82. Rheumatoid factor reacts with:

a. inert substances such as latex
b. Rh-positive erythrocytes
c. kinetoplasts of *Crithidia luciliae*
d. gamma globulin–coated particles

83. Which of the following immunoglobulin classes is associated with a secretory component (transport piece)?

a. IgA
b. IgD
c. IgE
d. IgG

84. A substrate is first exposed to patient's serum, then after washing, anti–human immunoglobulin labeled with a fluorochrome is added. The procedure described is:

   a. fluorescent quenching
   b. direct fluorescence
   c. indirect fluorescence
   d. fluorescence inhibition

85. Which of the following is DECREASED in serum during the active stages of systemic lupus erythematosus?

   a. antinuclear antibody
   b. immune complexes
   c. complement (C3)
   d. anti-DNA

86. Rheumatoid factor in a patient's serum may cause a false:

   a. positive test for the detection of IgM class antibodies
   b. negative test for the detection of IgM class antibodies
   c. positive test for the detection of IgG class antibodies
   d. negative test for the detection of IgG class antibodies

87. Antibodies are produced by:

   a. killer cells
   b. marrow stem cells
   c. mast cells
   d. B cells

88. The following pattern of agglutination was observed in an antibody titration:

| Tube | 1 | 2 | 3 | 4 | 5 | 6 | 7 | 8 | 9 | 10 | 11 |
|------|-----|-----|-----|-----|-----|-----|-----|-----|-----|-----|-----|
|      | 1+  | 2+  | 4+  | 4+  | 3+  | 3+  | 2+  | 1+  | 1+  | 0   | 0  |

This set of reactions most likely resulted from:

   a. faulty pipetting technique
   b. postzoning
   c. prozoning
   d. the presence of a high-titer, low-avidity antibody

89. Which of the following forms of exposure places a technologist at the highest risk for infection with human immunodeficiency virus (HIV)?

   a. aerosol inhalation (eg, AIDS patient's sneeze)
   b. ingestion (eg, mouth pipetting of positive serum)
   c. needlestick (eg, from AIDS-contaminated needle)
   d. splash (eg, infected serum spill onto intact skin)

90. Treatment of IgG with papain results in how many fragments?

   a. 2
   b. 3
   c. 4
   d. 5

91. Which of the following chemical classes of antigens is most likely to activate the alternative pathway of complement?

   a. proteins
   b. lipids
   c. polysaccharides
   d. haptens

92. In a complement fixation test, all reagent control tubes give the expected reactions. Both the unknown test and its serum control fail to hemolyze. What is the most likely explanation?

   a. old sheep red blood cells
   b. absence of antibody in the serum
   c. heat inactivated serum
   d. anticomplementary serum

93. A false-negative cold agglutinin test may result if:

   a. the specimen is centrifuged at room temperature
   b. the cold agglutinin demonstrates anti-I specificity
   c. the specimen is refrigerated prior to serum separation
   d. adult human O red cells are used in the assay

94. Following repeat exposure to an antigen, rapid antibody production to an elevated level that persists for a long period of time is called:

   a. hypersensitivity
   b. an Arthus reaction
   c. an anamnestic response
   d. a primary response

95. Which of the following immunoglobulins is the most efficient agglutinin?

    a. IgG
    b. IgA
    c. IgM
    d. IgE


96. Which of the following is an organ-specific autoimmune disease?

    a. myasthenia gravis
    b. rheumatoid arthritis
    c. Addison's disease
    d. progressive systemic sclerosis


97. Which immunologic mechanism is usually involved in bronchial asthma?

    a. immediate hypersensitivity
    b. antibody-mediated cytotoxicity
    c. immune complex
    d. delayed hypersensitivity


98. Antihistamines:

    a. stimulate IgE antibody production
    b. stimulate IgG blocking antibodies
    c. bind histamine
    d. block histamine receptors


99. Detection of which of the following substances is most useful to monitor the course of a patient with testicular cancer?

    a. alpha-fetoprotein
    b. carcinoembryonic antigen
    c. prolactin
    d. testosterone


100. Which laboratory technique is most frequently used to diagnose and follow the course of therapy of a patient with secondary syphilis?

    a. flocculation
    b. precipitation
    c. complement fixation
    d. indirect immunofluorescence

101. The visible serologic reaction between soluble antigen and its specific antibody is:

    a. sensitization
    b. precipitation
    c. agglutination
    d. opsonization

102. Substances that are antigenic only when coupled to a protein carrier are:

    a. opsonins
    b. haptens
    c. adjuvants
    d. allergens

103. A haptenic determinant will react with:

    a. both T cells and antibody
    b. T cells but not antibody
    c. neither T cells nor antibody
    d. antibody but not T cells

104. What is the immunologic method utilized in the flow cytometer?

    a. latex agglutination
    b. enzyme linked immunoassay
    c. immunofluorescence
    d. radioimmunoassay

105. Calculate the absolute CD4 from the data given below:

| WBC | $5.0 \times 10^3/\mu L$ |
|-----|------|
| Lymphs | 15% |
| CD4 | 8% |

    a. 40
    b. 60
    c. 400
    d. 750

106. What is the correct interpretation of the following data?

| WBC | $5.0 \times 10^3/\mu L$ |
|-----|------|
| Lymphs | 15% |
| CD4 | 8% |

a. CD4% and absolute CD4 normal
b. consistent with an intact immune system
c. consistent with a viral infection such as HIV
d. technical error

107. When testing a patient for HIV antibody, which of the following is used to confirm a positive screening test?

a. radioimmunoassay
b. Western blot
c. immunofluorescence
d. ELISA

108. For a thorough evaluation of the possibility of *Toxoplasma* in the AIDS patient, which is/are the most appropriate specimen(s) for testing?

a. CSF
b. urine
c. CSF and serum
d. urine and serum

109. Which serological marker of HBV (hepatitis B virus) infection indicates recovery and immunity?

a. viral DNA polymerase
b. $HB_e$ antigen
c. anti-HBs
d. HBsAg

110. Precautions for health care workers dealing with patients or patient specimens include:

a. mouth pipetting when specimens lack a "Precaution" label
b. reinserting needles into their original sheaths after drawing blood from a patient
c. wearing a mask and disposable gown to draw blood
d. prompt cleaning of blood spills with a disinfectant solution, such as sodium hypochlorite

111. The assembly of the complement "membrane attack unit" is initiated with the binding of:

a. C1
b. C3
c. C4
d. C5

112. A patient was tested for rubella antibody 21 days after the appearance of a rash. The result of the assay for rubella antibody was a titer of 1:32. This result indicates:

a. active rubella infection
b. susceptibility to rubella
c. absence of rubella infection
d. probable immunity

113. In the anti–double-stranded DNA procedure the antigen most commonly utilized is:

a. rat stomach tissue
b. mouse kidney tissue
c. *Crithidia luciliae*
d. *Toxoplasma gondii*

114. The air temperature throughout the serology laboratory is 20°C. How will this effect RPR test results?

a. no effect—the acceptable test range is 20°C-24°C
b. weaken reactions so that false negatives occur
c. strengthen reactions so that positive titers appear elevated
d. increase the number of false positives from spontaneous clumping

115. T cells are incapable of:

a. collaborating with B cells in some antibody responses
b. secretion of immunoglobulins
c. secretion of lymphokines
d. producing positive skin tests

116. T lymphocytes are incapable of functioning as:

a. cytotoxic cells
b. helper cells
c. phagocytic cells
d. suppressor cells

117. Refer to the following data from a peripheral blood sample:

| Total WBC | 10.0 x 10³/µL |
| --- | --- |
| Differential | |
| Neutros | 68% |
| Lymphs | 25% (40% T cells) |
| Monos | 4% |
| Eos | 2% |
| Basos | 1% |

The expected total number of T cells is:

a. 200
b. 1000
c. 2000
d. 2500

118. Nonspecific killing of tumor cells is carried out by:

a. cytotoxic T cells
b. helper T cells
c. natural killer cells
d. antibody and complement

119. Tumor markers found in the circulation are most frequently measured by:

a. immunoassays
b. thin-layer chromatography
c. high-pressure liquid chromatography
d. colorimetry

120. Which of the following is a major advantage of the ELISA vs the RIA procedure?

a. A gamma counter is used for quantitation.
b. A radioactive waste disposal system is required.
c. Enzyme labels are used instead of radioactive labels.
d. The enzyme tag is attached to a radioactive label.

121. Which of the following represents the relative concentration of immunoglobulins in decreasing order in normal serum?

a. IgG, IgM, IgA, IgD
b. IgG, IgA, IgM, IgD
c. IgG, IgD, IgA, IgM
d. IgG, IgA, IgD, IgM

122. In the indirect immunofluorescence method of antibody detection the labeled antibody is:

a. human anti–goat immunoglobulin
b. rheumatoid factor
c. goat anti–human immunoglobulin
d. complement

123. Antibodies directed at native DNA are most frequently associated with which pattern of fluorescence in the IFA-ANA test?

    a. rim
    b. diffuse
    c. speckled
    d. centromere

124. A consistently and repeatedly negative IFA-ANA is:

    a. strong evidence against untreated SLE
    b. associated with active SLE
    c. characteristic of SLE with renal involvement
    d. associated with lupus inhibitor

125. In an indirect (sandwich) ELISA method designed to detect antibody to the rubella virus in patient serum, the conjugate used should be:

    a. anti–human IgG conjugated to an enzyme
    b. antirubella antibody conjugated to an enzyme
    c. rubella antigen conjugated to an enzyme
    d. antirubella antibody conjugated to a substrate

126. An immunofluorescence test using reagent antibody directed against the CD3 surface marker would identify which of the following cell types in a sample of human peripheral blood?

    a. most circulating T lymphocytes
    b. T helper lymphocytes only
    c. T suppressor lymphocytes only
    d. natural killer cells only

127. The technologist observes apparent homogeneous staining of the nucleus of interphase cells while performing an IFA-ANA, as well as staining of the chromosomes in mitotic cells. This result is:

    a. indicative of two antibodies that should be separately reported after titration
    b. expected for anti-DNA antibodies
    c. inconsistent; the test should be reported with new reagent
    d. expected for anticentromere antibodies

128. Immunoglobulin production begins:

    a. in early fetal life
    b. at birth
    c. early in neonatal life
    d. at about 2 years of age

129. A concentrate of lymphocytes is most likely to be prepared from peripheral blood by:

    a. density gradient centrifugation
    b. ultracentrifugation
    c. zone electrophoresis
    d. freeze fractionation


130. Macrophages are characterized by:

    a. cytoplasmic receptors for C3 complement
    b. surface CD3 expression
    c. in vitro synthesis of immunoglobulin
    d. large amounts of rough endoplasmic reticulum


131. Macrophage phagocytosis of bacteria is enhanced by which of the following:

    a. opsonin
    b. antigen
    c. hapten
    d. secretory piece


132. Potent chemotactic activity is associated with which of the following components of the complement system:

    a. C1q
    b. C5a
    c. C3b
    d. IgG


133. Immunoassays are based on the principle of:

    a. separation of bound and free analyte
    b. antibody recognition of homologous antigen
    c. protein binding to isotopes
    d. production of antibodies against drugs


134. Which of the following describes an antigen-antibody reaction?

    a. the reaction is reversible
    b. the reaction is the same as a chemical reaction
    c. a lattice is formed at prozone
    d. a lattice is formed at postzone

135. The result of an antinuclear antibody test was a titer of 1:320 with a peripheral pattern. Which of the following sets of results best correlates with these results?

    a. anti-dsDNA titer 1:80, and a high titer of antibodies to Sm
    b. antimitochondrial antibody titer 1:160, and antibodies to RNP
    c. anti–Scl-70, and antibodies to single stranded DNA
    d. high titers of anti–SS-A and anti–SS-B

136. Refer to the following illustration:

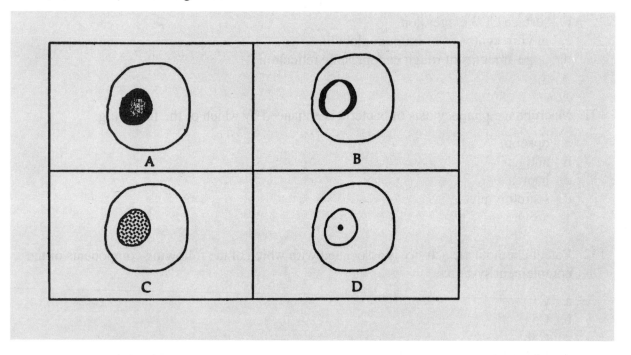

Which of the ANA patterns shown above would be associated with high titers of antibodies to the Sm antigen?

    a. Diagram A
    b. Diagram B
    c. Diagram C
    d. Diagram D

137. In most flow cytometers, labeled cells:

    a. scatter the light and absorb fluorescence
    b. absorb fluorescence and emit electronic impulses
    c. scatter the light and emit fluorescence
    d. absorb both fluorescence and light

...fi... or chronic active hepatitis due to hepatitis B virus is:

| ...ti-HBc | Anti-HBc | Anti-HBs |
|---|---|---|
| − | − | − |
| + | − | − |
| − | + | − |
| − | − | + |

...e from a rubella titer performed on acute and convalescent sera
...lution:

| ...e Serum Titer | Convalescent Serum Titer |
|---|---|
| | Negative |
| | 1:32 |

...e results, the best interpretation is:

... with active infection with rubella
... serum titers invalidates these results
... d by a different technologist
...nt... ed with rubella

...tr...olysin O enzyme inhibition test, the patient's:

... e in the patient serum neutralizes the antistreptolysin O reagent,
...m... ysis
... red blood cells are hemolyzed by the streptolysin O enzyme in the reagent
c.  antistreptolysin O neutralizes the streptolysin O reagent, resulting in hemolysis
d.  antistreptolysin O inhibits the reagent's streptolysin O, resulting in no hemolysis

141. After a penicillin injection, a patient rapidly develops respiratory distress, vomiting, and hives. This reaction is primarily mediated by:

a.  IgG
b.  IgA
c.  IgM
d.  IgE

142. Excess antigen in precipitation gel reactions will:

a.  have no effect on the precipitate reaction
b.  not dissolve precipitate after formation
c.  enhance the precipitate reaction
d.  dissolve the precipitate after formation

143. Soluble immune complexes are formed under the condition of:

    a. antigen deficiency
    b. antigen excess
    c. antibody excess
    d. complement


144. For diagnosis of late latent or tertiary syphilis, the most appropriate assay is:

    a. RPR
    b. VDRL
    c. FTA-ABS
    d. FTA-ABS IgM


145. The most common label in direct fluorescent antibody technique (DFA) is:

    a. alkaline phosphatase
    b. horseradish peroxidase
    c. fluorescein isothiocyanate
    d. calcofluor white


146. The most commonly used serologic indicator of recent streptococcal infection is the antibody to:

    a. an oxygen labile enzyme
    b. an oxygen stabile enzyme
    c. a spreading factor
    d. an enzyme that dissolves clots


147. An example of an organ-specific disease with autoimmune antibodies is:

    a. Wegener's granulomatosus
    b. rheumatoid arthritis
    c. Hashimoto's thyroiditis
    d. systemic lupus erythematosus


148. What kind of antigen-antibody reaction is expected if soluble antigen is added to homologous antibody?

    a. precipitation
    b. agglutination
    c. complement fixation
    d. hemagglutination

149. Avidity may be defined as the:

   a. degree of hemolysis
   b. titer of an antigen
   c. dilution of an antibody
   d. strength of a reacting antibody

150. The rapid plasma reagin test:

   a. is useful in screening for syphilis
   b. is useful in diagnosing syphilis
   c. does not give false positives
   d. uses heated plasma

151. Which of the following is the best indicator of an acute infection with the hepatitis A virus?

   a. the presence of IgG antibodies to hepatitis A virus
   b. the presence of IgM antibodies to hepatitis A virus
   c. a sharp decline in the level of IgG antibodies to hepatitis A virus
   d. a rise in both IgM and IgG levels of antibody to hepatitis A virus

152. Antibodies composed of IgG immunoglobulin:

   a. occur during the primary response to antigen
   b. are larger molecules than IgM antibodies
   c. can cross the placenta from mother to fetus
   d. can be detected in saline crossmatches

153. Biologic false-positive VDRL reactions are frequently encountered in patients with:

   a. lupus erythematosus
   b. acquired immune deficiency syndrome (AIDS)
   c. gonorrhea
   d. tertiary syphilis

154. In an antistreptolysin O titration, all the tubes including red cell and reagent controls showed hemolysis, indicating that:

   a. a high level of antistreptolysin is present
   b. no streptolysin is present
   c. the test results are reliable and should be reported as negative
   d. the test results should be repeated

155. Antinuclear antibody tests are performed to help diagnose:

   a. acute leukemia
   b. lupus erythematosus
   c. hemolytic anemia
   d. rheumatoid arthritis

156. Cholesterol is added to the antigen used in flocculation tests for syphilis to:

   a. destroy tissue impurities present in the alcoholic beef heart extract
   b. sensitize the sheep RBCs
   c. decrease specificity of the antigen
   d. increase sensitivity of the antigen

157. The strength of a visible reaction is known as:

   a. prozone reaction
   b. absorption
   c. avidity
   d. elution

158. The immunoglobulin that is passively transferred through the placenta to the fetus is:

   a. IgE
   b. IgG
   c. IgA
   d. IgM

159. A patient suspected of having typhoid fever has a titer of 1:160 with typhoid antigen and a rise in titer in a subsequent sample. This is indicative of:

   a. past infection
   b. present infection
   c. allergic response
   d. DPT vaccination

160. Of the following, the most sensitive and specific treponemal test is the:

   a. ART
   b. RPR
   c. FTA-ABS
   d. VDRL

161. Flocculation tests for syphilis detect the presence of:

    a. reagin
    b. cardiolipin
    c. hemolysin
    d. Forssman antigen

162. Measurement of serum levels of which of the following immunoglobulins can serve as a screening test for multiple allergies?

    a. IgA
    b. IgE
    c. IgG
    d. IgM

163. While performing a test for rheumatoid factor, the technician inactivated the test serum at 56°C for 30 minutes. This action would most likely result in:

    a. a false-negative test result
    b. hemolysis in the test reaction
    c. a prozone reaction
    d. total agglutination of the test reagents

164. In the cold agglutinin test, the tubes containing the serum and erythrocytes are allowed to stand overnight in the refrigerator and the results are read the next morning. If a disk of erythrocytes floats up from the bottom of the tube with only the flick of the finger, this is read as a:

    a. 4+ reaction
    b. 2+ reaction
    c. 1+ reaction
    d. negative reaction

165. The antigens used in the Weil-Felix agglutination test are derived from strains of which of the following organisms?

    a. *Proteus vulgaris*
    b. *Pseudomonas aeruginosa*
    c. *Escherichia coli*
    d. *Salmonella typhimurium*

166. IgM antibodies are frequently hemolytic because of:

    a. their dimeric structure
    b. the molecule's five-antigen binding sites
    c. their sedimentation coefficient of 7-15 S
    d. their efficient ability to fix complement

167. Humoral antibodies are produced by which cells?

    a. macrophages
    b. T lymphocytes
    c. B lymphocytes
    d. neutrophils

168. To which of the following classes do red cell immune antibodies usually belong?

    a. IgA
    b. IgE
    c. IgG
    d. IgD

169. Which of the following describes an antigen-antibody precipitation reaction of nonidentity?

    a. precipitin lines cross, forming double spurs
    b. precipitin lines fuse, forming a single spur
    c. no precipitin lines are formed
    d. precipitin lines fuse, forming a single arc

170. The IgM molecule is a:

    a. dimer
    b. trimer
    c. tetramer
    d. pentamer

171. What assay would confirm the immune status to hepatitis B virus?

    a. HBsAg
    b. anti-HBsAg
    c. IgM anti-HBcAg
    d. hepatitis C Ag

172. Flocculation tests for syphilis use antigen composed of:

    a. *Treponema pallidum*
    b. reagin
    c. cardiolipin and lecithin
    d. charcoal

173. To make a presumptive diagnosis of rheumatoid arthritis, which of the following qualitative methods is most commonly selected?

    a. latex agglutination
    b. immunoelectrophoresis
    c. RID
    d. radioimmunoassay

174. Refer to the following flow cytometric data.

| Absolute WBC | 8930 |
|---|---|
| Total lymphocytes | 30% |
| B lymphocytes | 40% |
| T lymphocytes | 58% |

Calculate the absolute count for B lymphocytes:

    a. 1072
    b. 2679
    c. 3572
    d. 6251

175. A DPT vaccination is an example of:

    a. active humoral mediated immunity
    b. passive humoral mediated immunity
    c. cell-mediated immunity
    d. immediate hypersensitivity

176. The following cold agglutinin titer results are observed:

| Tube # | 1 | 2 | 3 | 4 | 5 | 6 | 7 | 8 | 9 | 10 |
|---|---|---|---|---|---|---|---|---|---|---|
| Dilution | 1:1 | 1:2 | 1:4 | 1:8 | 1:16 | 1:32 | 1:64 | 1:128 | 1:256 | 1:512 |
| 4°C | + | + | + | + | + | + | + | + | 0 | 0 |
| 37°C | 0 | 0 | 0 | 0 | 0 | 0 | 0 | 0 | 0 | 0 |

The best interpretation is:

    a. positive, 1:128
    b. negative
    c. invalid, because 37°C reading is negative
    d. repeat the 4°C readings

177. A cold agglutinin titer end point is 1:16 after incubating overnight in the refrigerator and remains 1:16 after warming. The best course of action is to:

   a. report the titer as negative
   b. report the titer as positive, 1:16
   c. repeat the titer with a fresh sample
   d. test for antibody specificity

178. Refer to the following results for peripheral blood samples:

|  | % T Lymphocytes |
| --- | --- |
| Patient 1 | 85 |
| Patient 2 | 23 |
| Patient 3 | 51 |
| Patient 4 | 82 |
| Normal control | 44 |

   The data above indicate:

   a. patient 1 has an abnormally high T-lymphocyte count
   b. patient 2 has a normal T-lymphocyte count
   c. patients 1 and 3 have normal T-lymphocyte counts
   d. the normal control is too low and another sample should be selected

179. Cells known to be actively phagocytic include:

   a. neutrophils, monocytes, basophils
   b. neutrophils, eosinophils, monocytes
   c. monocytes, lymphocytes, neutrophils
   d. lymphocytes, eosinophils, monocytes

180. A VDRL serum sample is heat inactivated then placed in a refrigerator for overnight storage. Before being tested, the serum must be:

   a. kept colder than 10°C
   b. allowed to equilibrate to room temperature
   c. warmed to 37°C
   d. reheated to 56°C for 10 minutes

*The remaining questions (\*) have been identified as more appropriate for the entry level medical technologist.*

\*181. Which of the following is the major difference between a fluorescent microscope with epi-illumination and a fluorescent microscope with transmitted light?

a. The transmitted light microscope has a barrier filter.
b. The transmitted light microscope has an exciter filter.
c. The transmitted light microscope uses a halogen light source.
d. The epi-illuminated microscope has a dichroic mirror.

*182. Which of the following is a true statement about autoimmune diseases?

a. They are associated with HLA-B and HLA-D antigens.
b. They are B cell disorders.
c. All autoimmune disorders are drug induced.
d. Most autoimmune diseases are caused by viral infections.

*183. Which of the following is a true statement about selective IgA deficiency?

a. It is associated with a decreased incidence of allergic manifestations.
b. There is a high concentration of secretory component in the saliva.
c. It is associated with an increased incidence of autoimmune diseases.
d. It is found in approximately 1 of every 50 persons.

*184. Which of the following is a true statement about Bruton's agammaglobulinemia?

a. It is found only in females.
b. There are normal numbers of circulating B cells.
c. There are decreased to absent concentrations of immunoglobulins.
d. The disease presents with pyogenic infections one week after birth.

*185. Patients who appear to be high risk for the development of chronic hepatitis are those who maintain high titers of antibody to the:

a. core antigen
b. surface antigen
c. e antigen
d. alpha antigen

*186. Tissue injury in systemic rheumatic disorders such as systemic lupus erythematosus is thought to be caused by:

a. cytotoxic T cells
b. IgE activity
c. deposition of immune complexes
d. cytolytic antibodies

*187. A bacterial protein used to bind human immunoglobulins is:

    a. HAV antibody, IgA type
    b. *Escherichia coli* protein C
    c. staphylococcal protein A
    d. HAV antibody, IgG type

*188. Other hepatitis-causing viruses, such as cytomegalovirus and varicella-zoster virus, can be differentiated from HAV and HBV by:

    a. incubation period
    b. complement fixation
    c. immune electron microscopy
    d. tissue culture isolation

*189. The 20-nm spheres and filamentous structures of the HBV are:

    a. infectious
    b. circulating aggregates of HBcAg
    c. circulating aggregates of HBsAg
    d. highly infectious when present in great abundance

*190. The Raji cell line:

    a. has membrane receptors for C3b
    b. is used in an assay to measure insoluble immune complexes
    c. is a human T-type lymphoblastoid cell line
    d. has high affinity membrane receptors for IgG-Fc

*191. Which of the following immunologic abnormalities is associated with malabsorption syndrome?

    a. alpha chain disease
    b. gamma chain disease
    c. IgD myeloma
    d. IgE myeloma

*192. Which of the following immunologic abnormalities is associated with lymphadenopathy and fever?

    a. mu chain disease
    b. gamma chain disease
    c. alpha chain disease
    d. IgE myeloma

*193. Which of the following immunologic abnormalities is most likely associated with chronic lymphocytic leukemia?

a. IgE myeloma
b. IgD myeloma
c. mu chain disease
d. gamma chain disease

*194. Hereditary angioedema is characterized by:

a. decreased activity of C3
b. decreased activity of C1 esterase inhibitor
c. increased activity of C1 esterase inhibitor
d. increased activity of C2

*195. Which of the following is the most common humoral immune deficiency disease?

a. Bruton's agammaglobulinemia
b. IgG deficiency
c. selective IgA deficiency
d. Wiskott-Aldrich syndrome

*196. Which of the following is an important marker for the presence of immature T cells in patients with leukemia and lymphomas?

a. terminal deoxynucleotidyl transferase (TdT)
b. adenosine deaminase
c. glucose-6-phosphate dehydrogenase
d. purine nucleoside phosphorylase

*197. T-cell lymphocytes that possess Fc receptors for aggregated IgM have been found to be specific for which of the following types of T cell functions?

a. suppressor
b. prosuppressor
c. cytotoxic
d. helper

*198. Which T-cell malignancy may retain "helper" activity with regard to immunoglobulin synthesis by B cells?

a. Hodgkin's lymphoma
b. acute lymphocytic leukemia (ALL)
c. Sézary syndrome
d. chronic lymphocytic leukemia (CLL)

*199. Which of the following has been associated with patients who have homozygous C3 deficiency?

a. undetectable hemolytic complement activity in the serum
b. systemic lupus erythematosus
c. no detectable disease
d. a lifelong history of life-threatening infections


*200. Immunologic surveillance of tumors is thought to be affected by:

a. B lymphocytes and T lymphocytes
b. B lymphocytes and macrophages
c. T lymphocytes and macrophages
d. macrophages and lymphokines


*201. A benign monoclonal gammopathy:

a. usually is associated with a decrease in other immunoglobulins
b. occasionally is associated with radiographic bone lesions
c. occurs in approximately 10% of people over the age of 70
d. usually is of the IgM class


*202. Incompatibility by which of the following procedures is an absolute contraindication to allotransplantation?

a. MLC
b. HLA typing
c. Rh typing
d. ABO grouping


*203. Cells from a patient with hairy cell leukemia have immunologic and functional features of:

a. mast cells and B lymphocytes
b. B lymphocytes and T lymphocytes
c. granulocytes and monocytes
d. B lymphocytes and monocytes


*204. A 25-year-old woman is seen by a physician because of Raynaud's phenomenon, myalgias, arthralgias, and difficulty in swallowing. There is no evidence of renal disease. An ANA titer is 1:8000 with a speckled pattern. Which of the following are also likely to be found in this patient?

a. high-level nDNA antibody and a low $CH_{50}$ level
b. high-level Sm antibody
c. high-titer rheumatoid factor
d. high-level ribonucleoprotein (RNP) antibody

*205. A 28-year-old man is seen by a physician because of several months of intermittent low back pain. The patient's symptoms are suggestive of ankylosing spondylitis. Which of the following laboratory studies would support this diagnosis?

    a. a decreased synovial fluid $CH_{50}$ level
    b. low serum $CH_{50}$ level
    c. positive HLA-B27 antigen test
    d. rheumatoid factor in the synovial fluid

*206. True statements about the antibody response to infection with group A, beta-hemolytic streptococci include:

    a. 80% to 90% of patients with streptococcal pharyngitis who are treated will have significant increases (greater than two tubes) of antistreptolysin O (ASO) titers
    b. the anti-DNase B titer is a less sensitive index of nephritogenic skin infection than the ASO titer
    c. rheumatic fever is more likely to be present in individuals who have strong antibody responses than in those who have weak responses
    d. the anti-DNase B antibody titer is a more sensitive indicator than anti-group A specific carbohydrate titers for the detection of rheumatic fever

*207. True statements about antithyroid antibodies include:

    a. They may be directed against thyroglobulin or microsomal antigens.
    b. Their presence is a reliable diagnostic indicator in children with suspected thyroiditis.
    c. They are rarely present in patients with Graves' disease.
    d. They are rarely present in patients with parietal cell antibodies.

*208. Antibody idiotype is dictated by the:

    a. constant region of heavy chain
    b. constant region of light chain
    c. variable regions of heavy and light chains
    d. constant regions of heavy and light chains

*209. Antibody allotype is determined by the:

    a. constant region of heavy chain
    b. constant region of light chain
    c. variable regions of heavy and light chains
    d. constant regions of heavy and light chains

*210. Hereditary deficiency of early complement components (C1, C4, and C2) is associated with:

   a. pneumococcal septicemia
   b. small bowel obstruction
   c. systemic lupus erythematosus
   d. gonococcemia


*211. Which of the following findings is associated with a hereditary deficiency of C3?

   a. pneumococcal septicemia
   b. small bowel obstruction
   c. systemic lupus erythematosus
   d. gonococcemia


*212. Hereditary deficiency of late complement components (C5, C6, C7, or C8) can be associated with which of the following conditions?

   a. pneumococcal septicemia
   b. small bowel obstruction
   c. systemic lupus erythematosus
   d. gonococcemia


*213. In most individuals, edema is most likely the result of the activation of which complement component?

   a. C1
   b. C4
   c. C2
   d. C3

*214. Which of the following cells respond best to concanavalin A in culture?

   a. T lymphocytes
   b. B lymphocytes
   c. macrophages
   d. eosinophils


*215. C3b and Fc receptors are present on:

   a. B lymphocytes
   b. monocytes
   c. B lymphocytes and monocytes
   d. neither B lymphocytes nor monocytes

*216. A patient's abnormal lymphocytes form rosettes with sheep red blood cells, are positive for CD2 antigen, lack C3 receptors, and are negative for surface immunoglobulin. This can be classified as a disorder of:

a. T cells
b. B cells
c. monocytes
d. null cells


*217. A patient demonstrating abnormal cerebriform lymphocytes that form rosettes with sheep red blood cells and lack C3 receptors as well as surface membrane markers most likely has:

a. Hodgkin's disease
b. acute lymphocytic leukemia
c. chronic lymphocytic leukemia
d. Sézary syndrome


*218. Infantile X-linked agammaglobulinemia is referred to as:

a. Bruton's agammaglobulinemia
b. DiGeorge's syndrome
c. Swiss-type agammaglobulinemia
d. ataxia telangiectasia


*219. Immunodeficiency with thrombocytopenia and eczema is often referred to as:

a. DiGeorge's syndrome
b. Bruton's agammaglobulinemia
c. ataxia telangiectasia
d. Wiskott-Aldrich syndrome


*220. The autosomal recessive form of severe combined immunodeficiency disease is also referred to as:

a. Bruton's agammaglobulinemia
b. Swiss-type lymphopenic agammaglobulinemia
c. DiGeorge's syndrome
d. Wiskott-Aldrich syndrome


*221. Combined immunodeficiency disease with loss of muscle coordination is referred to as:

a. DiGeorge's syndrome
b. Bruton's agammaglobulinemia
c. ataxia telangiectasia
d. Wiskott-Aldrich syndrome

*222. HLA-B8 antigen has been associated with which of the following pairs of diseases?

    a. ankylosing spondylitis and myasthenia gravis
    b. celiac disease and ankylosing spondylitis
    c. myasthenia gravis and celiac disease
    d. Reiter's disease and multiple sclerosis


*223. Systemic lupus erythematosus patients with active disease often have which of the following test results?

    a. high titers of antimicrosomal antibodies
    b. high titers of anti–smooth muscle antibodies
    c. marked decrease in serum $CH_{50}$
    d. decreased serum immunoglobulin levels


*224. Anti–extractable nuclear antigens are most likely associated with which of the following antinuclear antibody immunofluorescent patterns?

    a. speckled
    b. rim
    c. diffuse
    d. nucleolar


*225. Anti–glomerular basement membrane antibody is most often associated with this condition:

    a. systemic lupus erythematosus
    b. celiac disease
    c. chronic active hepatitis
    d. Goodpasture's disease


*226. HLA typing of a family yields the following results:

| | Locus A | Locus B |
|---|---|---|
| Father | (8, 12) | (17, 22) |
| Mother | (7, 12) | (13, 27) |

On the basis of these genotypes, ankylosing spondylitis is possible in what percentage of their children:

    a. 25%
    b. 50%
    c. 75%
    d. 100%

*227. Bence Jones protein is:

    a. immunoglobulin catabolic fragments in the urine
    b. monoclonal light chains synthesized de novo
    c. bound light chains in the urine
    d. Fab fragments of a monoclonal protein


*228. A patient's serum IgA as measured by radial immunodiffusion (RID) was 40 mg/dL. Another laboratory reported IgA absent. A possible explanation for this discrepancy is that the:

    a. rabbit antiserum was used in the RID plates
    b. IgA has an Fc deletion
    c. IgA antiserum has kappa specificity
    d. patient serum has antibodies against a protein in the antiserum


*229. Which of the following lymphoproliferative disorders is often associated with autoimmune phenomenon and hypergammaglobulinemia?

    a. Burkitt's lymphoma
    b. immunoblastic lymphadenopathy
    c. acute lymphoblastic leukemia
    d. histiocytic lymphoma


*230. For several months a 31-year-old woman has had migratory polyarthritis and a skin rash. Upon admission to the hospital, the following laboratory data were obtained:

|  | Patient | Normal |
|---|---|---|
| Leukocyte count | $4.7 \times 10^3/\mu L$ | $5.0\text{-}10.0 \times 10^3/\mu L$ |
| Differential | Normal |  |
| Serum hemolytic complement | < 22 U | 80-150 U |
| C3 (by RID) | 117 U | 96-148 U |
| C4 (by RID) | 31 U | 14-40 U |
| ANA | Positive in a homogeneous pattern |  |
| Rheumatoid factor test | Negative |  |
| Urinalysis | Protein 1+, occasional RBCs |  |

This patient's test results are consistent with:

    a. dermatomyositis
    b. C2 deficiency
    c. systemic lupus erythematosus
    d. mixed connective tissue disease

*231. Immunologic enhancement of tumors and renal allografts is thought to be mediated by:

   a. T lymphocytes
   b. antibodies and antigen-antibody complexes
   c. B lymphocytes
   d. C3 and C5

*232. The serologic test that can be modified to selectively detect only specific IgM antibody in untreated serum is:

   a. complement fixation
   b. immunofluorescence
   c. hemagglutination inhibition
   d. passive hemagglutination

*233. Increased concentrations of alpha-fetoprotein (AFP) in adults are most characteristically associated with:

   a. hepatocellular carcinoma
   b. alcoholic cirrhosis
   c. chronic active hepatitis
   d. multiple myeloma

*234. In pernicious anemia, which of the following antibodies is characteristically detected?

   a. anti-mitochondrial
   b. anti–smooth muscle
   c. anti-DNA
   d. anti–parietal cell

*235. A child has severe hay fever. A total IgE measurement was performed by the Ouchterlony immunodiffusion method. No lines of precipitation appeared on the immunodiffusion plate. The most likely explanation is:

   a. IgE antibodies are not produced in children who have hay fever.
   b. Hay fever is mediated by the cellular system.
   c. IgE is in too low a concentration to be detected by this method.
   d. IgA is the antibody commonly produced in people with hay fever.

*236. The most sensitive procedure for detection of hepatitis B surface antigen (HBsAg) is:

   a. hemagglutination
   b. counterimmunoelectrophoresis
   c. radial immunodiffusion
   d. ELISA

*237. A patient has had a febrile illness of unknown origin for 6 weeks. Which complement fixing antibody titer(s) would most likely assist in determining the etiology of his disease?

a. 1:64 on week six
b. 1:512 on weeks one and six
c. 1:8 on week one and 1:256 on week six
d. 1:16 on weeks one and six

*238. In serologic tests for rubella using latex agglutination testing, rheumatoid factor has been shown to interfere, giving erroneous results. To prevent this interference, which action should be taken to remove the responsible immunoglobulin?

a. heating the serum to remove IgG
b. heating the serum to remove IgM
c. protein A adsorption to remove IgG
d. gel filtration to remove IgM

*239. HLA antibodies are generally obtained from which of the following?

a. multiparous women
b. nonidentical siblings
c. sheep
d. rabbits

*240. The enzyme control tube in an ASO hemolytic assay exhibits no cell lysis. What is the most likely explanation for this?

a. incorrect pH of buffer
b. low ionic strength buffer
c. oxidation of the enzyme
d. reduction of the enzyme

*241. Goat anti–human IgG is a:

a. monoclonal reagent that reacts with gamma heavy chains
b. monoclonal reagent that reacts with light chains
c. polyclonal reagent that reacts with gamma heavy chains
d. polyclonal reagent that reacts with light chains

*242. The ratio of kappa to lambda light chains in normal individuals is:

a. 1:1
b. 2:1
c. 3:1
d. 4:1

*243. What is the cluster of differentiation (CD) designation for the E-rosette receptor?

    a. CD2
    b. CD3
    c. CD8
    d. CD21


*244. Rheumatoid factors are immunoglobulins with specificity for allotypic determinants located on the:

    a. Fc fragment of IgG
    b. Fab fragment of IgG
    c. J chain of IgM
    d. secretory component of IgA


*245. In an antinuclear antibody indirect immunofluorescence test, a sample of patient serum shows a positive, speckled pattern. Which would be the most appropriate additional test to perform?

    a. antimitochondrial antibody
    b. immunoglobulin quantitation
    c. screen for Sm and RNP antibodies
    d. anti-DNA antibody using *C luciliae*


*246. Polyclonal B-cell activation:

    a. inhibits antibody production
    b. requires the participation of T-helper cells
    c. results from the activation of suppressor T-cells
    d. can induce autoantibody production


*247. Immunoglobulin idiotypic diversity is best explained by the theory of:

    a. somatic mutation
    b. germ line recombination
    c. antigen induction
    d. clonal selection


*248. The key structural difference that distinguishes immunoglobulin subclasses is the:

    a. number of domains
    b. stereometry of the hypervariable region
    c. number and arrangement of interchain disulfide bridges
    d. covalent linkage of the light chains

*249. Membrane-bound immunoglobulin molecules:

    a. have an additional amino-terminal sequence of about 40 residues
    b. are not anchored in a transmembrane configuration
    c. are anchored by a hydrophobic sequence of about 26 residues
    d. form a membrane spanning double beta helix


*250. Which is a recognized theory of the origin of autoimmunity?

    a. enhanced suppressor T-cell function
    b. diminished helper T-cell activity
    c. defects in the idiotype–anti-idiotype network
    d. deficient B-cell activation


*251. A positive ANA with the pattern of anticentromere antibodies is most frequently seen in patients with:

    a. rheumatoid arthritis
    b. systemic lupus erythematosus
    c. CREST syndrome
    d. Sjögren's syndrome


*252. Components of the complement system most likely to coat a cell are:

    a. C1 and C2
    b. C3 and C4
    c. C6 and C7
    d. C8 and C9


*253. Which of the following fungal agents is a frequent complication of AIDS?

    a. *Sporothrix* species
    b. *Blastomyces* species
    c. *Histoplasma* species
    d. *Pneumocystis* species


*254. A peripheral blood total leukocyte count is $10.0 \times 10^3/\mu L$. The differential reveals 55% neutrophils, 2% eosinophils, 40% lymphocytes, and 3% monocytes. Assuming a lymphocyte recovery of 85% to 95%, what is the expected number of T cells in a normal individual?

    a. $750/\mu L$
    b. $2500/\mu L$
    c. $4000/\mu L$
    d. $8000/\mu L$

*255. A monoclonal spike of IgG, Bence Jones proteinuria, and bone pain are usually associated with:

   a. Burkitt's lymphoma
   b. Burton's disease
   c. severe combined immunodeficiency disease
   d. multiple myeloma


*256. In laser flow cytometry, applying a voltage potential to sample droplets as they stream past the light beam and using charged deflector plates results in:

   a. an emission of red fluorescence from cells labeled with fluorescein isothiocyanate
   b. an emission of green fluorescence from cells labeled with rhodamine
   c. a 90° light scatter related to cell size
   d. the separation of cells into subpopulations based on their charge


*257. The correct sequence of events in successful phagocytosis is:

   a. chemotaxis, opsonization, phagosome formation, and the action of antibacterial substances
   b. destruction of bacteria or particulate matter, movement of phagocytes, engulfment, and digestion
   c. opsonization, chemotaxis, phagosome formation, and the action of antibacterial substances
   d. engulfment, opsonization, digestion, and destruction of bacteria or particulate matter


*258. Long-acting thyroid stimulator (LATS) is a(n):

   a. slow release capsule preparation implanted subdermally in patients with idiopathic hypothyroidism
   b. autoantibody that causes excess secretion of thyroid hormone in patients with Graves' disease
   c. polypeptide hormone secreted by the posterior pituitary
   d. marker for carcinoma of the thyroid


*259. Which test has the greatest sensitivity for antigen detection?

   a. precipitin
   b. agglutination
   c. ELISA
   d. complement fixation


*260. Positive rheumatoid factor is generally associated with:

   a. hyperglobulinemia
   b. anemia
   c. decreased erythrocyte sedimentation rate
   d. azotemia

*261. Sera to be tested for IFA-ANA 6 days after drawing is best stored at:

    a.  room temperature
    b.  5°C ± 2°C
    c.  –70°C in a constant temperature freezer
    d.  –20°C in a self-defrosting freezer

*262. The specificity of an immunoassay is determined by the:

    a.  label used on the antigen
    b.  method used to separate the bound from free antigen
    c.  antibody used in the assay
    d.  concentration of unlabeled antigen

*263. The immunoglobulin classes most commonly found on the surface of circulating B lymphocytes in the peripheral blood of normal persons are:

    a.  IgM, IgA
    b.  IgM, IgG
    c.  IgM, IgD
    d.  IgM, IgE

*264. The sensitivity of the RAST test is such that:

    a.  false-positive results are frequent
    b.  it is not helpful with common pollen allergens
    c.  false-negative results are frequent
    d.  it is most useful in proving drug allergens

*265. In hybridoma technology, the desirable fused cell is the:

    a.  myeloma-myeloma hybrid
    b.  myeloma-lymphocyte hybrid
    c.  lymphocyte-lymphocyte hybrid
    d.  lymphocyte-granulocyte hybrid

*266. A patient with a B-cell deficiency will most likely exhibit:

    a.  decreased phagocytosis
    b.  increased bacterial infections
    c.  decreased complement level
    d.  increased complement levels

*267. A patient with a T-cell deficiency will most likely exhibit:

    a. increased immune complex formation
    b. increased parasitic infections
    c. decreased IgE-mediated responses
    d. decreased complement levels

*268. A marked decrease in the CD4 lymphocytes and decrease in the CD4/CD8 ratio:

    a. is diagnostic for bacterial septicemia
    b. may be seen in hereditary and acquired immunodeficiency disorders
    c. is not associated with viral induced immunodeficiency
    d. is only seen in patients with advanced disseminated cancer

*269. One of the first steps in performing a quantitative analysis method study is to:

    a. select the most capable individuals to perform the evaluation
    b. eliminate specimens with possible interference from bilirubin, hemolysis, and turbidity
    c. determine recovery by adding known amounts of the analyte to actual specimens
    d. determine within-run precision by analyzing duplicates or several aliquots of a specimen

*270. Bone marrow transplant donors and their recipients must be matched for which antigen system(s)?

    a. ABO-Rh
    b. HLA
    c. CD4/CD8
    d. $Pl^{A1}$

*271. In assessing the usefulness of a new laboratory test, sensitivity is defined as the percentage of:

    a. positive specimens correctly identified
    b. falsely positive specimens
    c. negative specimens correctly identified
    d. falsely negative specimens

*272. In the interpretation of agglutination tests for febrile diseases, which of the following is of the greatest diagnostic importance?

    a. anamnestic reactions caused by heterologous antigens
    b. rise in titer of the patient's serum
    c. history of previous vaccination
    d. naturally occurring antibodies prevalent where the disease is endemic

*273. Which course of action is most appropriate when a control serum shows a titer twofold lower than expected in a test for *Brucella* antibody?

    a. The results should be reported because this represents expected variability.

    b. The results should not be reported; the tests should be repeated with the original and another control serum.

    c. The results should be corrected by reporting titers of clinical specimens twofold higher than observed values.

    d. The results should be reported with the qualifying remark, "reliability of results questionable, please repeat."


*274. Cells that are precursors of plasma cells and also produce immunoglobulins are:

    a. macrophages

    b. B lymphocytes

    c. T lymphocytes

    d. monocytes


*275. Examination of a nasal smear reveals moderate cellularity with 5% granulocytes, 75% eosinophils, and 20% lymphocytes. This is characteristic of:

    a. pneumonia

    b. allergic rhinitis

    c. a sinus infection

    d. a normal smear


*276. The simplest test to evaluate the cellular immune system in a patient is a(n):

    a. skin test for commonly encountered antigens

    b. protein electrophoresis of serum

    c. immunoelectrophoresis of serum

    d. measurement of anti-HBsAg after immunization


*277. The normal controls for a quantitative B-lymphocyte assay should have a value of:

    a. 21% B cells counted

    b. 48% B cells counted

    c. 76% B cells counted

    d. 89% B cells counted

# Immunology Answer Key

| | | | | |
|---|---|---|---|---|
| 1. c | 42. d | 83. a | 124. a | 165. a |
| 2. a | 43. a | 84. c | 125. a | 166. d |
| 3. b | 44. d | 85. c | 126. a | 167. c |
| 4. c | 45. a | 86. a | 127. b | 168. c |
| 5. b | 46. c | 87. d | 128. a | 169. a |
| 6. a | 47. a | 88. c | 129. a | 170. d |
| 7. d | 48. b | 89. c | 130. a | 171. b |
| 8. a | 49. b | 90. b | 131. a | 172. c |
| 9. c | 50. d | 91. c | 132. b | 173. a |
| 10. c | 51. c | 92. d | 133. b | 174. a |
| 11. c | 52. b | 93. c | 134. a | 175. a |
| 12. c | 53. c | 94. c | 135. a | 176. a |
| 13. d | 54. a | 95. c | 136. c | 177. d |
| 14. a | 55. a | 96. c | 137. c | 178. d |
| 15. d | 56. b | 97. a | 138. a | 179. b |
| 16. c | 57. b | 98. d | 139. a | 180. d |
| 17. b | 58. c | 99. a | 140. d | 181. d |
| 18. b | 59. a | 100. a | 141. d | 182. a |
| 19. b | 60. c | 101. b | 142. d | 183. c |
| 20. b | 61. d | 102. b | 143. b | 184. c |
| 21. c | 62. d | 103. d | 144. c | 185. d |
| 22. d | 63. c | 104. c | 145. c | 186. c |
| 23. a | 64. a | 105. b | 146. a | 187. c |
| 24. d | 65. c | 106. c | 147. c | 188. d |
| 25. c | 66. b | 107. b | 148. a | 189. c |
| 26. a | 67. d | 108. c | 149. d | 190. a |
| 27. b | 68. a | 109. c | 150. a | 191. a |
| 28. b | 69. a | 110. d | 151. b | 192. b |
| 29. b | 70. b | 111. d | 152. c | 193. c |
| 30. b | 71. d | 112. d | 153. a | 194. b |
| 31. a | 72. b | 113. c | 154. d | 195. c |
| 32. c | 73. c | 114. b | 155. b | 196. a |
| 33. b | 74. a | 115. b | 156. d | 197. d |
| 34. a | 75. d | 116. c | 157. c | 198. c |
| 35. b | 76. a | 117. b | 158. b | 199. d |
| 36. c | 77. a | 118. c | 159. b | 200. c |
| 37. d | 78. c | 119. a | 160. c | 201. c |
| 38. a | 79. a | 120. c | 161. a | 202. d |
| 39. b | 80. b | 121. b | 162. b | 203. d |
| 40. d | 81. d | 122. c | 163. a | 204. d |
| 41. a | 82. d | 123. a | 164. a | 205. c |

| 206. c | 221. c | 236. d | 251. c | 266. b |
|--------|--------|--------|--------|--------|
| 207. a | 222. c | 237. c | 252. b | 267. b |
| 208. c | 223. c | 238. d | 253. c | 268. b |
| 209. d | 224. a | 239. a | 254. b | 269. c |
| 210. c | 225. d | 240. c | 255. d | 270. b |
| 211. a | 226. b | 241. c | 256. d | 271. a |
| 212. d | 227. b | 242. b | 257. a | 272. b |
| 213. c | 228. d | 243. a | 258. b | 273. b |
| 214. a | 229. b | 244. a | 259. c | 274. b |
| 215. c | 230. b | 245. c | 260. a | 275. b |
| 216. a | 231. b | 246. d | 261. c | 276. a |
| 217. d | 232. b | 247. b | 262. c | 277. a |
| 218. a | 233. a | 248. c | 263. c | |
| 219. d | 234. d | 249. c | 264. c | |
| 220. b | 235. c | 250. c | 265. b | |

# CHAPTER 13

## Laboratory Management

*The following items have been identified as being appropriate for the entry level medical technologist.*

1. On repeated occasions, the day shift supervisor has observed a technologist on the night shift sleeping. Which of the following is the most appropriate INITIAL course of action for the day supervisor?

   a. Ignore the repeated incidents.
   b. Discuss the incidents with the technologist's immediate supervisor.
   c. Notify the personnel department.
   d. Advise the laboratory director.

2. A major laboratory policy change is going to take place that will affect a significant number of the laboratory employees. In order to minimize the resistance to change the supervisor should:

   a. announce the change one day after it goes into effect
   b. discuss the change in detail with all concerned, well in advance
   c. announce only the positive aspects in advance
   d. discuss only the positive aspects with those concerned

3. Employees are guaranteed the right to engage in self-organization and collective bargaining through representatives of their choice or to refrain from these activities by which of the following?

   a. Civil Rights Act
   b. Freedom of Information Act
   c. Clinical Laboratory Improvements Act (CLIA)
   d. National Labor Relations Act

4. A workload reporting system is an important part of laboratory management because it:

    a. tells exactly how much should be charged per test
    b. keeps personnel busy in their free time
    c. counts only tests done and specimens received in the laboratory without inflating these figures by adding in quality control and standardization efforts
    d. helps in planning, developing, and maintaining efficient laboratory services with administrative and budget controls

5. A good way to monitor precision is by:

    a. running duplicate assays
    b. repeated serial testing
    c. processing unknown specimens
    d. running normal and abnormal controls

6. A supervisor notices that a technologist continues to mouth-pipet liquids when making reagents. The supervisor's best course of action is to:

    a. allow the technologist to continue this practice as long as it is not done when dealing with specimens
    b. discuss this problem with the employee immediately
    c. order a mechanical device (bulb-pipet) for employee to use
    d. compliment the employee on his rapid pipetting technique

7. What action should be taken when dealing with a long-term problem?

    a. ignore the problem
    b. seek more information
    c. base decision on available information
    d. refer the problem to another level of management

8. Evaluating the performance of employees should be done:

    a. annually
    b. semiannually
    c. as needed in the judgment of management
    d. in the form of immediate feedback and at regular intervals

9. Which one of the following is NOT a reason for doing a performance evaluation?

    a. give employee performance feedback
    b. determine training needs
    c. help the employee improve performance
    d. criticize a problem employee

10. A new clinic in the area is sending a very large number of additional chemistry tests to the laboratory. The existing chemistry instrument is only 2 years old and works well; however, there is a need to acquire a high throughput instrument. Which one of the following is the appropriate "Justification Category"?

    a. replacement
    b. volume increase
    c. reduction of FTEs
    d. new service

11. Package inserts may be used:

    a. instead of a typed procedure
    b. as a reference in a procedure
    c. at the bench but not in the procedure manual
    d. if initialed and dated by the laboratory director

12. Which one of the following questions can be legally asked on an employment application?

    a. Are you a U.S. citizen?
    b. What is your date of birth?
    c. Is your wife/husband employed full-time?
    d. Do you have any dependents?

13. The ability to make good decisions often depends on the use of a logical sequence of steps, which includes:

    a. defining problem, considering options, implementing decisions
    b. obtaining facts, considering alternatives, reviewing results
    c. defining problem, obtaining facts, considering options
    d. obtaining facts, defining problem, implementing decision

14. In the context of the planning process, the term "goal" has been defined as a:

    a. plan for reaching certain objectives
    b. set of specific tasks
    c. set of short- and long-term plans
    d. major purpose or final desired result

15. As information is reported upward through an organization, the amount of detail communicated will generally:

    a. decrease to facilitate the flow of information
    b. increase to allow consideration of all options
    c. remain the same to ensure consistency in reporting
    d. remain the same to ensure goal accomplishment

16. Delegation is a process in which:

    a. interpersonal influence is redefined
    b. authority of manager is surrendered
    c. power is given to others
    d. responsibility for specific tasks is given to others


17. The most important part of any effective behavior modification system is:

    a. feedback to employees
    b. salary structure
    c. job enrichment
    d. tactful discipline


18. Which of the following is considered to be a variable cost in a clinical laboratory?

    a. overtime pay
    b. health insurance premiums
    c. FICA
    d. pension contributions


19. An effective program of continuing education for medical laboratory personnel should first:

    a. find a good speaker
    b. motivate employees to attend
    c. determine an adequate budget
    d. identify the needs


20. Disciplinary policy is generally developed as a series of steps, each one being more strict than the preceding one. Normally, the first step in the process is to:

    a. send the employee a warning letter
    b. send the employee a counseling memo
    c. counsel the employee verbally
    d. dismiss less serious infractions


21. Matching the content and requirements of the task with the skills, abilities, and needs of the worker is a function of:

    a. leadership
    b. job design
    c. recruitment
    d. reward systems

22. Which of the following organizations was formed to encourage the voluntary attainment of uniformly high standards in institutional medical care?

    a. Centers for Disease Control (CDC)
    b. Health Care Finance Administration (HCFA)
    c. Joint Commission on Accreditation of Healthcare Organizations (JCAHO)
    d. Federal Drug Administration (FDA)


23. The reliability of a test to be positive in the presence of the disease it was designed to detect is known as:

    a. accuracy
    b. sensitivity
    c. precision
    d. specificity


24. Which of the following actions will facilitate group interactions at staff meetings?

    a. adhering strictly to an agenda
    b. treating every problem consistently
    c. encouraging input from all staff
    d. announcing the assignments for upcoming projects


25. Which of the following topic areas should NOT be discussed with a prospective employee during a job interview?

    a. location of clinical education program
    b. number of dependents
    c. previous employment that the applicant disliked
    d. specific details in the job description


26. A general term for the formal recognition of professional or technical competence is:

    a. regulation
    b. licensure
    c. accreditation
    d. credentialing


27. The process by which an agency or organization uses predetermined standards to evaluate and recognize a program of study in an institution is called:

    a. regulation
    b. licensure
    c. accreditation
    d. credentialing

28. Which of the following parameters of a diagnostic test will vary with the prevalence of a given disease in a population?

   a. precision
   b. sensitivity
   c. accuracy
   d. specificity


29. The major workload in most hospital laboratories is generated in:

   a. hematology
   b. chemistry
   c. microbiology
   d. immunohematology


30. In general, 60%-70% of the operating expenses of laboratories are:

   a. labor or labor related
   b. reagents and supplies
   c. equipment replacement and maintenance
   d. safety supplies and disposables


31. Direct, indirect, and overhead costs incurred during the production of tests per unit time are classified as:

   a. total costs
   b. actual costs
   c. standard costs
   d. controllable costs


32. The number of hours used to calculate the annual salary of a full-time employee is:

   a. 1920
   b. 1950
   c. 2080
   d. 2800


33. The overtime budget for the laboratory is $38,773, but $50,419 has already been spent. What percent over budget does this represent?

   a. 30%
   b. 70%
   c. 77%
   d. 100%

34. A new laboratory is being designed to include a stat lab with a method of specimen transport from critical care areas. What laboratory services should be provided in the stat lab?

    a. microbiology and hematology
    b. chemistry and serology
    c. hematology and chemistry
    d. chemistry and microbiology


35. An advantage of reagent lease/rental agreements is:

    a. less time spent by laboratory manager justifying new instrumentation
    b. increased flexibility to adjust to changes in workload
    c. flexibility in reagent usage from one manufacturer to another
    d. less expenditures over life expectancy of instrument


36. Legal preemployment questions on an application are:

    a. medical history of an employee
    b. place of birth
    c. felonies unrelated to job requirements
    d. name and address of person to notify in case of emergency


37. The laboratory information system has been turned off for routine maintenance. To restore the system the operator must:

    a. initiate a service call
    b. reenter all transactions since last routine backup
    c. perform a simple reboot of the system
    d. reprogram the operating system


38. Several parents of children in the pediatric wing have voiced concern over the anxiety that venipuncture causes their children. An informal staff meeting with the phlebotomists reveals that they feel both parents and pediatric nurses are less than supportive and frequently make the task of venipuncture in children worse with their own anxiety. The best course of action would be to:

    a. have pediatric nurses do venipuncture on children, as they are more familiar with the children
    b. limit physicians to only one draw per day on children
    c. prepare written pamphlets for parents and in-service education for nursing personnel
    d. take no action, as parents will always overreact where their children are concerned

39. A technologist has an idea that would possibly decrease the laboratory turnaround time for reporting results. In order to begin implementation of this idea, he/she should:

    a. encourage the staff to utilize the idea
    b. discuss it with his/her immediate supervisor
    c. try out the idea on himself/herself on an experimental basis
    d. present the idea to the lab director


40. To be effective, criticism should be:

    a. specific to the behavior
    b. related to general laboratory performance
    c. focused on the person, not the behavior
    d. repeatedly discussed for reinforcement


41. The most important aspect of supervision is:

    a. balancing the budget
    b. performing technical procedures
    c. writing accurate job descriptions
    d. dealing with people


42. A patient has complained to the administration that a bruise was left after a "brutal" venipuncture. What should be done first?

    a. Ask the patient's nurse if the patient is just seeking additional attention.
    b. Ask the phlebotomy supervisor to investigate the incident.
    c. Ignore the complaint, a bruise is insignificant.
    d. Have the phlebotomy supervisor check the phlebotomist's technique.


43. When employees are going to be responsible for implementing a change in procedure or policy, the manager should:

    a. make the decision and direct the employees to implement it
    b. solicit the employee input but do what he/she thinks should be done
    c. involve the employees in the decision-making process from the very beginning
    d. involve only those employees in the decision-making process who will benefit from the change


44. The best way to motivate an ineffective employee would be to:

    a. confirm low performance with subjective data
    b. set short-term goals for the employee
    c. transfer the employee to another department
    d. ignore failure to meet goals

45. Data for a new procedure are as follows:

| | |
|---|---|
| No. of procedures per year | 10,000 |
| Equipment cost | $97,000 |
| Expected useful life | 7 years |
| Reagent cost per year | $20,000 |
| CAP units per procedure | 30.0 |
| Average wage | $10.75/hr |

The cost per procedure is:

a. $2.00
b. $5.38
c. $7.38
d. $8.77

# Laboratory Management **Answer Key**

| | | | | |
|---|---|---|---|---|
| 1. b | 10. b | 19. d | 28. c | 37. c |
| 2. b | 11. b | 20. c | 29. b | 38. c |
| 3. d | 12. a | 21. b | 30. a | 39. b |
| 4. d | 13. c | 22. c | 31. b | 40. a |
| 5. a | 14. d | 23. b | 32. c | 41. d |
| 6. b | 15. a | 24. c | 33. a | 42. b |
| 7. b | 16. d | 25. b | 34. c | 43. c |
| 8. d | 17. a | 26. d | 35. b | 44. b |
| 9. d | 18. a | 27. c | 36. d | 45. d |

# CHAPTER 14

## *Microbiology*

*The following items have been identified as appropriate for both entry level medical technologists and medical laboratory technicians.*

1. Children who have infections with beta-hemolytic streptococci can develop:

   a. acute pyelonephritis
   b. acute glomerulonephritis
   c. chronic glomerulonephritis
   d. nephrosis

2. *Haemophilus influenzae* becomes resistant to ampicillin when the organism produces a(n):

   a. capsule of polysaccharide material
   b. affinity for the beta-lactam ring of the ampicillin
   c. requirement for hemin
   d. beta-lactamase

3. Thioglycollate broth is stored at room temperature and in the dark so that:

   a. ureases are not formed
   b. the cysteine is not decomposed
   c. sunlight does not hydrolyze the glucose in the medium
   d. there is a decreased absorption of oxygen by the medium

4. A liquid fecal specimen from a three-month-old infant is submitted for microbiologic examination. In addition to culture on routine media for *Salmonella* and *Shigella*, this specimen routinely should be:

a. examined for the presence of *Entamoeba hartmanni*
b. examined for the presence of *Campylobacter* sp
c. screened for the detection of enterotoxigenic *Escherichia coli*
d. placed in thioglycollate broth to detect *Clostridium botulinum*

5. An unusual number of methicillin-resistant *Staphylococcus aureus* (determined by the Bauer-Kirby method) were isolated in the laboratory in the past month. Which of the following is the most likely explanation?

a. incubation of the susceptibility plates at 35°C
b. deterioration of the methicillin disks
c. inoculation of plates 10 minutes after standardizing the inoculum
d. standardization of the inoculum to a 0.5 McFarland turbidity standard

6. A Gram-stained sputum smear revealed 25-50 squamous epithelial cells and 10-25 poly-morphonuclear leukocytes per 100x field, as well as many lancet-shaped, gram-positive cocci; many gram-negative rods; and many gram-positive cocci in pairs, clumps, and long chains. The technologist's best course of action would be to:

a. inoculate appropriate media and incubate anaerobically
b. inoculate appropriate media and incubate aerobically
c. call the physician and notify him of this "life-threatening" situation
d. call the nursing station and request a new specimen

7. Which one of the following specimen requests is acceptable?

a. feces submitted for anaerobic culture
b. Foley catheter tip submitted for aerobic culture
c. rectal swab submitted for direct smear for gonococci
d. urine for culture of acid-fast bacilli

8. A gram-positive coccus isolated from a blood culture has the following characteristics:

| | |
|---|---|
| Optochin susceptibility | Negative |
| Bacitracin (0.04 U) susceptibility | Negative |
| Bile esculin hydrolysis | Negative |
| Hippurate hydrolysis | Positive |
| Catalase | Negative |

This organism is most likely:

a. *Staphylococcus aureus*
b. *Streptococcus pneumoniae*
c. *Streptococcus pyogenes* (group A)
d. *Streptococcus agalactiae* (group B)

9. A gram-negative rod was isolated from a wound infection caused by a bite from a pet cat. The following characteristic reactions were seen:

| | |
|---|---|
| Oxidase | Positive |
| Glucose OF | Fermentative |
| Catalase | Positive |
| Motility | Negative |
| MacConkey agar | No growth |

Which of the following is the most likely organism?

a. *Pseudomonas aeruginosa*
b. *Pasteurella multocida*
c. *Aeromonas hydrophila*
d. *Vibrio cholerae*

10. A 10-year-old boy was admitted to the emergency room with lower right quadrant pain and tenderness. The following laboratory results were obtained:

| | Patient | Normal |
|---|---|---|
| Segs | 75% | 16%-60% |
| WBC | 200 x 10³/µL | 13.0 x 10³/µL |

The admitting diagnosis was appendicitis. During surgery the appendix appeared normal; an enlarged node was removed and cultured. Small gram-negative rods were isolated from the room temperature plate. The organism most likely is:

a. *Prevotella (Bacteroides) melaninogenica*
b. *Shigella sonnei*
c. *Listeria monocytogenes*
d. *Yersinia enterocolitica*

11. Which of the following is most often used to prepare a slide from a plate culture of a dermatophyte for microscopic observation?

a. lactophenol cotton blue
b. potassium hydroxide
c. iodine solution
d. Gram stain

12. Which of the following is the most useful morphological feature in identifying the mycelial phase of *Histoplasma capsulatum*?

    a. arthrospores every other cell
    b. microspores, 2-5 μm
    c. tuberculate macroconidia, 8-14 μm
    d. nonseptate macroconidia of 5-7 cells


13. The function of N-acetyl-L-cysteine required in the NALC-NaOH reagent for acid-fast digestion-decontamination procedures is to:

    a. inhibit growth of normal respiratory flora
    b. inhibit growth of fungi
    c. neutralize the sodium hydroxide
    d. liquify the mucus


14. Middlebrook 7H10 and 7H11 media must be refrigerated in the dark and incubated in the dark as well. If these conditions are not met, the media may prove toxic for mycobacteria because:

    a. carbon dioxide will be released, retarding growth
    b. growth factors will be broken down
    c. sunlight destroys the ammonium sulfate necessary in the mycobacterial metabolism
    d. formaldehyde may be produced


15. *Ureaplasma urealyticum* are difficult to grow in the laboratory on routine media because of their requirement for:

    a. sterols
    b. horse blood
    c. ferric pyrophosphate
    d. surfactant such as Tween 80


16. The cyst stage may be recovered from formed fecal specimens submitted for parasitic examination if the specimen:

    a. is incubated at 37°C for 24 hours
    b. is the result of a saline enema
    c. is stored at refrigerator temperature
    d. contains barium


17. The stock cultures needed for quality control testing of deoxyribonuclease (DNAse) production are:

    a. *Salmonella typhimurium/Escherichia coli*
    b. *Escherichia coli/Pseudomonas aeruginosa*
    c. *Proteus mirabilis/Escherichia coli*
    d. *Serratia marcescens/Escherichia coli*

18. The stock cultures needed for quality control testing of deamination activity are:

    a. *Escherichia coli/Klebsiella pneumoniae*
    b. *Salmonella typhimurium/Escherichia coli*
    c. *Escherichia coli/Pseudomonas aeruginosa*
    d. *Proteus mirabilis/Escherichia coli*

19. The stock cultures needed for quality control testing of oxidase production are:

    a. *Escherichia coli/Klebsiella pneumoniae*
    b. *Salmonella typhimurium/Escherichia coli*
    c. *Escherichia coli/Pseudomonas aeruginosa*
    d. *Proteus mirabilis/Escherichia coli*

20. The stock cultures needed for quality control testing of motility are:

    a. *Salmonella typhimurium/Escherichia coli*
    b. *Escherichia coli/Pseudomonas aeruginosa*
    c. *Serratia marcescens/Escherichia coli*
    d. *Klebsiella pneumoniae/Escherichia coli*

21. An antibiotic that inhibits cell wall synthesis is:

    a. chloramphenicol
    b. penicillin
    c. sulfonamide
    d. colistin

22. Group B, beta-hemolytic streptococci may be distinguished from other hemolytic strepto-cocci by which of the following procedures?

    a. coagglutination
    b. growth in 6.5% NaCl broth
    c. growth on bile esculin medium
    d. bacitracin susceptibility

23. A gram-negative diplococcus that grows on modified Thayer-Martin medium can be further confirmed as *Neisseria gonorrhoeae* if it is:

    a. oxidase positive, glucose positive, and maltose positive
    b. oxidase positive and glucose positive, maltose negative
    c. oxidase positive and maltose positive, glucose negative
    d. glucose positive, oxidase negative, and maltose negative

24. Organisms that may be mistaken for *Neisseria gonorrhoeae* in Gram-stained smears of uterine cervix exudates include:

    a. *Lactobacillus* species
    b. *Streptococcus agalactiae*
    c. *Pseudomonas aeruginosa*
    d. *Moraxella osloensis*

25. Coagglutination is associated with:

    a. *Chlamydia trachomatis*
    b. *Neisseria gonorrhoeae*
    c. *Streptococcus pneumoniae*
    d. *Klebsiella pneumoniae*

26. Chocolate agar base containing vancomycin, colistin, nystatin, and trimethoprim is also known as:

    a. EMB agar
    b. modified Thayer-Martin agar
    c. Columbia CNA agar
    d. KV-laked blood agar

27. Sodium bicarbonate and sodium citrate are components of which of the following?

    a. JEMBEC system
    b. MTM agar
    c. NYC medium
    d. ML agar

28. One advantage of the antimicrobial dilution tests is that:

    a. it is based on a predetermined breakpoint
    b. contamination can be detected easily
    c. it provides categorical reports
    d. it can detect varying degrees of organism sensitivity and resistance

29. Clinical resistance to penicillin dosages appears to correlate with beta-lactamase production in:

    a. *Neisseria gonorrhoeae*
    b. *Neisseria meningitidis*
    c. *Streptococcus agalactiae*
    d. *Streptococcus pyogenes*

30. Which of the following organisms is, to date, considered universally susceptible to penicillin:

    a. *Haemophilus influenzae*
    b. *Neisseria gonorrhoeae*
    c. *Streptococcus pyogenes*
    d. *Corynebacterium diphtheriae*


31. First-generation cephalosporins can be adequately represented by:

    a. streptomycin
    b. chloramphenicol
    c. cephalothin
    d. colistin


32. Which of the following media is routinely used to culture *Campylobacter jejuni*?

    a. Skirrow's medium
    b. CIN agar
    c. anaerobic CNA agar
    d. bismuth sulfite


33. Which one of the following results is typical of *Campylobacter jejuni*?

    a. optimal growth at 42°C
    b. oxidase negative
    c. catalase negative
    d. nonmotile


34. Which of the following organisms must be incubated in a microaerophilic environment for optimal recovery of the organism?

    a. *Campylobacter fetus*
    b. *Escherichia coli*
    c. *Pseudomonas aeruginosa*
    d. *Proteus mirabilis*


35. The recovery of some *Cryptococcus* species may be compromised if the isolation media contains:

    a. cycloheximide
    b. gentamicin
    c. chloramphenicol
    d. penicillin

36. The one characteristic by which an unknown *Cryptococcus* species can be identified as *Cryptococcus neoformans* is:

a. appearance of yellow colonies
b. positive urease test
c. presence of a capsule
d. positive Niger seed agar test

37. A cell culture line commonly used for the recovery of *Chlamydia trachomatis* from clinical specimens is:

a. HeLa 229
b. Hep-2
c. BHK-21
d. McCoy's

38. Fluid from a cutaneous black lesion was submitted for routine bacteriological culture. After 18 hours of incubation at 35°C there was no growth on MacConkey agar, but 3+ growth on sheep blood agar. The colonies were nonhemolytic, 4 to 5 mm in diameter, and off-white with a ground-glass appearance. Each colony had an irregular edge with comma-shaped outgrowths that stood up like "beaten egg whites" when gently lifted with an inoculating needle. A Gram-stained smear of a typical colony showed large, gram-positive, rectangular rods. The organism is most likely:

a. *Clostridium perfringens*
b. *Aeromonas hydrophila*
c. *Bacillus anthracis*
d. *Mycobacterium marinum*

39. An 8-year-old girl was admitted to the hospital with a 3-day history of fever, abdominal pain, diarrhea, and vomiting. A stool culture grew many lactose-negative colonies that yielded the following test results:

| | |
|---|---|
| Oxidase | Negative |
| TSI | Acid slant/acid butt |
| Indole | Negative |
| Urease | Positive |
| Ornithine decarboxylase | Positive |
| Sucrose | Positive |
| $H_2S$ | Negative |
| Motility at 22°C | Positive |

The most probable identification of this organism is:

a. *Providencia alcalifaciens*
b. *Providencia stuartii*
c. *Yersinia enterocolitica*
d. *Providencia rettgeri*

40. An autopsy performed on an 8-year-old child revealed Waterhouse-Friderichsen syndrome. Blood and throat cultures taken just prior to death were positive for which organism?

   a. *Neisseria gonorrhoeae*
   b. *Neisseria meningitidis*
   c. *Haemophilus influenzae*
   d. *Klebsiella pneumoniae*

41. An anaerobic gram-negative bacillus isolated from a blood culture following bowel surgery grew smooth, white, nonhemolytic colonies. A Gram stain showed a pale, bipolar-staining rod with rounded ends. Bile stimulated growth of the organism and catalase was produced. The isolate was not inhibited by colistin, kanamycin, or vancomycin; indole was not produced. The most likely identification of this isolate is:

   a. *Bacteroides fragilis*
   b. *Prevotella (Bacteroides) melaninogenica*
   c. *Fusobacterium nucleatum*
   d. *Fusobacterium varium*

42. Relapsing fever in humans is caused by:

   a. *Borrelia recurrentis*
   b. *Brucella abortus*
   c. *Leptospira interrogans*
   d. *Spirillum minor*

43. A suspension of organisms suspected to be *Shigella* based on biochemical reactions did not agglutinate with *Shigella* antisera subgroups A, B, C, and D. The technologist would conclude that:

   a. this particular *Shigella* possesses a capsular antigen that blocks agglutination in O antiserum and must first be destroyed by heating
   b. this organism is not a *Shigella*
   c. the bacterial suspension was not dense enough, resulting in a false-negative reaction
   d. a rough colony was used for the serotyping procedure

44. Which of the following tests is used to monitor bactericidal activity during antimicrobic therapy in cases of endocarditis?

   a. Elek
   b. tolerance
   c. Sherris synergism
   d. Schlichter

45. In a disk diffusion susceptibility test, which of the following can result if disks are placed on the inoculated media and left at room temperature for an hour before incubation?

    a. the antibiotic would not diffuse into the medium, resulting in no zone
    b. zones of smaller diameter would result
    c. zones of larger diameter would result
    d. there would be no effect on the final zone diameter

46. Which one of the following combinations of organisms would be appropriate as controls to test the functions listed?

    a. beta hemolysis—*Escherichia coli* and *Streptococcus pyogenes*
    b. catalase—*Staphylococcus aureus* and *Staphylococcus epidermidis*
    c. hydrogen sulfide production—*Proteus mirabilis* and *Salmonella typhi*
    d. indole—*Escherichia coli* and *Proteus mirabilis*

47. Which one of the following organisms could be used as the positive quality control test for lecithinase on egg yolk agar?

    a. *Bacteroides fragilis*
    b. *Fusobacterium necrophorum*
    c. *Clostridium perfringens*
    d. *Clostridium sporogenes*

48. The porphyrin test was devised to detect strains of *Haemophilus* capable of:

    a. ampicillin degradation
    b. capsule production
    c. synthesis of porphobilinogen
    d. chloramphenicol resistance

49. Failure to obtain anaerobiosis in anaerobe jars is most often due to the:

    a. inactivation of the palladium-coated alumina catalyst pellets
    b. condensation of water on the inner surface of the jar
    c. instability of reactants in the disposable hydro–carbon dioxide generator envelope
    d. expiration of the methylene blue indicator strip that monitors oxidation

50. A 1- to 2-mm translucent, nonpigmented colony, isolated from an anaerobic culture of a lung abscess after 72 hours, was found to fluoresce brick-red under ultraviolet light. A Gram-stained smear of the organism revealed a coccobacillus that had the following characteristics:

| | |
|---|---|
| Growth in bile | Inhibited |
| Vancomycin | Resistant |
| Catalase | Negative |
| Esculin hydrolysis | Negative |
| Indole | Negative |
| Nitrate | Negative |
| Glucose, lactose, and sucrose | Acid produced |

The most likely identification of this isolate is:

a. *Bacteroides ovatus*
b. *Prevotella (Bacteroides) oralis*
c. *Prevotella (Bacteroides) melaninogenica*
d. *Porphyromonas (Bacteroides) asaccharolyticus*

51. A thin, anaerobic, gram-negative bacillus with tapered ends isolated from an empyema was found to be indole positive, lipase negative, and inhibited by 20% bile. Colonies were described as "speckled" or resembling "ground glass" and fluoresced weakly when exposed to ultraviolet light. The most probable identification of this isolate would be:

a. *Bacteroides ureolyticus*
b. *Prevotella (Bacteroides) melaninogenica*
c. *Fusobacterium nucleatum*
d. *Fusobacterium mortiferum*

52. Which of the following anaerobes is inhibited by sodium polyanethol sulfonate (SPS)?

a. *Peptostreptococcus magnus*
b. *Peptostreptococcus prevotii*
c. *Peptostreptococcus anaerobius*
d. *Veillonella parvula*

53. A beta-hemolytic, catalase positive, gram-positive coccus is coagulase-negative by the slide coagulase test. Which of the following is the most appropriate action in identification of this organism?

a. report a coagulase-negative *Staphylococcus*
b. report a coagulase-negative *Staphylococcus aureus*
c. reconfirm the hemolytic reaction on a fresh 24-hour culture
d. do a tube coagulase test to confirm the slide test

54. Which of the following is the most reliable test to differentiate *Neisseria lactamica* from *Neisseria meningitidis*?

    a. acid from maltose
    b. growth on modified Thayer-Martin
    c. lactose degradation
    d. nitrite reduction to nitrogen gas


55. Which of the following sets of tests best differentiate *Salmonella* and *Citrobacter* species?

    a. KCN, malonate, beta-galactosidase, lysine decarboxylase
    b. dulcitol, citrate, indole, $H_2S$ production
    c. lactose, adonitol, KCN, motility
    d. lysine decarboxylase, lactose, sucrose, malonate, indole


56. Which characteristic best differentiates *Acinetobacter* species from *Moraxella* species?

    a. production of indophenol oxidase
    b. growth on MacConkey agar
    c. motility
    d. susceptibility to penicillin


57. Recent evidence has shown that specimens to be inoculated for the recovery of acid-fast bacilli should be centrifuged at approximately:

    a. 2000*g*
    b. 2500*g*
    c. 3000*g*
    d. 3500*g*


58. The most important constituent of the tubercle bacillus for the activity of the various tuberculins is the:

    a. phospholipid
    b. protein
    c. wax D
    d. polysaccharide


59. An antibiotic used to suppress or kill contaminating fungi in media is:

    a. penicillin
    b. cycloheximide
    c. streptomycin
    d. amphotericin B

60. Which of the following statements concerning the germ tube test is true?

  a. Using a heavy inoculum enhances the rapid production of germ tubes.
  b. Germ tubes should be read after 2 hours' incubation at 25°C.
  c. *Candida albicans* and *Candida tropicalis* can be used as positive and negative controls, respectively.
  d. Serum will be stable for 1 year if stored at 4°C prior to use.

61. The term "internal autoinfection" is generally used in referring to infections with:

  a. *Ascaris lumbricoides*
  b. *Necator americanus*
  c. *Trichuris trichiura*
  d. *Strongyloides stercoralis*

62. When stool examination is negative, the preferred specimen for the diagnosis of paragonimiasis is:

  a. bile drainage
  b. duodenal aspirate
  c. sputum
  d. rectal biopsy

63. Protozoan cysts are found in a wet mount of sediment from ethyl-acetate concentrated material. The cysts are without peripheral chromatin on the nuclear membrane. Each cyst has four nuclei and each nucleus has a large karyosome that appears as a refractive dot. These oval-shaped cysts are most likely:

  a. *Endolimax nana*
  b. *Chilomastix mesnili*
  c. *Entamoeba histolytica*
  d. *Entamoeba hartmanni*

64. A batch of trichrome-stained slides for ova and parasite examination contains numerous minute crystals that totally obscure the microscopic field. Which of the following measures is the most appropriate remedial action?

  a. Change the Schaudinn's fixative, remove coverslips, and restain.
  b. Change the acid alcohol and restain.
  c. Remove coverslips and remount using fresh Permount or similar medium.
  d. Change the iodine alcohol solution to obtain a strong tea–colored solution, restrain.

65. Which of the following would you LEAST expect to culture from a case of otitis media?

    a. *Moraxella (Branhamella) catarrhalis*
    b. *Neisseria meningitidis*
    c. *Haemophilus influenzae*
    d. *Streptococcus pneumoniae*

66. Which one of the following species of *Mycobacterium* does NOT usually fluoresce on fluorochrome stain?

    a. *Mycobacterium fortuitum*
    b. *Mycobacterium tuberculosis*
    c. *Mycobacterium ulcerans*
    d. *Mycobacterium bovis*

67. Which of the following organisms can grow in the small bowel and cause diarrhea in children, traveler's diarrhea, or a severe cholera-like syndrome through the production of enterotoxins?

    a. *Yersinia enterocolitica*
    b. *Escherichia coli*
    c. *Salmonella typhi*
    d. *Shigella dysenteriae*

68. When combined antimicrobial drugs are clearly less effective than the most active drug alone, the condition is described as:

    a. minimal inhibitory concentration
    b. synergism
    c. minimum bactericidal concentration
    d. antagonism

69. The smallest concentration of antimicrobial agent that prevents growth in subculture or results in a 99.9% decrease of the initial inoculum is the definition of:

    a. minimum bactericidal concentration
    b. indifference of additive
    c. minimal inhibitory concentration
    d. synergism

70. If the effect of combined antimicrobials is greater than the sum of the effects observed with the two drugs independently, the condition is described as:

    a. indifference of additive
    b. inhibition
    c. synergism
    d. antagonism

71. The smallest amount of test antimicrobial that will inhibit visible growth of a microbe is the definition of:

a. synergism
b. minimal inhibitory concentration
c. indifference of additive
d. minimum bactericidal concentration

72. Beta-hemolytic streptococci that are bacitracin-resistant and CAMP-positive are:

a. group A or B
b. group A
c. group B
d. beta-hemolytic, group D

73. Beta-hemolytic streptococci that are bacitracin-sensitive and CAMP-negative are:

a. group B
b. group A
c. beta-hemolytic, not group A, B, or D
d. beta-hemolytic, group D

74. A TSI tube inoculated with an organism gave the following reactions:

Alkaline slant
Acid butt
No $H_2S$
No gas produced

This organism is most likely:

a. *Yersinia enterocolitica*
b. *Salmonella typhi*
c. *Salmonella enteritidis*
d. *Shigella dysenteriae*

75. Which of the following reagents should be used as a mucolytic, alkaline reagent for digestion and decontamination of a sputum for mycobacterial culture?

a. N-acetyl-L-cystine and NaOH
b. NaOH alone
c. Zephiran-trisodium phosphate
d. oxalic acid

76. An organism was inoculated to a TSI tube and gave the following reactions:

Acid slant
Acid butt
No H$_2$S
Gas produced

This organism most likely is:

a. *Klebsiella pneumoniae*
b. *Shigella dysenteriae*
c. *Salmonella typhimurium*
d. *Salmonella typhi*

77. An organism was inoculated into a TSI tube and gave the following reactions:

Alkaline slant
Acid butt
H$_2$S
Gas produced

This organism most likely is:

a. *Klebsiella pneumoniae*
b. *Shigella dysenteriae*
c. *Salmonella typhimurium*
d. *Escherichia coli*

78. An organism was inoculated into a TSI tube and gave the following reactions:

Acid slant
Acid butt
No H$_2$S
No gas

This organism most likely is:

a. *Yersinia enterocolitica*
b. *Salmonella typhi*
c. *Salmonella typhimurium*
d. *Shigella dysenteriae*

79. It is important to identify individual members of the group D streptococci because:

a. viridans streptococci are often confused with enterococci
b. several enterococci cause severe puerperal sepsis
c. nonenterococcal group D streptococci are avirulent
d. enterococci often show more antibiotic resistance than other group D streptococci

80. When testing for oxidase activity, for which of the following organisms is it recommended that a 5% aqueous solution of tetramethyl-phenylenediamine dihydrochloride be used, rather than commercially available strips?

    a. *Eikenella corrodens*
    b. *Haemophilus aphrophilus*
    c. *Flavobacterium meningosepticum*
    d. *Pasteurella multocida*


81. Anaerobic infections differ from aerobic infections in which of the following?

    a. They usually respond favorably with aminoglycoside therapy.
    b. They usually arise from exogenous sources.
    c. They are usually polymicrobic.
    d. Gram-stained smears of specimens are less helpful in diagnosis.


82. The presence of 20% bile in blood agar would probably enhance the growth of:

    a. *Fusobacterium nucleatum*
    b. *Bacteroides ovatus*
    c. *Prevotella (Bacteroides) melaninogenica*
    d. *Prevotella (Bacteroides) disiens*


83. Which of the following organisms may exhibit a brick red fluorescence?

    a. *Prevotella (Bacteroides) melaninogenica* and *Clostridium difficile*
    b. *Clostridium difficile* and *Fusobacterium* sp
    c. *Veillonella parvula* and *Prevotella (Bacteroides) melaninogenicus*
    d. *Fusobacterium* sp and *Veillonella parvula*


84. When a *Brucella* species is suspected in a blood culture, the bottle should be held for a minimum of:

    a. 5 days
    b. 7 days
    c. 14 days
    d. 21 days


85. An organism has been identified as a member of the fluorescent group of *Pseudomonas*. Which of the following sets of tests should be used to determine the species of the organism?

    a. growth at 42°C, pyocyanin production, gelatinase production
    b. pyocyanin production, gelatinase production, OF glucose
    c. growth at 37°C, pyocyanin production, OF glucose
    d. gelatinase production, growth at 52°C, $H_2S$

86. The ONPG test allows organisms to be classified as a lactose fermenter by testing for which of the following?

   a. permease
   b. beta-galactosidase
   c. beta-lactamase
   d. phosphatase


87. Which of the following combinations of media provides an egg base, agar base, and a selective egg or agar base media?

   a. Lowenstein-Jensen, American Thoracic Society (ATS), Middlebrook 7H11
   b. Lowenstein-Jensen, Middlebrook 7H11, Lowenstein-Jensen (Gruft Modification)
   c. Middlebrook 7H10, Petragnani, Lowenstein-Jensen
   d. Middlebrook 7H10, Middlebrook 7H11, 7H11 (Mitchison's)


88. Organisms that can be easily identified to the species level from the ova in fecal specimens include:

   a. *Metagonimus yokogawai, Heterophyes heterophyes*
   b. *Taenia solium, Taenia saginata*
   c. *Necator americanus, Ancylostoma duodenale*
   d. *Paragonimus westermani, Hymenolepis nana*


89. A stool specimen for ova and parasite examination contained numerous rhabditiform larvae. Which factor does NOT aid in the identification of larvae?

   a. length of the buccal cavity
   b. age of the specimen
   c. appearance of the genital primordium
   d. endemic area traveled


90. Nonmetallic surfaces contaminated with blood should be disinfected with:

   a. a phenol solution
   b. 5% bleach (sodium hypochlorite)
   c. 70% isopropyl alcohol
   d. green soap


91. Tests for beta-lactamase production in *Haemophilus influenzae*:

   a. are not commercially available
   b. include tests that measure a change to an alkaline pH
   c. should be performed on all blood and CSF isolates
   d. are not valid for any other bacterial species

92. Definitive identification of *Neisseria gonorrhoeae* is made with the:

   a. Gram stain
   b. oxidase test
   c. degradation of amino acids
   d. hydrolysis of carbohydrates

93. *Listeria* can be confused with some streptococci because of its hemolysis and because it is:

   a. nonmotile
   b. catalase negative
   c. oxidase positive
   d. esculin positive

94. At the present time *Clostridium difficile* toxin can be detected by:

   a. fluorescent staining
   b. EIA
   c. growth on culture media
   d. high-pressure liquid chromatography

95. Most of the automated microbiology equipment currently available has been designed to replace:

   a. manual susceptibility procedures
   b. manual methods that are infrequently performed but are time consuming
   c. repetitive manual methods that are performed daily on a large number of specimens
   d. all manual methods used in the clinical microbiology laboratory

96. The most critical distinction between *Staphylococcus aureus* and other staphylococci is:

   a. phosphatase reaction
   b. DNA production
   c. coagulase production
   d. hemolysis

97. One of the enterotoxins produced by enterotoxigenic *Escherichia coli* in traveler's diarrhea is similar to a toxin produced by:

   a. *Clostridium perfringens*
   b. *Clostridium difficile*
   c. *Vibrio cholerae*
   d. *Yersinia enterocolitica*

98. Optimum growth of *Campylobacter jejuni* is obtained on suitable media incubated at 42°C in an atmosphere containing:

    a. 6% $O_2$, 10%-15% $CO_2$, 85%-90% nitrogen
    b. 10% $H_2$, 5% $CO_2$, 85% nitrogen
    c. 10% $H_2$, 10% $CO_2$, 80% nitrogen
    d. 25% $O_2$, 5% $CO_2$, 70% nitrogen

99. *Vibrio parahaemolyticus* can be isolated best from feces on:

    a. eosin methylene blue (EMB) agar
    b. Hektoen enteric (HE) agar
    c. *Salmonella-Shigella* (SS) agar
    d. thiosulfate citrate bile salts (TCBS) agar

100. Of the following bacteria, the most frequent cause of prosthetic heart valve infections occurring within two to three months after surgery is:

    a. *Streptococcus pneumoniae*
    b. *Streptococcus pyogenes*
    c. *Staphylococcus aureus*
    d. *Staphylococcus epidermidis*

101. The bacterium most often responsible for acute epiglottitis is:

    a. *Bordetella pertussis*
    b. *Haemophilus influenzae*
    c. *Haemophilus aphrophilus*
    d. Group A beta-hemolytic streptococci

102. Diagnosis of typhoid fever during the first two days of illness can be confirmed best by:

    a. stool culture
    b. urine culture
    c. blood culture
    d. demonstration of antibodies against O antigen in the patient's serum

103. *Streptococcus pneumoniae* can be differentiated best from the viridans group of streptococci by:

    a. Gram stain
    b. the type of hemolysis
    c. colonial morphology
    d. bile solubility

104. A culture from an infected dog bite yields a gram-negative, bipolar-staining bacillus. The organism is cytochrome oxidase and indole test positive. The most likely identification of this isolate is:

a. *Aeromonas hydrophila*
b. *Pasteurella haemolytica*
c. *Pasteurella multocida*
d. *Vibrio parahaemolyticus*

105. Biochemical reactions of an organism are consistent with *Shigella*. A suspension is tested in polyvalent antiserum without resulting agglutination. However, after 15 minutes of boiling, agglutination occurs in polyvalent and group D antisera. This indicates that the:

a. organism contains a blocking O antigen
b. antiserum is of low potency
c. organism possesses capsular antigens
d. antiserum is of low specificity

106. Which of the following would best differentiate *Streptococcus agalactiae* (Group B) from *Streptococcus pyogenes* (Group A)?

a. ability to grow in sodium azide broth
b. a positive bile-esculin reaction
c. hydrolysis of sodium hippurate
d. beta-hemolysis on sheep blood agar

107. Staib's medium (Niger seed agar) is useful in the identification of which of the following?

a. *Candida albicans*
b. *Candida (Torulopsis) glabrata*
c. *Saccharomyces cerevisiae*
d. *Cryptococcus neoformans*

108. A urine culture from a patient with a urinary tract infection yields a yeast with the following characteristics:

Failure to produce germ tubes
Hyphae not formed on cornmeal agar
Urease-negative
Assimilates trehalose

The most likely identification is:

a. *Saccharomyces cerevisiae*
b. *Cryptococcus laurentii*
c. *Candida pseudotropicalis*
d. *Candida (Torulopsis) glabrata*

109. Which one of the following organisms does not require susceptibility testing when isolated from a clinically significant source?

  a. *Staphylococcus aureus*
  b. *Proteus mirabilis*
  c. group A streptococci
  d. *Escherichia coli*


110. Psittacosis is transmissible to man via contact with:

  a. insects
  b. birds
  c. cattle
  d. dogs


111. *Shigella* species characteristically are:

  a. urease positive
  b. nonmotile
  c. oxidase positive
  d. lactose fermenters


112. Characteristically, group D enterococci are:

  a. unable to grow in 6.5% NaCl
  b. relatively resistant to penicillin
  c. sodium hippurate positive
  d. bile esculin negative


113. The best medium for culture of *Francisella tularensis* is:

  a. Bordet-Gengou
  b. cystine blood agar
  c. Loeffler's
  d. Lowenstein-Jensen's


114. The best medium for culture of *Bordetella pertussis* is:

  a. Bordet-Gengou
  b. cystine blood agar
  c. Thayer-Martin
  d. Loeffler's

115. The best medium for culture of *Mycobacterium tuberculosis* is:

    a. Bordet-Gengou
    b. Loeffler's
    c. Lowenstein-Jensen's
    d. cystine blood agar

116. *Haemophilus influenzae* is most likely considered normal indigenous flora in the:

    a. oropharynx
    b. female genital tract
    c. large intestine
    d. small intestine

117. A nonphotochromogen that grows best at 42°C and is highly resistant to antibiotics is *Mycobacterium*:

    a. *chelonei*
    b. *marinum*
    c. *tuberculosis*
    d. *xenopi*

118. A positive niacin test is most characteristic of *Mycobacterium*:

    a. *chelonei*
    b. *marinum*
    c. *tuberculosis*
    d. *xenopi*

119. A 27-year-old scuba diver has an abrasion on his left thigh. A culture of this wound grew an acid-fast organism at 30°C. This isolate most likely is *Mycobacterium*:

    a. *chelonei*
    b. *marinum*
    c. *tuberculosis*
    d. *xenopi*

120. Encephalitis is most commonly associated with which of the following viruses?

    a. Epstein-Barr
    b. herpes simplex
    c. coxsackie B
    d. varicella zoster

121. Colds and other acute respiratory diseases are most often associated with:

a. Epstein-Barr virus
b. adenovirus
c. coxsackie B
d. reovirus


122. If present, a characteristic that is helpful in separating *Pseudomonas aeruginosa* from other members of the *Pseudomonas* family is:

a. a positive test for cytochrome oxidase
b. oxidative metabolism in the O/F test
c. production of fluorescein pigment
d. production of pyocyanin pigment


123. An important cause of acute exudative pharyngitis is:

a. *Staphylococcus aureus* (beta-hemolytic)
b. *Streptococcus pneumoniae*
c. *Streptococcus agalactiae*
d. *Streptococcus pyogenes*


124. The organism most commonly associated with neonatal purulent meningitis is:

a. *Neisseria meningitidis*
b. *Streptococcus pneumoniae*
c. group B streptococci
d. *Haemophilus influenzae*


125. Which of the following is a synergistic bacterial infection?

a. scarlet fever
b. strep throat
c. erythrasma
d. Vincent's angina


126. Which of the following is a dimorphic fungus?

a. *Sporothrix schenckii*
b. *Candida albicans*
c. *Cryptococcus neoformans*
d. *Aspergillus fumigatus*

127. Chlamydial infections have been implicated in:

a. urethritis and conjunctivitis
b. gastroenteritis and urethritis
c. neonatal pneumonia and gastroenteritis
d. neonatal meningitis and conjunctivitis

128. A catheterized urine specimen from an 82-year-old woman with recurrent infections is submitted for culture. The Gram stain reveals:

Many WBCs
No epithelial cells
Many gram-negative rods
Many gram-positive cocci in chains

The physician requests that sensitivities be performed on all pathogens isolated. In addition to the sheep blood agar and EMB plates routinely used for urine cultures, the technologist might also process a(n):

a. CNA agar plate
b. chocolate agar plate
c. XLD agar plate
d. chopped meat glucose

129. Cerebrospinal fluid from a febrile 25-year-old man with possible meningitis is rushed to the laboratory for a stat Gram stain and culture. While performing the Gram stain, the technologist accidentally spills most of the specimen. The smear shows many neutrophils and no microorganisms. Since there is only enough CSF to inoculate one plate, the technologist should use a:

a. blood agar plate
b. chopped meat glucose
c. chocolate agar plate
d. Thayer-Martin plate

130. A small gram-negative rod isolated from an eye culture has the following test results:

| X factor requirement | Yes |
| V factor requirement | Yes |
| Hemolysis on rabbit blood agar | No |

This organism is most probably *Haemophilus*:

a. *influenzae*
b. *parainfluenzae*
c. *haemolyticus*
d. *parahaemolyticus*

131. When processing throat swabs for a strep culture, the medium of choice is:

    a. sheep blood agar plates
    b. rabbit blood agar plates
    c. human blood agar plates
    d. horse blood agar plates


132. When performing a Kovac's indole test, the substrate must contain:

    a. indole
    b. tryptophane
    c. ornithine
    d. paradimethylaminobenzaldehyde


133. A throat swab is submitted for anaerobic culture. This specimen should be:

    a. set up immediately
    b. rejected
    c. inoculated into thioglycollate broth
    d. sent to a reference laboratory


134. A vaginal smear is submitted for a Gram stain for *Neisseria gonorrhoeae*. The technologist finds the following results on the Gram stain:

    Many white blood cells
    Few epithelial cells
    Many gram-positive rods
    Few gram-negative diplococci
    Few gram-positive cocci in chains

    The technologist should:

    a. report out smear positive for gonorrhea
    b. report out smear negative for gonorrhea
    c. request a new specimen due to number of white blood cells
    d. not read or report a Gram stain on a vaginal specimen


135. The causative agent of cysticercosis is:

    a. *Taenia solium*
    b. *Taenia saginata*
    c. *Ascaris lumbricoides*
    d. *Trichuris trichiura*

136. A liquid stool specimen is collected at 10:00 PM and brought to the laboratory for culture, ova and parasites. It is refrigerated until 10:10 AM the next day when the physician requests that the technologist look for amebic trophozoites. The best course of action would be to:

    a. request a fresh specimen
    b. perform a concentration on the original specimen
    c. perform a trichrome stain on the original specimen
    d. perform a saline wet mount on the original specimen


137. The optimal wound specimen for culture of anaerobic organisms should be:

    a. a swab of lesion obtained before administration of antibiotics
    b. a swab of lesion obtained after administration of antibiotics
    c. a syringe filled with pus, obtained before administration of antibiotics
    d. a syringe filled with pus, obtained after administration of antibiotics


138. Lab workers should always work under a biological safety hood when working with cultures of:

    a. *Streptococcus pyogenes*
    b. *Staphylococcus aureus*
    c. *Candida albicans*
    d. *Coccidioides immitis*


Questions 139-142 refer to the following illustration:

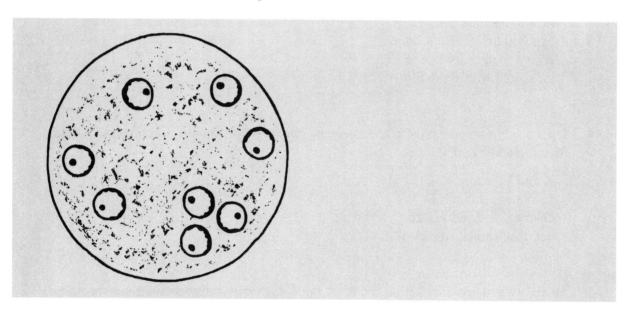

139. Trophozoites of the cyst shown above are likely to:

    a. contain red blood cells
    b. have clear, pointed pseudopodia
    c. contain few if any vacuoles
    d. have slow, undefined motility

140. Upon finding the depicted in a fecal concentrate, the technologist should:

    a. telephone the report of this pathogen to the physician immediately
    b. review the fecal concentration carefully for the presence of other microorganisms which may be pathogenic
    c. look for motile trophozoites
    d. request a new specimen because of the presence of excessive pollen grains

141. An inexperienced parasitology student may confuse the depicted organism with:

    a. *Entamoeba histolytica*
    b. *Dientamoeba fragilis*
    c. *Giardia lamblia*
    d. *Trichomonas vaginalis*

142. This structure depicts a:

    a. cyst of a nonpathogenic ameba
    b. trophozoite of a nonpathogenic ameba
    c. cyst of a pathogenic ameba
    d. trophozoite of a pathogenic ameba

143. Photochromogens produce pigment when:

    a. kept in the dark at 22°C
    b. exposed to light for 1 hour
    c. grown in the presence of $CO_2$
    d. incubated with x-ray film

144. Media used to support growth of *Legionella pneumophila* should contain which of the following additives?

    a. X and V factors
    b. hemin and vitamin K
    c. charcoal and yeast extract
    d. dextrose and laked blood

145. The ability to detect methicillin-resistant *Staphylococcus aureus* may be enhanced by:

    a. shortening incubation of standard susceptibility plates
    b. incubating susceptibility plates at 39°C-41°C
    c. using Mueller-Hinton agar with 4% NaCl
    d. adjusting inoculum to 0.1 McFarland before inoculating susceptibility plates

146. A request is received in the laboratory for assistance in selecting the appropriate test(s) for detecting Lyme disease. Which of the following would be suggested?

a. Stool culture should be done to isolate the causative organism.
b. The organism is difficult to isolate, and antibody titers will provide the most help.
c. *Borrelia burgdorferi* is easily isolated from routine blood cultures.
d. This is an immunologic syndrome, and cultures are not indicated.

147. A *Campylobacter* species has been isolated from a blood culture. The organism is susceptible to nalidixic acid and resistant to cephalothin. Which of the following tests would aid in the differentiation between *Campylobacter jejuni* and *Campylobacter coli*?

a. raffinose fermentation
b. hippurate hydrolysis
c. optochin susceptibility
d. 5% NaCl tolerance

148. A *Campylobacter* species isolated from a stool culture gives the following biochemical reactions:

| | |
|---|---|
| Nalidixic acid | Susceptible |
| Cephalothin | Resistant |
| Hippurate hydrolysis | Positive |
| Oxidase | Positive |
| Catalase | Positive |

This biochemical profile is consistent with *Campylobacter*:

a. *fetus*
b. *jejuni*
c. *coli*
d. *laridis*

149. A catheterized urine is inoculated onto blood and MacConkey agar using a 0.01 mL loop. After 48 hours, 68 colonies of a small translucent nonhemolytic organism grew on blood agar but not MacConkey. Testing reveals small gram-positive, catalase-negative cocci. The preliminary report and follow-up testing would be:

a. growth of 680 CFU/mL of gram-positive cocci, optochin and bacitracin susceptibility tests to follow
b. growth of 6800 CFU/mL of a *Staphylococcus* species, coagulase test to follow
c. growth of 6800 CFU/mL of a *Streptococcus* species, esculin hydrolysis and NaCl growth to follow
d. growth of 6800 CFU/mL of a *Streptococcus* species, no further testing

150. Which of the following gram-negative bacilli ferments carbohydrates?

    a. *Alcaligenes faecalis*
    b. *Pseudomonas cepacia*
    c. *Acinetobacter lwoffi*
    d. *Yersinia enterocolitica*

151. A cerebrospinal fluid has been inoculated onto sheep blood and chocolate agar plates and into a tube of trypticase soy broth. All media were incubated in an atmosphere of 5% $CO_2$. Which of the following organisms would usually be isolated by this procedure?

    a. *Francisella tularensis*
    b. *Haemophilus influenzae*
    c. *Bordetella pertussis*
    d. *Bacteroides fragilis*

152. The examination of human feces is no help in the detection of:

    a. *Strongyloides stercoralis*
    b. *Entamoeba histolytica*
    c. *Echinococcus granulosus*
    d. *Ancylostoma duodenale*

153. The scolex of *Taenia saginata* has:

    a. 4 suckers
    b. no suckers and 14 hooklets
    c. 24 hooklets
    d. 26 to 28 sucking disks

154. Structures important in the microscopic identification of *Coccidioides immitis* are:

    a. irregular staining, barrel-shaped arthrospores
    b. tuberculate, thick-walled macroconidia
    c. thick-walled sporangia containing sporangiospores
    d. small pyriform microconidia

155. An aspirate of a deep wound was plated on blood agar plates aerobically and anaerobically. At 24 hours there was growth on the anaerobic plate only. The next step in the evaluation of this culture is to:

    a. reincubate for another 24 hours
    b. begin organism identification
    c. issue the final report
    d. set up a Bauer-Kirby sensitivity

156. A medium that is used for primary isolation and enhances the growth of a particular organism is called:

   a. enrichment
   b. simple
   c. differential
   d. nutrient

157. Upon review of a sputum Gram stain, the technician notes that the nuclei of all of the neutrophils present in the smear are staining dark blue. The best explanation for this finding is:

   a. the slide was inadequately decolorized with acetone/alcohol
   b. the sputum smear was prepared too thin
   c. the cellular components have stained as expected
   d. the iodine was omitted from the staining procedure

158. Which of the following factors would make an organism appear to be more resistant on a disk diffusion susceptibility test?

   a. too little agar in the plate
   b. too many organisms in the inoculum
   c. the presence of 0.5% NaCl in the medium
   d. a medium with a pH of 7.4

159. The most rapid means of detecting herpes virus in clinical specimens is:

   a. serologic testing
   b. Gram stain
   c. cell culture
   d. direct immunofluorescence

160. SPS is used as an anticoagulant for blood cultures because it:

   a. inactivates penicillin and cephalosporins
   b. prevents clumping of red cells
   c. inactivates neutrophils and components of serum complement
   d. facilitates growth of anaerobes

161. Darkfield microscopy is commonly used to visualize:

   a. *Pseudomonas aeruginosa*
   b. *Streptococcus pneumoniae*
   c. *Treponema pallidum*
   d. *Legionella pneumophila*

162. A digested and decontaminated sputum is inoculated into a Bactec 12B bottle and incubated in air at 37°C. On day 14 a positive growth index is obtained and the auramine-rhodamine stain is positive. Broth from the initial bottle is inoculated into one Bactec 12B bottle and one Bactec 12B bottle with NAP. After reincubation, the uninoculated growth bottle shows an increase in growth index, while the bottle containing NAP shows no increase. The organism cultured from the sputum is *Mycobacterium*:

a. *marinum*
b. *kansasii*
c. *tuberculosis*
d. *avium-intracellulare*

163. A fibrous skin nodule is removed from the back of a patient from Central America. A microfilaria seen upon microscopic exam of the nodule would be:

a. *Wuchereria bancrofti*
b. *Brugia malayi*
c. *Onchocerca volvulus*
d. *Loa loa*

164. A patient with a nosocomial pneumonia has a sputum Gram stain that shows many white blood cells and numerous small gram-negative coccobacilli. The organism grew in 24 hours as a mucoid, hemolytic colony on blood agar, and a colorless colony on a MacConkey agar. The organism had the following characteristics:

Oxidase-negative
Arginine-negative
Catalase-positive
Ornithine-negative
Nitrate-negative
Lysine-negative
ONPG-negative

The organism is:

a. *Xanthomonas maltophilia*
b. *Alcaligenes xylosoxidans*
c. *Moraxella lacunata*
d. *Acinetobacter calcoaceticus*

165. Which organism commonly causes food poisoning from consumption of foods containing excessive populations of organisms or preformed enterotoxin?

a. *Salmonella enteritidis*
b. *Shigella sonnei*
c. *Bacillus cereus*
d. *Escherichia coli*

166. Multifocal brain lesion in AIDS patients is commonly caused by:

    a. *Toxoplasma gondii*
    b. *Pneumocystis carinii*
    c. *Cryptosporidium* sp
    d. *Giardia lamblia*

167. In the Kirby-Bauer disk diffusion susceptibility test, which variable is critical when testing *Pseudomonas* species for antibiotic susceptibility?

    a. incubation temperature
    b. duration of incubation
    c. cation content of media
    d. depth of agar

168. Patient specimens are being tested for *Brucella* antibody. Which course of action is most appropriate when the control serum displays a titer that is fourfold lower than expected?

    a. The results should be reported; this represents expected variability.
    b. The results should not be reported; the test should be repeated on the original specimen and a new control.
    c. The results should be corrected by reporting titers fourfold higher than observed values.
    d. The results should be reported as "results questionable, please repeat."

169. The Gram stain procedure in the procedure manual calls for acetone-alcohol decolorization for 2 minutes. The best course of action for a newly employed technologist would be to:

    a. perform the stain according to the manual's directions
    b. perform the stain according to the manufacturer's directions
    c. ask the supervisor if this is indeed the timing to be followed
    d. change the timing in the manual and initial the change with the date

170. A gram-negative rod has been isolated from feces, and the confirmed biochemical reactions fit those of *Shigella*. The organism does not agglutinate in *Shigella* antisera. What should be done next?

    a. test the organism with a new lot of antisera
    b. test with Vi antigen
    c. repeat the biochemical tests
    d. boil the organism and retest with the antisera

171. The diagnosis of *Neisseria gonorrhoeae* in females is best made from:

    a. clinical history
    b. a cervical culture
    c. a Gram stain of cervical secretions
    d. examination for clue cells

172. The reverse CAMP test, lecithinase production, double zone hemolysis, and Gram stain morphology are all useful criteria in the identification of:

    a. *Clostridium perfringens*
    b. *Streptococcus agalactiae*
    c. *Streptococcus pyogenes*
    d. *Clostridium tetani*

173. Which disinfectant inactivates HIV and HBV?

    a. alcohol
    b. iodine
    c. phenol
    d. sodium hypochlorite

174. Used needles from blood collection should be:

    a. recapped and placed in a biohazard bag
    b. placed in a biohazard bag and autoclaved
    c. placed in a biohazard bag with bleach
    d. placed in a puncture-proof container

175. A Gram stain from a swab of a hand wound reveals:

> Moderate gram-positive cocci in chains
> Moderate large gram-negative bacilli

Select the appropriate media that will selectively isolate each organism.

    a. KV-laked agar, Thayer-Martin
    b. sheep blood, MacConkey
    c. Columbia CNA, chocolate
    d. Columbia CNA, MacConkey

176. All species of the genus *Neisseria* have the enzyme to oxidize:

    a. naphthylamine
    b. dimethylaminobenzaldehyde
    c. glucopyranoside
    d. tetramethyl-phenylenediamine

177. A media for selective isolation of *Neisseria* from a cervical exudate is:

    a. chocolate
    b. Columbia CNA
    c. Thayer-Martin
    d. CTA

178. A sputum culture from an alcoholic seen in the ER grows gray, mucoid, stringy colonies on sheep blood. The isolate grows readily on MacConkey agar and forms mucoid, dark pink colonies. The colonies yield the following test results:

| | |
|---|---|
| ONPG | Positive |
| Indole | Negative |
| Glucose | Positive |
| Oxidase | Negative |
| Citrate | Positive |
| VP | Positive |

The organism is most likely:

a. *Edwardsiella tarda*
b. *Klebsiella pneumoniae*
c. *Escherichia coli*
d. *Proteus vulgaris*

179. An organism previously thought to be nonpathogenic, *Moraxella (Branhamella) catarrhalis*, is now known to be associated with infection and nosocomial transmission. Characteristic identification criteria include:

a. oxidase negative
b. carbohydrates negative
c. beta-lactamase negative
d. gram-negative bacilli

180. A control strain of *Clostridium* should be used in the GasPak™ anaerobe jar to ensure:

a. that plate media is working
b. that anaerobic environment is achieved
c. the jar is filled with a sufficient number of plates
d. the indicator strip is working

181. Which of the following groups of specimens would be acceptable for anaerobic culture?

a. vaginal, eye
b. ear, nose
c. pleural fluid, brain abscess
d. urine, sputum

182. Antibiotics tested for isolates of *Pseudomonas* species include:

a. penicillin
b. erythromycin
c. clindamycin
d. gentamicin

183. Refer to the following illustration:

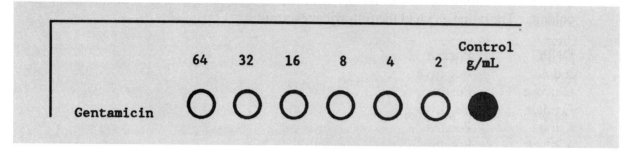

Examine the minimum inhibitory concentration (MIC) tray shown above and determine the MIC for gentamicin.

a. ≥ 64 g/mL
b. 32 g/mL
c. 16 g/mL
d. ≤ 2 g/mL

184. More than 100,000 CFU/mL of gram-negative bacilli were isolated on MacConkey from a urine specimen. Biochemical results are as follows:

| | |
|---|---|
| Glucose | Acid, gas produced |
| Indole | Negative |
| Urea | Positive |
| TDA | Positive |
| H$_2$S | Positive |

The organism is most likely:

a. *Morganella morganii*
b. *Proteus mirabilis*
c. *Proteus vulgaris*
d. *Providencia stuartii*

185. A urine culture had the following culture results:

| | |
|---|---|
| Sheep blood | Swarming |
| Columbia CNA | No growth |
| MacConkey | 1. > 100,000 CFU/mL nonlactose-fermenter |
| | 2. > 100,000 CFU/mL red, nonlactose-fermenter |

The isolates from MacConkey agar had the following biochemical reactions:

| | Isolate 1 | Isolate 2 |
|---|---|---|
| Glucose | Positive | Positive |
| Urea | Positive | Negative |
| TDA | Positive | Negative |
| H$_2$S | Positive | Negative |

The organisms are most likely:

a. *Proteus vulgaris* and *Enterobacter cloacae*
b. *Proteus mirabilis* and *Serratia marcescens*
c. *Morganella morganii* and *Klebsiella pneumoniae*
d. *Providencia stuartii* and *Serratia liquefaciens*

186. An isolate on chocolate agar from a patient with epiglottitis was suggestive of *Haemophilus* species. Additional testing showed that the isolate required NAD for growth and was non-hemolytic. The organism is most likely *Haemophilus*:

a. *haemolyticus*
b. *ducreyi*
c. *influenzae*
d. *parainfluenzae*

187. Which of the following is the most appropriate organism and media combination?

a. *Legionella* species - Mueller-Hinton
b. *Clostridium difficile* - phenylethyl alcohol (PEA)
c. *Campylobacter* species - charcoal yeast extract
d. *Yersinia enterocolitica* - cefsulodin-irgasan-novobiocin (CIN)

188. Which of the following is the most appropriate specimen source and primary media battery?

a. endocervical - chocolate, Thayer-Martin
b. sputum - sheep blood, Thayer-Martin, KV-laked blood
c. CSF - Columbia CNA, MacConkey
d. urine - sheep blood, chocolate, Columbia CNA

189. Gram stain examination of a CSF specimen indicates the presence of yeast-like cells with gram-positive granular inclusions. Which of the following techniques should be used next to assist in the identification of this organism?

a. 10% KOH
b. lactophenol cotton blue
c. India ink
d. periodic acid–Schiff

190. When performing a stool culture, a colony type typical of an enteric pathogen is subcultured on a blood agar plate. The resulting pure culture is screened with several tests to obtain the following results:

| | |
|---|---|
| TSI | Acid butt, alkaline slant, no gas, no $H_2S$ |
| Phenylalanine deaminase | Negative |
| Motility | Positive |
| Serological typing | *Shigella flexneri* (*Shigella* subgroup B) |

The serological typing is verified with new kit and controls. The best course of action would be to:

a. report the organism as *Shigella flexneri* without further testing
b. verify reactivity of motility medium with positive and negative controls
c. verify reactivity of the TSI slants with positive and negative controls for $H_2S$ production
d. verify reactivity of phenylalanine deaminase with positive and negative controls

191. A first-morning sputum is received for culture of mycobacteria. It is digested and concentrated by the N-acetyl-L-cysteine alkali method. Two Lowenstein-Jensen slants are incubated in the dark at 35°C with 5%-10% $CO_2$. The smears reveal acid-fast bacilli, and after 7 days no growth appears on the slants. The best explanation is:

a. improper specimen submitted
b. incorrect concentration procedure
c. exposure to $CO_2$ prevents growth
d. cultures held for insufficient length of time

192. A first-morning sputum specimen is received for acid-fast culture. The specimen is centrifuged, and the sediment is inoculated on two Lowenstein-Jensen slants that are incubated at 35°C in 5%-10% $CO_2$. After 1 week, the slants show abundant growth over the entire surface. Stains reveal gram-negative bacilli. To avoid this problem:

a. utilize a medium that inhibits bacterial growth
b. add sodium-hypochlorite to the sediment before inoculation
c. incubate the tubes at room temperature to retard bacterial growth
d. decontaminate the specimen with NALC-sodium hydroxide mixture

193. The characteristic MOST commonly associated with the presence of strict anaerobic bacteria and that can be taken as presumptive evidence of their presence in a clinical specimen is the:

a. presence of bacterial pleomorphism
b. production of abundant gas in a thioglycollate broth culture
c. abundant growth on a blood agar plate incubated in an anaerobic jar
d. presence of a foul, putrid odor from tissue specimens and cultures

194. A beta-hemolytic streptococcus that has been isolated from an ear culture grows up to the edge of a 0.04-unit bacitracin disk. Which of the following tests would determine if the organism is an enterococcus?

    a. growth in 6.5% NaCl broth
    b. growth in the presence of penicillin
    c. optochin susceptibility
    d. fermentation of 10% lactose

195. Gram stain of a deep wound showed many gram-positive spore-forming rods. The specimen was placed on brain-heart infusion blood agar and incubated aerobically at 35°C for 3 days. At the end of that time, the plates showed no growth. The most likely explanation is that the culture should have been incubated:

    a. on chocolate agar
    b. for 5 days
    c. under 5% $CO_2$
    d. anaerobically

196. *Acinetobacter lwoffi* differs from *Neisseria gonorrhoeae* in that the former:

    a. exhibits a gram-negative staining reaction
    b. will grow on MacConkey and EMB media
    c. is indophenol oxidase-positive
    d. produces hydrogen sulfide on a TSI slant

197. A gram-negative rod that does not grow on MacConkey or sheep blood agars but grows well on chocolate agar has been isolated from sputum. Which of the following tests should be done next to identify the organism?

    a. determination of X and V factor requirements
    b. ONPG
    c. catalase
    d. carbohydrate reactions

198. Mycobacteria that produce pigment only after exposure to light are classified as:

    a. photochromogens
    b. scotochromogens
    c. rapid growers
    d. nonphotochromogens

199. In a suspected case of Hansen's disease (leprosy), a presumptive diagnosis is established by:

   a. isolation of organisms on Lowenstein-Jensen medium
   b. detection of weakly acid-fast rods in infected tissue
   c. isolation of organisms in a cell culture
   d. detection of niacin production by the isolated bacterium


200. On a culture suspected to be *Mycobacterium tuberculosis*, the MOST important test to perform is:

   a. catalase production
   b. tellurite reduction
   c. Tween 80 hydrolysis
   d. niacin


201. A patient is suspected of having amebic dysentery. Upon microscopic examination of a fresh fecal specimen for ova and parasites, the following data were obtained:

   A trophozoite of 25 μm
   Progressive, unidirectional crawl
   Evenly distributed peripheral chromatin
   Finely granular cytoplasm

   This information probably indicates:

   a. *Entamoeba coli*
   b. *Entamoeba histolytica*
   c. *Endolimax nana*
   d. *Iodamoeba bütschlii*


202. In a quality control procedure on a new batch of Mueller-Hinton plates using a stock culture of *Staphylococcus aureus* (ATCC 25923), all the disk zone sizes are too small. The most likely reason for this is that the:

   a. Mueller-Hinton plates were poured too thin
   b. potency of the antibiotic disks is too high
   c. bacterial suspension was not diluted to the proper concentration
   d. disks should have been set up on mannitol salt


203. The best procedure to differentiate *Listeria monocytogenes* from *Corynebacterium* species is:

   a. catalase
   b. motility at 25°C
   c. motility at 35°C
   d. Gram stain

204. Establishing the pathogenicity of a microorganism isolated from a child's throat and identified as *Corynebacterium diphtheriae* would depend on:

a. the morphological appearance as revealed by Gram stain
b. the type of hemolysis on blood agar
c. a positive toxigenicity test
d. the appearance of growth on Tinsdale tellurite agar

205. The MOST common cause for failure of a GasPak™ anaerobic jar to establish an adequate environment for anaerobic incubation is:

a. the failure of the oxidation-reduction potential indicator system due to deterioration of methylene blue
b. the failure of the packet to generate adequate $H_2$ and/or $CO_2$
c. the failure of the O-ring gas-tight seal, resulting in a leak of oxygen into the jar
d. catalysts that have become inactivated after repeated use

206. The direct quellung reaction using specific antiserum is useful in the bacteriologic examination of which of the following specimens?

a. cerebrospinal fluid for *Haemophilus influenzae*
b. synovial fluid for *Neisseria gonorrhoeae*
c. sputum for *Cryptococcus neoformans*
d. cerebrospinal fluid for *Streptococcus pneumoniae*

207. A first-morning sputum is received for culture of acid-fast bacilli. It is digested and concentrated by the N-acetyl-L-cysteine alkali method. Two Sabouraud dextrose slants are incubated in the dark at 35°C with 5%-10% $CO_2$. The smears reveal acid-fast bacilli, but the slants show no growth after 8 weeks. The explanation is:

a. improper media used
b. incorrect concentration procedure used
c. improper specimen submitted
d. exposure to $CO_2$ prevents growth

208. Three sets of blood cultures were obtained. The aerobic bottle of one set had growth of *Staphylococcus epidermidis* on the 7-day subculture. This indicates that:

a. there was low-grade bacteremia
b. the organism is most likely a contaminant
c. the subculture plates were defective
d. the subculture should have been done at 5 days

209. A bronchial washing is processed for acid-fast bacilli. Which of the following precautions should be taken to prevent infection of laboratory personnel?

  a. Add an equal amount of NALC to the specimen.
  b. Process all specimens under ultraviolet light.
  c. Centrifuge specimen only after the addition of preservative.
  d. Process all specimens in a biological safety hood.

210. In order to isolate *Campylobacter coli/jejuni*, the fecal specimen should be:

  a. inoculated onto selective plating media and incubated in reduced oxygen with added $CO_2$ at 42°C
  b. stored in tryptic soy broth before plating to ensure growth of the organism
  c. inoculated onto selective plating media and incubated at both 35°C and room temperature
  d. incubated at 35°C for 2 hours in Cary-Blair media before inoculating onto selective plating media

211. A 4-year-old is admitted with symptoms of meningitis, and a Gram stain of the cerebrospinal fluid reveals small, pleomorphic, gram-negative coccobacilli. After 24 hours' incubation at 35°C, small, moist, gray colonies, which are oxidase negative, are found on the chocolate agar plate only. Which of the following biochemical data would be consistent with this isolate:

  a. CTA dextrose      Positive
      CTA maltose      Positive
      ONPG      Negative

  b. Sodium hippurate hydrolysis      Positive
      A disk      Negative
      CAMP test      Positive

  c. X factor      No growth
      V factor      No growth
      XV factor      Growth
      Horse blood      No hemolysis

  d. Catalase      Positive
      Esculin hydrolysis      Positive
      Methyl red      Positive
      "Umbrella" motility at room temperature

212. An expectorated sputum from a patient with respiratory distress is sent to the laboratory for culture. The Gram stain of the specimen shows many squamous epithelial cells (more than 25 per low power field) and only rare WBCs. The microscopic appearance of the organisms present include gram-positive cocci in chains and diplococci, gram-negative diplococci, and palisading gram-positive rods, all in moderate numbers. This Gram stain is most indicative of:

  a. a pneumococcal pneumonia
  b. an anaerobic infection
  c. a *Haemophilus* pneumonia
  d. oropharyngeal flora

213. Which type of microscope would be most useful in examining viruses and the structure of microbial cells?

    a. electron
    b. phase-contrast
    c. dark-field
    d. bright-field

214. An organism was isolated on kanamycin-vancomycin agar from a peritoneal abscess. The genus of this organism most likely is:

    a. *Veillonella*
    b. *Bacteroides*
    c. *Fusobacterium*
    d. *Peptostreptococcus*

215. Polyvinyl alcohol used in the preparation of permanently stained smears of fecal material:

    a. concentrates eggs
    b. dissolves artifacts
    c. serves as an adhesive
    d. enhances stain penetration

216. The procedure that ensures the most accurate results of oxacillin (methicillin) susceptibility testing against staphylococci is:

    a. addition of 4% NaCl
    b. incubation at 30°C
    c. incubation for 48 hours
    d. addition of 2% bile

217. A Wright's stain on a conjunctival smear from a neonate shows granular cytoplasmic perinuclear inclusions. This is most indicative of:

    a. *Chlamydia trachomatis*
    b. herpes simplex virus
    c. cytomegalovirus
    d. varicella-zoster virus

218. A Gram stain performed on a sputum specimen revealed gram-negative diplococci within PMNs. Oxidase testing is positive and carbohydrate degradation tests are inert. The organism is:

    a. *Neisseria lactamica*
    b. *Moraxella catarrhalis*
    c. *Neisseria meningitidis*
    d. *Neisseria sicca*

219. A gastroenterologist submits a gastric biopsy from a patient with a peptic ulcer. To obtain presumptive evidence of *Helicobacter pylori*, a portion of the specimen should be added to which media?

   a. urea broth
   b. tetrathionate
   c. selenite
   d. tryptophane

220. A gastric biopsy from a patient with severe gastritis and peptic ulcer is submitted to the laboratory with requests for Gram-stained touch preps and culture for *Helicobacter (Campylobacter) pylori*. The gram-negative rod is:

   a. slender and uniform
   b. thick and uniform
   c. slender and curved
   d. pleomorphic and curved

221. In an outbreak of nosocomial infection, the data readily available for epidemiologic investigation include:

   a. phage and bacteriocin typing
   b. antibiograms and biochemical profiles
   c. Western blot and serotyping
   d. colonial morphology and serogrouping

222. Which of the following groups of viruses are BEST diagnosed by serologic methods:

   a. hepatitis A, herpes simplex, and respiratory syncytial viruses
   b. herpes simplex, rubella viruses, and adenovirus
   c. respiratory syncytial virus, cytomegalovirus, and adenovirus
   d. human immunodeficiency virus, Epstein-Barr virus, and hepatitis B

223. Which compound, detected by Lugol's iodine, is used in the nonimmunologic detection of *Chlamydia trachomatis* in cell culture?

   a. DNA
   b. RNA
   c. glycogen
   d. DNA polymerase

224. Which of the following genera is among the least biochemically reactive members of the Enterobacteriaceae?

 a. *Proteus*
 b. *Pseudomonas*
 c. *Citrobacter*
 d. *Shigella*

225. An HIV-positive patient began to show signs of meningitis. Spinal fluid was collected and cultured for bacteria and fungus. A budding, encapsulated yeast was recovered. Which organism is consistent with this information?

 a. *Cryptococcus neoformans*
 b. *Aspergillus fumigatus*
 c. *Microsporum audouinii*
 d. *Sporothrix schenckii*

226. A urine specimen was submitted for isolation of cytomegalovirus. The urine was inoculated into human fibroblast tissue culture tubes. After 72 hours, no cytopathic effect was observed in the culture tubes. The most appropriate course of action is to:

 a. incubate the culture tubes for 2 to 3 weeks longer
 b. request a fecal specimen, as urine is inappropriate
 c. repeat the test using monkey kidney cell culture tubes
 d. request CMV serology, as CMV cannot be isolated

227. In the detection of *Chlamydia trachomatis*, culture on McCoy cells is:

 a. more sensitive than EIA methods
 b. less sensitive than EIA methods
 c. more specific than EIA
 d. as sensitive as EIA

228. Which technique can identify HSV, CMV, and adenovirus infection within 24 hours?

 a. tube monolayers
 b. shell vial
 c. electron microscopy
 d. polymerase chain reaction

229. Infection rate is highest for laboratory professionals exposed to blood and body fluids containing:

 a. hepatitis A
 b. hepatitis B
 c. CMV
 d. HIV

230. In agar disk susceptibility testing, as an antimicrobic agent diffuses away from the disk, the concentration gradient is:

    a. increased
    b. decreased
    c. unchanged
    d. inoculum dependent


231. The most sensitive substrate for the detection of $\beta$-lactamases is:

    a. penicillin
    b. ampicillin
    c. cefoxitin
    d. nitrocefin


232. In the USA, the most common organism causing eumycetic mycetoma is:

    a. *Pseudallescheria boydii*
    b. *Nocardia brasiliensis*
    c. *Blastomyces dermatitidis*
    d. *Aspergillus fumigatus*


233. The system that optimizes recovery of fungi from blood is:

    a. Bactec 460™
    b. biphasic bottles
    c. Dupont Isolator™
    d. Bactec NR680™


234. The genus of virus associated with anogenital warts, cervical dysplasia, and neoplasia is:

    a. herpes
    b. papillomavirus
    c. cytomegalovirus
    d. coxsackie


235. The method of choice to detect *Acanthamoeba* sp from corneal ulcer scrapings is:

    a. Nory, MacNeal, and Nicolle (NNN) medium
    b. culture on McCoy cells
    c. direct exam
    d. BAP flooded with a 24-hour growth of *E coli*

236. "Nutritionally deficient" streptococci are:

   a. enterococci
   b. group D nonenterococci
   c. cell wall–deficient streptococci
   d. viridans streptococci

237. Iodine staining of a McCoy cell monolayer culture of a cervical swab reveals a large brown intracytoplasmic inclusion. What is the MOST likely infecting organism?

   a. cytomegalovirus
   b. *Ehrlichia canis*
   c. *Chlamydia trachomatis*
   d. *Rickettsia prowazekii*

238. The preferred carbon source for mycobacteria is:

   a. glycerol
   b. glucose
   c. fatty acids
   d. casein hydrolysate

239. *Propionibacterium acnes* is most often associated with:

   a. normal oral flora
   b. postantibiotic diarrhea
   c. tooth decay
   d. blood culture contamination

240. Quality control of the spot indole test requires the use of ATCC cultures of:

   a. *Pseudomonas aeruginosa* and *Proteus mirabilis*
   b. *Salmonella typhi* and *Shigella sonnei*
   c. *Escherichia coli* and *Proteus vulgaris*
   d. *Escherichia coli* and *Enterobacter cloacae*

241. The Gram stain from a blood culture shows gram-positive cocci in chains. No growth occurs on blood agar plates incubated both aerobically and anaerobically. Additional testing should be done to detect the presence of:

   a. *Staphylococcus saprophyticus*
   b. nonpathogenic streptococci
   c. nutritionally deficient streptococci
   d. *Streptococcus pneumoniae*

242. The primary isolation of *Neisseria gonorrhoeae* requires:

    a. anaerobic conditions
    b. starch media
    c. carbon dioxide
    d. blood agar


243. *Streptococcus viridans* can be differentiated from *Streptococcus pneumoniae* by:

    a. alpha hemolysis
    b. morphology
    c. catalase reaction
    d. bile solubility


244. A reliable test for distinguishing pathogenic strains from nonpathogenic strains of staphylococci is:

    a. oxidase
    b. coagulase
    c. catalase
    d. optochin susceptibility


245. The optochin (ethylhydrocupreine hydrochloride) disk is used for the identification of:

    a. *Haemophilus influenzae*
    b. group A beta-hemolytic streptococci
    c. *Streptococcus pneumoniae*
    d. alpha-hemolytic streptococci


246. In the optochin (ethylhydrocupreine hydrochloride) susceptibility test, if there is a zone of inhibition of 19 to 30 mm surrounding the disk following overnight incubation at 37°C, the colony most likely consists of:

    a. staphylococci
    b. streptococci
    c. pneumococci
    d. intestinal bacilli


247. Proper media for culture of a urethral discharge from a man include:

    a. sheep blood and phenylethyl alcohol agars
    b. eosin-methylene blue and sheep blood agars
    c. thioglycollate broth and chocolate agar
    d. chocolate and modified Thayer-Martin agars

248. Assuming the agent isolated from a patient's spinal fluid produces a positive oxidase test, the most likely diagnosis is:

a. tuberculous meningitis
b. meningococcal meningitis
c. viral meningitis
d. pneumococcal meningitis

249. A sheep blood agar plate inoculated with 0.001 mL of urine grows 70 colonies of *Staphylococcus aureus*. How many colonies per mL of urine should be reported?

a. 70
b. 700
c. 7000
d. 70,000

250. A Gram stain of organisms on Loeffler agar showed pleomorphic gram-positive bacilli. The organism should be subcultured to:

a. blood
b. chocolate
c. MacConkey
d. potassium tellurite

251. Material from a brain abscess is suspected to contain *Bacteroides* species. Isolation of this organism is best accomplished on:

a. sheep blood agar in a candle jar
b. chocolate agar in a candle jar
c. eosin-methylene blue agar in an anaerobic jar
d. sheep blood agar in anaerobic conditions

252. Which of the following genera include anaerobic, gram-negative, nonsporulating bacilli?

a. *Brucella*
b. *Pasteurella*
c. *Actinomyces*
d. *Bacteroides*

253. Tubercle bacilli are specifically stained by:

a. crystal violet
b. 1% acid fuchsin
c. methylene blue
d. Kinyoun carbol fuchsin

254. The species of mycobacteria that will give a positive niacin test is *Mycobacterium*:

    a. *leprae*
    b. *kansasii*
    c. *fortuitum*
    d. *tuberculosis*

255. An organism that demonstrates budding yeast cells with wide capsules in an India ink preparation of spinal fluid is probably:

    a. *Cryptococcus neoformans*
    b. *Histoplasma capsulatum*
    c. *Blastomyces dermatitidis*
    d. *Candida albicans*

256. The best method to demonstrate the ova of *Enterobius vermicularis* is:

    a. acid-ether concentration
    b. cellophane tape preparation
    c. formalin-ether concentration
    d. zinc sulfate flotation

257. Artifacts found in a stool specimen that can be confused with ova or cysts are:

    a. partially digested meat fibers
    b. degenerated cells from the gastrointestinal mucosa
    c. dried chemical crystals
    d. pollen grains

258. The end point of the tube dilution test for antibiotic susceptibility is the:

    a. minimal inhibitory concentration
    b. optimal blood level equivalent
    c. maximum combining proportion
    d. optimum proportion point

259. Which two diseases are usually preceded by infection with beta-hemolytic streptococci?

    a. rheumatic fever, undulant fever
    b. glomerulonephritis, rheumatic fever
    c. rheumatic fever, tularemia
    d. glomerulonephritis, undulant fever

260. Infection of the urinary tract is most frequently associated with:

  a. *Staphylococcus aureus*
  b. *Escherichia coli*
  c. *Enterococcus* species
  d. *Serratia* species


261. The etiologic agent of botulism is:

  a. highly motile
  b. non–spore-forming
  c. *Clostridium perfringens*
  d. an exotoxin producer


262. The enterotoxin produced by certain strains of hemolytic, coagulase positive *Staphylococcus aureus*:

  a. is destroyed by boiling for 15-30 minutes
  b. is identical to the dermonecrotic toxin
  c. causes one type of bacterial food poisoning
  d. is highly antigenic


263. Which of the following clean voided urine culture counts indicates the patient probably has a urinary tract infection?

  a. 10 CFU/mL
  b. $10^3$ CFU/mL
  c. $10^5$ CFU/mL
  d. no growth


264. An organism that exhibits the satellite phenomenon around colonies of staphylococci is:

  a. *Haemophilus influenzae*
  b. *Neisseria meningitidis*
  c. *Neisseria gonorrhoeae*
  d. *Klebsiella pneumoniae*


265. The autoclave method of sterilization:

  a. uses 15 lb of pressure for 15 minutes
  b. utilizes dry heat for 20 minutes
  c. produces a maximum temperature of 100°C
  d. requires a source of ethylene oxide

266. An organism isolated from the surface of a skin burn is found to produce a diffusible green pigment on a blood agar plate. Further studies of the organism would most likely show the organism to be:

a. *Staphylococcus aureus*
b. *Serratia marcescens*
c. *Flavobacterium meningosepticum*
d. *Pseudomonas aeruginosa*

267. A strict anaerobe that produces terminal spores is:

a. *Clostridium tetani*
b. *Corynebacterium diphtheriae*
c. *Bacillus anthracis*
d. *Propionibacterium acnes*

268. The following results were obtained from a culture of unknown origin:

| | |
|---|---|
| Gram stain | Gram-negative diplococci |
| Indophenol oxidase | Positive |
| Glucose | Positive |
| Maltose | Negative |
| Sucrose | Negative |

The most likely source of the specimen would be the:

a. respiratory tract
b. blood
c. genitourinary tract
d. cerebrospinal fluid

269. An anaerobic, spore-forming, nonmotile, gram-positive bacillus isolated from a deep wound of the leg is most probably:

a. *Francisella tularensis*
b. *Clostridium perfringens*
c. *Bacillus subtilis*
d. *Bacillus anthracis*

270. In concentration methods for acid-fast bacilli, the sputum must be:

a. digested then centrifuged
b. centrifuged then digested
c. treated with phenol
d. digested then inoculated

271. Blood is drawn from a patient for serological tests for a viral disease at the time of onset and again 4 weeks later. The results of the tests are considered diagnostic if the:

    a. first antibody titer is twice the second
    b. first and second antibody titers are equal
    c. second antibody titer is one half the first
    d. second antibody titer is at least four times the first

272. Which of the following is most useful in establishing a diagnosis in the convalescence phase of a viral infection?

    a. slide culture
    b. serological techniques
    c. shell vial
    d. culture on McCoy's media

273. The IMViC reaction differentiates:

    a. *Streptococcus* from *Staphylococcus*
    b. bacillus from coccus
    c. *Escherichia coli* from *Enterobacter*
    d. *Enterobacter* from *Pseudomonas*

274. A nonfermenting gram-negative bacillus is isolated from a wound. The nitrate and oxidase are strongly positive. The organism produces a shiny blue-green pigment on sheep blood agar. The organism is a species of:

    a. *Alcaligenes*
    b. *Moraxella*
    c. *Flavobacterium*
    d. *Pseudomonas*

275. A gamma-hemolytic *Streptococcus*, which blackens bile esculin but does not grow in 6.5% NaCl broth, is most likely group:

    a. B
    b. group D enterococci
    c. group D nonenterococci
    d. G

276. *Penicillium* can best be separated from *Aspergillus* by:

    a. color of the colonies
    b. optimum growth temperature
    c. presence of rhizoids
    d. arrangement of the conidia on the conidiophore

277. A small, gram-negative rod is isolated from an eye culture. It grows only on chocolate agar and is oxidase-negative. The most likely organism is:

a. *Neisseria gonorrhoeae*
b. *Haemophilus influenzae*
c. *Corynebacterium diphtheriae*
d. *Pseudomonas aeruginosa*

278. Gram stain examination from a blood culture bottle shows dark blue, spherical organisms in clusters. Growth on sheep blood agar shows small, round, pale yellow colonies. Further tests should include:

a. catalase production and coagulase test
b. bacitracin susceptibility and serological typing
c. oxidase and deoxyribonuclease reactions
d. Voges-Proskauer and methyl red reactions

279. The formation of germ tubes presumptively identifies:

a. *Candida tropicalis*
b. *Candida parapsilosis*
c. *Candida glabrata*
d. *Candida albicans*

280. A blood culture bottle with macroscopic signs of growth is Gram stained and the technician notes small, curved, gram-negative rods resembling "gull wings." It is subcultured to blood and chocolate agar and incubated aerobically and anaerobically. After 24 hours no growth is apparent. The next step should be to:

a. subculture the bottle and incubate in microaerophilic conditions
b. assume the organism is nonviable
c. utilize a pyridoxal disk to detect nutritionally deficient streptococci
d. subculture the bottle to a medium containing X and V factors

281. The expected colony count in a suprapubic urine from a healthy individual is:

a. 0 CFU/mL
b. 100 CFU/mL
c. 1000 CFU/mL
d. 100,000 CFU/mL

282. Gram-positive cocci in chains are seen on a Gram stain from a blood culture. Further tests should include:

a. bile esculin, bacitracin, and hippurate
b. catalase and coagulase
c. oxidase and deoxyribonuclease
d. Voges-Proskauer and methyl red

283. Which of the following is the best choice for decontaminating bench tops contaminated by the AIDS virus?

   a. sodium hypochlorite bleach
   b. formalin
   c. a quaternary ammonium compound
   d. 100% alcohol


284. An aspirate of a deep wound was plated on blood agar plates aerobically and anaerobically. At 24 hours there was growth on both plates. This indicates that the organism is:

   a. a nonfermenter
   b. strictly anaerobic
   c. aerobic
   d. facultatively anaerobic


285. A urethral swab obtained from a man with a urethral exudate was plated directly on chocolate agar and modified Thayer-Martin (MTM) agar, and a Gram stain was made. The Gram stain showed gram-negative diplococci. The culture plates were incubated at 35°C but had no growth at 48 hours. The most likely failure for organism growth is that the:

   a. wrong media were used
   b. Gram stain was misread
   c. organism grows only at room temperature
   d. organism requires $CO_2$ for growth


286. In processing clinical specimens and fungal isolates, laboratory workers may contract systemic fungal infections through:

   a. inhalation
   b. ingestion
   c. skin contact
   d. insect vector


287. Virus transport medium containing penicillin, gentamicin, and amphotericin is used to collect and transport specimens for virus culture because this medium:

   a. enables rapid viral growth during the transport time
   b. inhibits bacterial and fungal growth
   c. destroys nonpathogenic viruses
   d. inhibits complement-fixing antibodies

288. A urine Gram stain shows gram-positive cocci in clusters. To SPECIATE this organism from culture, the technician should perform a coagulase test and a(n):

    a. catalase
    b. novobiocin inhibition
    c. oxidase
    d. β-lactamase


289. The microscopic structures most useful in the identification of dermatophytes are:

    a. septate and branching hyphae
    b. racquet and pectinate hyphae
    c. chlamydospores and microconidia
    d. macroconidia and microconidia


290. A direct smear of a sputum specimen that demonstrated acid-fast bacilli would:

    a. not need further cultures unless specifically ordered
    b. be diagnostic of *Mycobacterium tuberculosis*
    c. be reported and cultures done for isolation
    d. be of little value without including Gram stain results


291. In preparing an India ink slide, the technician should ensure that the:

    a. CSF is unspun
    b. sputum is well mixed
    c. proper amount of reagent is added
    d. slide is properly dried first


292. The advantage of thick blood smears for malarial parasites is to:

    a. improve staining of the organisms
    b. improve detection of the organisms
    c. remove RBC artifacts
    d. remove platelets


293. The optimal incubator temperature for isolation of the *Campylobacter jejuni/coli* group is:

    a. 4°C
    b. 20°C
    c. 25°C
    d. 42°C

294. Respiratory syncytial virus (RSV) is best isolated using a:

a. nasopharyngeal aspirate
b. cough plate
c. expectorated sputum
d. throat swab

295. Which of the following indicates the presence of a viral infection in tissue smears or biopsies?

a. cytopathic effect
b. intranuclear inclusions
c. cell lysis
d. mononuclear inflammatory cells

296. The safest method of disposing of hypodermic needles is:

a. recap the needle with its protective sheath prior to discarding
b. cut the needle with a special device before disposal
c. discard the needle in an impermeable container without other handling immediately after use
d. drop the needle in the waste basket immediately after use

297. Proper collection of a sample for recovery of *Enterobius vermicularis* includes:

a. a 24-hour urine collection
b. a first-morning stool collection with proper preservative
c. a swab from the perianal region before bathing or bowel movement
d. peripheral blood from a finger

298. A gram-negative rod growing on BAP has colonies with feathered edges and the following characteristics:

| | |
|---|---|
| O-F glucose | Oxidizer |
| Growth on MacConkey | Positive |
| Oxidase | Positive |
| Odor | Grape-like |

The organism is most likely:

a. *Acinetobacter* sp
b. *Aeromonas hydrophila*
c. *Pasteurella multocida*
d. *Pseudomonas aeruginosa*

299. A penicillin-resistant *Neisseria gonorrhoeae* produces:

 a. alpha-hemolysin
 b. beta-lactamase
 c. enterotoxin
 d. coagulase

300. A technician is asked to clean out the chemical reagent storeroom and discard any reagents not used in the past 5 years. How should the technician proceed?

 a. Discard chemicals into biohazard containers, where they will later be autoclaved.
 b. Pour reagents down the drain, followed by flushing of water.
 c. Consult MSDS sheets for proper disposal.
 d. Pack all chemicals for incineration.

301. Media for screening suspected cases of hemorrhagic *E coli* 0157:H7 must contain:

 a. indole
 b. citrate
 c. sorbitol
 d. lactose

302. Which selective medium is used for the isolation of gram-positive microorganisms?

 a. Columbia CNA with 5% sheep blood
 b. trypticase soy agar with 5% sheep blood
 c. eosin methylene blue
 d. modified Thayer-Martin

303. With few exceptions, all members of the family *Enterobacteriaceae* show which of the following characteristics?

 a. produce cytochrome oxidase
 b. ferment lactose
 c. produce β-hemolysis
 d. reduce nitrate to nitrite

*The remaining questions (\*) have been identified as more appropriate for the entry level medical technologist.*

*304. Which of the following characteristics best distinguishes *Mycobacterium scrofulaceum* from *Mycobacterium gordonae*?

 a. iron uptake
 b. Tween hydrolysis
 c. good growth at 25°C
 d. niacin production

*305. A specimen of hair that fluoresced under a Wood's lamp was obtained from a child with low-grade scaling lesions of the scalp. Cultures revealed a fungus with mycelium and very few macroconidia or microconidia. This fungus is most likely:

a. *Microsporum gypseum*
b. *Microsporum audouinii*
c. *Trichophyton tonsurans*
d. *Epidermophyton floccosum*

*306. Primary amebic-encephalitis may be caused by:

a. *Entamoeba coli*
b. *Dientamoeba fragilis*
c. *Endolimax nana*
d. *Naegleria* sp

*307. The usefulness of counterimmunoelectrophoresis (CIE) in the diagnosis of meningitis is limited because:

a. commercial antisera are not available for the detection of the organisms that commonly cause meningitis
b. cross-reactions commonly occur between *Streptococcus pneumoniae, Haemophilus influenzae,* and *Neisseria meningitidis*
c. antigens are detected in less than 50% of bacteriologically proven cases of meningitis
d. a concentration of $10^5$ CFU/mL is required before sufficient antigen can be detected

*308. All of the following are advantages of automated susceptibility testing EXCEPT:

a. end point objectivity
b. greater sensitivity of readings
c. cost reduction with small volumes
d. reduction of experimental error

*309. All of the following are in vitro methods of determining synergism EXCEPT:

a. kill-curve method
b. kill-curve using an MIC endpoint
c. checkerboard using an MIC endpoint
d. checkerboard using an MBC endpoint

*310. Production of beta-lactamase is inducible in which of the following?

a. *Haemophilus influenzae*
b. *Staphylococcus aureus*
c. *Corynebacterium diphtheriae*
d. *Streptococcus pyogenes*

*311. Anaerobic susceptibility tests are helpful in the management of patients with:

    a. synovial infections
    b. rectal abscesses
    c. streptococcal pharyngitis
    d. pilonidal sinuses

*312. When combination antibiotic therapy is used:

    a. antagonistic effects should exist between the antibiotics
    b. the combination effect of the drugs should be less than the sum of the independent effects of the two drugs
    c. the synergistic effects of the drugs should be assessed
    d. the killing power of the combination must be at least fourfold greater than the anti-microbic used alone

*313. The most appropriate clinical test for diagnosing *Clostridium difficile* is:

    a. tissue culture toxin assay
    b. gas-liquid chromatography
    c. routine fecal cultures
    d. anaerobic culture techniques

*314. Pseudomembranous colitis caused by *Clostridium difficile* toxin is BEST confirmed by which of the following laboratory findings?

    a. isolation of the causative agent
    b. Gram stain showing many gram-positive rods
    c. gas production in chopped meat glucose
    d. presence of toxin in stool

*315. Which one of the following results is typical of *Campylobacter fetus* subspecies *fetus*?

    a. optimal growth at 42°C
    b. oxidase negative
    c. growth at 37°C
    d. catalase negative

*316. Items to consider when using the staphylococcal coagglutination procedure include:

    a. Hyperproteinemia may cause autoagglutination and thus false-positive test results.
    b. Direct testing of group A, beta-hemolytic streptococci isolates from agar plates results in pseudoagglutination.
    c. Gonococcal isolates must be cold-treated to avoid pseudoagglutination.
    d. Cerebrospinal fluid must be heated to 56°C for 5 minutes before testing.

*317. A 25-year-old man who had recently worked as a steward on a transoceanic grain ship presented to the emergency room with high fever, diarrhea, and prostration. Axillary lymph nodes were hemorrhagic and enlarged. A Gram-stained smear was prepared from a lymph node aspirate and many gram-negative bacilli were noted. The bacilli demonstrated a marked bipolar staining reaction described as a "safety-pin appearance" with Wayson's stain. The most likely identification of this organism is:

a. *Brucella melitensis*
b. *Streptobacillus moniliformis*
c. *Spirillum minor*
d. *Yersinia pestis*


*318. A culture from an infected dog bite on a small boy's finger yielded a small, gram-negative coccobacillus that was smooth, raised, and beta-hemolytic on blood agar. The isolate was found to grow readily on MacConkey agar forming colorless colonies. The organism was motile with peritrichous flagella, catalase positive, oxidase positive, reduced nitrate, utilized citrate, and was urease positive within 4 hours. No carbohydrates were fermented. The most likely identification of this isolate is:

a. *Brucella canis*
b. *Yersinia pestis*
c. *Francisella tularensis*
d. *Bordetella bronchiseptica*


*319. Multiple blood cultures from a patient with endocarditis grew a facultatively anaerobic, pleomorphic gram-negative bacillus with the following characteristics:

| | |
|---|---|
| Hemolysis | Negative |
| MacConkey agar | No growth |
| Catalase | Negative |
| Oxidase | Negative |
| Nitrate | Positive, reduced to nitrites |
| Bile solubility | Insoluble |
| Indole | Negative |
| Glucose | Acid and gas produced |
| Enhanced growth on blood & chocolate agar in 5% $CO_2$ | |
| Required X factor under 5%-10% $CO_2$ atmosphere | |

The most likely identification is:

a. *Brucella abortus*
b. *Actinobacillus actinomycetemcomitans*
c. *Haemophilus aphrophilus*
d. *Cardiobacterium hominis*

*320. While swimming in a lake near his home, a young boy cut his foot as he stepped on a piece of glass from a broken bottle. An infection developed and the site was cultured. A nonfastidious gram-negative, oxidase-positive, beta-hemolytic, motile bacillus was recovered. The organism produced deoxyribonuclease and was most probably identified as:

    a. *Enterobacter cloacae*
    b. *Serratia marcescens*
    c. *Aeromonas hydrophila*
    d. *Escherichia coli*

*321. The most rapid and specific method for detection of *Francisella tularensis* is:

    a. serological slide agglutination utilizing specific antiserum
    b. dye-stained clinical specimens
    c. fluorescent antibody staining techniques on clinical specimens
    d. biotyping

*322. The macrobroth dilution method for determining antibiotic susceptibility of the *Enterobacteriaceae* cannot be used effectively for the sulfonamides or trimethoprim because:

    a. misleading results can occur due to inadequate concentrations of $Mg^{++}$ and $Ca^{++}$
    b. organisms are resistant at 35°C; at 37°C end points are less clear unless incubated for 48 hours
    c. definite end points have not yet been established
    d. end points are difficult to determine, as susceptible organisms can go through several generations before being inhibited

*323. Blood cultures from a case of suspected leptospiremia should be drawn:

    a. between 10 PM and 2 AM
    b. in the first 7-10 days of infection
    c. during febrile periods, late in the course of the disease
    d. after the first 10 days of illness

*324. Which of the following anaerobes would be positive for indole?

    a. *Bacteroides thetaiotaomicron*
    b. *Bacteroides fragilis*
    c. *Bacteroides distasonis*
    d. *Bacteroides ureolyticus*

*325. Which of the following is a growth requirement for the isolation of *Leptospira*?

    a. an atmosphere of 10% $CO_2$
    b. an incubation temperature of 4°C
    c. 4- to 5-day incubation
    d. medium containing 10% serum plus fatty acids

*326. An aerobic, gram-negative coccobacillus was isolated on blood agar from a nasopharyngeal swab 48 hours after culture from a 6-month-old infant with suspected pertussis. The organism exhibited the following characteristics:

| | |
|---|---|
| Urea | Negative at 4 hours, positive at 18 hours |
| Oxidase | Negative |
| Catalase | Positive |
| Citrate | Positive |
| Small zones of beta-hemolysis | |
| Slight brownish coloration of the medium | |

The most probable identification of this isolate is:

a. *Pasteurella multocida*
b. *Pasteurella ureae*
c. *Bordetella pertussis*
d. *Bordetella parapertussis*


*327. Which feature distinguishes *Erysipelothrix rhusiopathiae* from other clinically significant non–spore-forming, gram-positive, facultatively anaerobic bacilli?

a. "tumbling" motility
b. beta-hemolysis
c. more pronounced motility at 25°C than 37°C
d. H$_2$S production


*328. Which of the following characteristics best differentiates *Bordetella bronchiseptica* from *Alcaligenes* species?

a. flagellar pattern
b. growth at 24°C
c. oxidase activity
d. rapid hydrolysis of urea


*329. Which of the following results would you expect if motility agar was made with a 1% agar concentration?

a. false-negative for *Acinetobacter lwoffi*
b. false-positive for *Alcaligenes faecalis*
c. false-positive for *Moraxella osloensis*
d. false-negative for *Pseudomonas aeruginosa*

*330. A two-week-old culture of a urine specimen produced a few colonies of acid-fast bacilli, which were rough and nonpigmented. The niacin test was weakly positive and the nitrate test was positive. Which of the following is the most appropriate action when a presumptive identification has been requested as soon as possible?

    a. Report the organism as presumptive *Mycobacterium tuberculosis*.
    b. Wait a few days and repeat the niacin test; report presumptive *Mycobacterium tuberculosis* if the test is more strongly positive.
    c. Subculture the organism and set up the routine battery of biochemicals; notify the physician that results will not be available for 3 weeks.
    d. Set up a thiophene-2-carboxylic acid hydrazide ($T_2H$); if the organism is sensitive, report *Mycobacterium bovis*.

*331. An acid-fast bacillus recovered from an induced sputum had the following characteristics:

| | |
|---|---|
| Pigmentation | Yellow in the dark, turning a deeper yellow-orange after 2 weeks of light exposure |
| Nitrate reduction | Negative |
| Tween hydrolysis | Positive at 5-10 days |
| Urease | Negative |

Based on this information, the organism is most likely *Mycobacterium*:

    a. *scrofulaceum*
    b. *gordonae*
    c. *szulgai*
    d. *flavescens*

*332. When staining acid-fast bacilli with Truant's auramine-rhodamine stain, potassium permanganate is used as a:

    a. decolorizing agent
    b. quenching agent
    c. mordant
    d. dye

*333. Characteristics necessary for the definitive identification of *Mycobacterium tuberculosis* are:

    a. buff color, slow growth at 37°C, niacin production positive, nitrate reduction negative
    b. rough colony, slow growth at 37°C, nonpigmented
    c. rough, nonpigmented colony, cording positive, niacin production negative, catalase negative at pH 7/68°C
    d. rough, nonpigmented colony, slow growth at 37°C, niacin production positive, nitrate reduction positive

*334. Which of the following is a true statement about pigment production by *Mycobacterium kansasii*?

    a. It is a result of beta carotene formation and accumulation.
    b. It can be an indication of virulence.
    c. It can be inhibited by inclusion of albumin in growth medium.
    d. It is increased at 30°C incubation.


*335. Differentiation of *Mycobacterium avium* from *Mycobacterium intracellulare* can be accomplished by:

    a. nitrate reduction test
    b. Tween hydrolysis test
    c. resistance to 10 µg thiophene-2-carboxylic acid hydrazide (TCH)
    d. DNA probe


*336. Differential skin testing for mycobacteriosis has diagnostic value in young children because:

    a. immaturity of the immune system allows useful reactions
    b. infections develop more slowly, yielding more definitive immune response
    c. they have not yet become sensitized to many mycobacteria
    d. they develop hypersensitivity at an early age


*337. Because ultraviolet light is used to decontaminate the work surface inside a biological safety cabinet, the lamp should be replaced when the intensity compared to the original output reading differs by:

    a. 10%
    b. 20%
    c. 30%
    d. 40%


*338. A fungal isolate from the sputum of a patient with a pulmonary infection is suspected to be *Histoplasma capsulatum*. Tuberculate macroconidia were seen on the hyphae of the mold phase, which was isolated at room temperature on Sabouraud's dextrose agar containing chloramphenicol and cycloheximide (SDA-CC). A parallel set of cultures incubated at 35°C showed bacterial growth on SDA but no growth on SDA-CC. Which of the following is the appropriate course of action?

    a. Repeat subculture of the mold phase to tubes of moist SDA-CC, incubate at 35°C.
    b. Subculture the mold phase to tubes of moist BHI-blood media, incubate at 25°C.
    c. Subculture the mold phase to moist BHI-blood media, incubate at 35°C.
    d. Perform animal inoculation studies.

*339. Pus from a draining fistula on a foot was submitted for culture. Gross examination of the specimen revealed the presence of a small (0.8 mm in diameter), yellowish, oval granule. Direct microscopic examination of the crushed granule showed hyphae 3-4 μm in diameter and the presence of chlamydospores at the periphery. After 2 days a cottony, white mold was seen that turned gray with a gray to black reverse after a few days. When viewed microscopically, moderately large hyaline septate hyphae with long or short conidiophores, each single pear-shaped aleuriospore, 5-7 x 8-10 μm, were seen. The most likely identification is:

    a. *Exophiala jeanselmei*
    b. *Fonsecaea pedrosoi*
    c. *Pseudallescheria boydii*
    d. *Cladosporium carrionii*

*340. Crust from a cauliflower-like lesion on the hand exhibited brown spherical bodies 6-12 μm in diameter when examined microscopically. After 3 weeks of incubation at room temperature, a slow-growing black mold grew on Sabouraud's dextrose agar. Microscopic examination revealed *Cladosporium*, *Phialophora*, and *Acrotheca* types of sporulation. The probable identification of this organism is:

    a. *Fonsecaea pedrosoi*
    b. *Pseudallescheria boydii*
    c. *Phialophora verrucosa*
    d. *Cladosporium carrionii*

*341. A fungus superficially resembles *Penicillium* species but may be differentiated because its sterigmata are long and tapering and bend away from the central axis. The sterigmata also arise singly from the hyphae. The most probable identification is:

    a. *Exophiala* sp
    b. *Acremonium* sp
    c. *Cladosporium* sp
    d. *Paecilomyces* sp

*342. Culture of a strand of hair that fluoresced yellow-green when examined with a Wood's lamp produced a slow-growing, flat gray colony with a salmon-pink reverse. Microscopic examination demonstrated racquet hyphae, pectinate bodies, chlamydospores, and a few abortive or bizarre-shaped macroconidia. The most probable identification of this isolate is:

    a. *Microsporum gypseum*
    b. *Microsporum canis*
    c. *Microsporum audouinii*
    d. *Trichophyton rubrum*

*343. A mold grown at 25°C exhibited delicate septate hyaline hyphae and many conidiophores extending at right angles from the hyphae. Oval, 2- to 5-µm conidia were formed at the end of the conidiophores, giving a flowerlike appearance. In some areas "sleeves" of spores could be found along the hyphae as well. A 37°C culture of this organism produced small, cigar-shaped yeast cells. This organism is most likely:

    a. *Histoplasma capsulatum*
    b. *Sporothrix schenckii*
    c. *Blastomyces dermatitidis*
    d. *Acremonium falciforme*

*344. Which of the following is the best aid in the identification of *Epidermophyton floccosum* macroconidia?

    a. parallel side walls with at least 10 cells
    b. spindle-shaped spore with thin walls
    c. spindle-shaped spore, thick walls, and distinct terminal knob with echinulations
    d. smooth walls, club-shaped

*345. A 44-year-old man was admitted to the hospital following a 2-week history of low-grade fever, malaise, and anorexia. Examination of a Giemsa-stained blood film revealed many intraerythrocytic parasites. Further history revealed frequent camping trips near Martha's Vineyard and Nantucket Island, but no travel outside the continental United States. This parasite could easily be confused with:

    a. *Trypanosoma cruzi*
    b. *Trypanosoma rhodesiense/gambiense*
    c. *Plasmodium falciparum*
    d. *Leishmania donovani*

*346. What material should be used to prepare slides for direct smear examination for virus detection by special stains or FA technique?

    a. vesicular fluid
    b. leukocytes from the edge of the lesion
    c. the top portion of the vesicle
    d. epithelial cells from the base of the lesion

*347. Many fungal infections are transmitted to man via inhalation of infectious structures. Which of the following is usually NOT contracted in this manner?

    a. histoplasmosis
    b. blastomycosis
    c. coccidioidomycosis
    d. sporotrichosis

*348. The agent used for processing specimens for mycobacterial culture contaminated with *Pseudomonas* is:

a. N-acetyl-L-cysteine and NaOH
b. NaOH alone
c. Zephiran-trisodium phosphate
d. oxalic acid

*349. A branching gram-positive, partially acid-fast organism is isolated from a bronchial washing on a 63-year-old woman receiving chemotherapy. The organism does NOT hydrolyze casein, tyrosine, or xanthine. The most likely identification is:

a. *Actinomadura madurae*
b. *Nocardia caviae*
c. *Streptomyces somaliensis*
d. *Nocardia asteroides*

*350. Which of the following viruses may be detected only by use of an electron microscope or EIA methods?

a. respiratory syncytial virus
b. influenza A
c. rotavirus
d. herpes simplex 1

*351. It has been recommended that cephalexin instead of penicillin be incorporated into Bordet-Gengou agar because:

a. cephalexin is more stable at incubation temperature
b. cephalexin inhibits organisms indigenous to the nasopharynx
c. cephalexin may inactivate some inhibitory fatty acids and peroxides
d. penicillin may inhibit some strains of *Bordetella pertussis*

*352. *Legionella pneumophila* characteristically is:

a. oxidase positive
b. gelatin negative
c. nonmotile
d. gram-positive

*353. Skin scrapings obtained from the edge of a crusty wrist lesion were found to contain thick-walled, spherical yeast cells (8-15 µm in diameter) that had single buds with a wide base of attachment. Microscopic examination of the room temperature isolate from this specimen would probably reveal the presence of:

a. "rosette-like" clusters of pear-shaped conidia at the tips of delicate conidiophores
b. thick-walled, round to pear-shaped tuberculate macroconidia
c. numerous conidia along the length of hyphae in a "sleeve-like" arrangement
d. septate hyphae bearing round or pear-shaped small conidia attached to conidiophores of irregular lengths

*354. Microorganisms resembling L-forms have been isolated from the blood of patients treated with antibiotics that:

a. complex with flagellar protein
b. interfere with cell membrane function
c. inhibit protein synthesis
d. interfere with cell wall synthesis

*355. The Epstein-Barr virus is associated with which of the following?

a. chickenpox
b. Hodgkin's lymphoma
c. Burkitt's lymphoma
d. smallpox

*356. Which of the following is the most appropriate method for collecting a urine specimen from a patient with an indwelling catheter?

a. Remove the catheter, cut the tip, and submit it for culture.
b. Disconnect the catheter from the bag and collect urine from the terminal end of the catheter.
c. Collect urine directly from the bag.
d. Aspirate urine aseptically from the catheter tubing.

*357. Which of the two different antimicrobial agents listed below are commonly used and may result in synergistic action in the treatment of endocarditis caused by *Enterococcus faecalis*?

a. an aminoglycoside and a macrolide
b. a penicillin derivative and an aminoglycoside
c. a cell membrane active agent and nalidixic acid
d. a macrolide and a penicillin derivative

*358. The most meaningful laboratory procedure in confirming the diagnosis of clinical botulism is:

a. demonstration of toxin in the patient's serum
b. recovery of *Clostridium botulinum* from suspected food
c. recovery of *Clostridium botulinum* from the patient's stool
d. Gram stain of suspected food for gram-positive, sporulating bacilli

*359. The main reason for the administration of two or more drugs for the treatment of pulmonary tuberculosis is to:

    a. obtain a greater therapeutic effect
    b. prevent the emergence of bacilli resistant to the action of either or both drugs
    c. reduce the toxicity of either drug if used alone
    d. reduce the deleterious effect of tuberculin hypersensitivity

*360. The disease-producing capacity of *Mycobacterium tuberculosis* depends primarily upon:

    a. production of exotoxin
    b. production of endotoxin
    c. capacity to withstand intracellular digestion by macrophages
    d. lack of susceptibility to the myeloperoxidase system

*361. Assuming that the host has no known immunologic defect, which of the following is most likely to be associated with resistance to standard drug therapy?

    a. *Mycobacterium tuberculosis*
    b. BCG (*Mycobacterium bovis*)
    c. *Mycobacterium intracellulare-avium*
    d. *Mycobacterium scrofulaceum*

*362. The nitrate test for mycobacteria can be performed with a reagent-impregnated paper strip or by the use of standard reagents. In order to quality control the test properly, which of the following should be used for a positive control?

    a. *Mycobacterium bovis*
    b. *Mycobacterium gordonae*
    c. *Mycobacterium tuberculosis*
    d. *Mycobacterium intracellulare*

*363. Rickettsiae infecting man multiply preferentially within which of the following cells?

    a. reticuloendothelial
    b. hepatic
    c. renal tubule
    d. endothelial

*364. Mycoplasmas differ from bacteria in that they:

    a. do not cause disease in humans
    b. cannot grow in artificial inanimate media
    c. lack cell walls
    d. are not serologically antigenic

*365. The most reliable serologic test for the diagnosis of Q fever is the:

    a.  cold agglutinin test
    b.  heterophile antibody test
    c.  complement fixation test
    d.  Weil-Felix test

*366. The preferred specimen for laboratory diagnosis of acquired cytomegalovirus infection is:

    a.  blood
    b.  urine
    c.  stool
    d.  cutaneous vesicular fluid

*367. Routine quality control tests revealed that a batch of chocolate agar was able to support the growth of *Haemophilus influenzae* only as satellite colonies around *Staphylococcus aureus*. The most likely source of difficulty is:

    a.  excess heating in preparation of the medium
    b.  dehydration during storage of the medium
    c.  attenuation of the quality control organism
    d.  use of improperly cleaned glassware

*368. Which of the following statements is true regarding the diagnosis of herpes simplex encephalitis caused by herpes simplex 1?

    a.  The virus can usually be recovered from fluid during the first week of illness.
    b.  The virus can usually be recovered from feces during the first week of illness.
    c.  The virus is rarely recoverable from either spinal fluid or feces during herpes encephalitis.
    d.  Cytopathic effects are slow to develop in cell cultures compared with those induced by mumps virus.

*369. A 29-year-old man is seen for recurrence of a purulent urethral discharge 10 days after the successful treatment of culture-proven gonorrhea. The most likely etiology of his urethritis is:

    a.  *Mycoplasma hominis*
    b.  *Chlamydia trachomatis*
    c.  *Trichomonas vaginalis*
    d.  *Neisseria gonorrhoeae*

*370. Which species of *Mycobacterium* includes a BCG strain used for vaccination against tuberculosis?

    a.  *tuberculosis*
    b.  *bovis*
    c.  *kansasii*
    d.  *fortuitum/chelonei* complex

*371. Quality control results for disk diffusion susceptibility tests yield the aminoglycoside zones too small and the penicillin zones too large. This is probably due to the:

a. inoculum being too heavy
b. inoculum being too light
c. pH of Mueller-Hinton agar being too low
d. calcium and magnesium concentration in the agar being too high

*372. When using a control strain of *Staphylococcus aureus* the technologist notices that the zone around the methicillin disk is too small. This is probably due to the use of:

a. a Mueller-Hinton agar plate that was too thin
b. an inoculum that was too light
c. Mueller-Hinton agar that was overly acidic
d. outdated antibiotic disks

*373. How many hours after eating contaminated food do initial symptoms of staphylococcal food poisoning typically occur?

a. 5 to 7 hours
b. 12 to 18 hours
c. 24 to 48 hours
d. 72 hours to a week

*374. An example of a live attenuated vaccine used for human immunization is:

a. rabies
b. tetanus
c. influenza
d. measles

*375. A 73-year-old man diagnosed as having pneumococcal meningitis is not responding to his penicillin therapy. Which of the following tests should be performed on the isolate to best determine this organism's susceptibility to penicillin agents?

a. beta-lactamase
b. oxacillin disk diffusion
c. penicillin disk diffusion
d. Schlichter test

*376. A jaundiced 7-year-old boy, with a history of playing in a pond in a rat-infested area, has a urine specimen submitted for a direct dark-field examination. No organisms are seen in the specimen. Which medium should be inoculated in an attempt to isolate the suspected organism?

a. blood cysteine dextrose
b. PPLO agar
c. Fletcher's semisolid
d. chopped meat glucose

*377. A skin abscess is submitted for mycobacterial culture on a patient who scraped his hand while cleaning his fish aquarium. The technologist should:

a. inoculate one set of media at 30°C and one at 35°C-37°C
b. set up an anaerobic culture in addition to acid-fast culture
c. process the specimen immediately upon receipt
d. keep inoculated media under a constant light source

*378. A beta-hemolytic gram-positive coccus was isolated from the cerebrospinal fluid of a 2-day-old infant with signs of meningitis. The isolate grew on sheep blood agar under aerobic conditions and was resistant to a bacitracin disk. Which of the following should be performed for the identification of the organism?

a. oxidase production
b. catalase formation
c. CAMP test
d. esculin hydrolysis

*379. An outbreak of *Staphylococcus aureus* has occurred in a hospital nursery. In order to establish the epidemiological source of the outbreak, it is helpful to do:

a. plasmid fingerprinting
b. serological typing
c. coagulase testing
d. catalase testing

*380. An isolate from a stool culture gives the following growth characteristics and biochemical reactions:

| MacConkey agar | Colorless colonies |
| Hektoen agar | Yellow-orange colonies |
| TSI | Acid slant/acid butt, no gas, no H$_2$S |
| Urea | Positive |

These screening reactions are consistent with which of the following enteric pathogens?

a. *Yersinia enterocolitica*
b. *Shigella sonnei*
c. *Vibrio parahaemolyticus*
d. *Campylobacter jejuni*

*381. In the disk diffusion method of determining antibiotic susceptibility, the size of the inhibition zone used to indicate susceptibility has been determined by:

a. testing 30 strains of one genus of bacteria
b. correlating the zone size with minimum inhibitory concentrations
c. correlating the zone size with minimum bactericidal concentrations
d. correlating the zone size with the antibiotic content of the disk


*382. A formed stool is received in the laboratory at 3 AM for ova and parasite exam. The night shift technologist is certain that the workload will prevent examination of the specimen until 6 AM when the next shift arrives. The technologist should:

a. request that a new specimen be collected after 6 AM
b. perform a zinc sulfate flotation procedure for eggs and hold the remaining specimen at room temperature
c. examine a direct prep for trophozoites and freeze the remaining specimen
d. preserve the specimen in formalin until it can be examined


*383. Serum samples collected from a patient with pneumonia demonstrate a rising antibody titer to *Legionella*. A bronchoalveolar lavage (BAL) specimen from this patient had a positive antigen test for *Legionella*, but no organisms were recovered from this specimen on buffered charcoal yeast extract (CYE) medium after 2 days of incubation. The best explanation is that the:

a. antibody titer represents an earlier infection
b. positive antigen test is a false positive
c. specimen was cultured on the wrong media
d. culture was not incubated long enough


*384. After 24 hours a blood culture from a newborn grows catalase-negative, gram-positive cocci. The bacterial colonies are small, translucent and beta-hemolytic on a blood agar plate. Biochemical test results of a pure culture are:

| | |
|---|---|
| Bacitracin | Susceptible |
| CAMP reaction | Positive |
| Bile esculin | Not hydrolyzed |
| 6.5% NaCl broth | No growth |

Assuming that all controls react properly and reactions are verified, the next step would be to:

a. perform a *Streptococcus* group typing
b. report the organism as *Streptococcus pneumoniae*
c. report the organism as *Staphylococcus aureus*
d. report the organism as *Staphylococcus epidermidis*

*385. Which of the following may be used as a positive quality control organism for the bile esculin test?

   a. *Staphylococcus epidermidis*
   b. *Staphylococcus aureus*
   c. group A *Streptococcus*
   d. group D *Enterococcus*


*386. A sputum specimen from a patient with a known *Klebsiella pneumoniae* infection is received in the laboratory for fungus culture. The proper procedure for handling this specimen is to:

   a. reject the current specimen and request a repeat culture when the bacterial organism is no longer present
   b. incubate culture tubes at room temperature in order to inhibit the bacterial organism
   c. include media that have cycloheximide and chloramphenicol added to inhibit bacterial organisms and saprophytic fungi
   d. perform a direct PAS stain; if no fungal organisms are seen, reject the specimen


*387. During the past month, *Staphylococcus epidermidis* has been isolated from blood cultures at two to three times the rate from the previous year. The most logical explanation for the increase in these isolates is that:

   a. the blood culture media are contaminated with this organism
   b. the hospital ventilation system is contaminated with *Staphylococcus epidermidis*
   c. there has been a break in proper skin preparation before blood drawing
   d. a relatively virulent isolate is being spread from patient to patient


*388. Filters generally used in biological safety cabinets to protect the laboratory worker from particulates and aerosols generated by microbiology manipulations are:

   a. fiberglass
   b. HEPA
   c. APTA
   d. charcoal


*389. A jaundiced 7-year-old boy, with a history of playing in a pond in a rat-infested area, has a urine specimen submitted for a direct dark-field examination. Several spiral organisms are seen. Which of the following organisms would most likely be responsible for the patient's condition?

   a. *Spirillum minor*
   b. *Streptobacillus moniliformis*
   c. *Listeria monocytogenes*
   d. *Leptospira interrogans*

*390. An anaerobic gram-positive bacillus with subterminal spores was isolated from a peritoneal abscess. The most likely identification of this organism is:

a. *Bacillus cereus*
b. *Clostridium septicum*
c. *Eubacterium lentum*
d. *Bifidobacterium dentium*

*391. An aspirated specimen of purulent material was obtained from a brain abscess. After 24 hours' incubation, pinpoint colonies grew on sheep blood and small, yellowish colonies grew on chocolate. Gram stain of the organism showed gram-negative cocci. Results of carbohydrate degradation studies were as follows:

| Dextrose | Acid |
|----------|----------|
| Maltose | Acid |
| Sucrose | Acid |
| Lactose | Negative |

Additional testing revealed that the organism was oxidase positive and beta-galactosidase negative. The organism is most likely *Neisseria*:

a. *meningitidis*
b. *sicca*
c. *lactamica*
d. *gonorrhoeae*

*392. A fecal specimen inoculated to xylose lysine deoxycholate (XLD) and Hektoen enteric (HE) media produced colonies with black centers. Additional testing results are as follows:

| Biochemical Screen | | Serological Testing | |
|----------|----------|----------|----------|
| Glucose | Positive | Polyvalent | No agglutination |
| H₂S | Positive | Group A | No agglutination |
| Lysine decarboxylase | Positive | Group B₁ | No agglutination |
| Urea | Negative | Group C | No agglutination |
| ONPG | Negative | Group D | No agglutination |
| Indole | Positive | Group Vi | No agglutination |

The most probable identification is:

a. *Salmonella choleraesuis*
b. *Edwardsiella tarda*
c. *Salmonella typhi*
d. *Shigella sonnei*

*393. An organism frequently isolated from burn wounds and often associated with nosocomial infections has the following biochemical reactions:

| | |
|---|---|
| Oxidase | Positive |
| OF glucose | Oxidizer |
| Pyocyanin | Positive |

The organism is most likely:

a. *Enterobacter sakazakii*
b. *Pseudomonas aeruginosa*
c. *Serratia marcescens*
d. *Chromobacterium violaceum*

*394. A technologist is reading a Gram stain from a CSF and observes small structures suggestive of gram-negative coccobacilli. Chemistry and hematology CSF results that would indicate bacterial meningitis include:

| | WBC | Glucose | Protein |
|---|---|---|---|
| a. | increased | increased | increased |
| b. | decreased | decreased | decreased |
| c. | increased | decreased | increased |
| d. | decreased | increased | decreased |

*395. An isolate from a cornea infection had the following culture results:

| | |
|---|---|
| Sabouraud dextrose | White and cottony at 2 days, rose color at 6 days |
| Slide culture | Slender sickle shape micro- and macroconidia |

The most likely organism is:

a. *Acremonium* sp
b. *Petriellidium* sp
c. *Fusarium* sp
d. *Geotrichum* sp

*396. Of the following, the organism MOST commonly isolated from spinal fluid of children less than 5 years of age is:

a. *Listeria monocytogenes*
b. *Haemophilus influenzae*
c. *Neisseria gonorrhoeae*
d. *Neisseria meningitidis*

*397. A yeast isolate from a CSF specimen produced the following results:

| | |
|---|---|
| India ink | No encapsulated yeast cells |
| Cryptococcal antigen | Negative |
| Urea | Negative |
| Germ tube | Negative |

What should the technologist do next to identify this organism?

a.  inoculate Niger seed agar
b.  ascospore stain
c.  cycloheximide susceptibility
d.  carbohydrate assimilation


*398. An organism recovered from a sputum specimen has the following characteristics:

| | |
|---|---|
| Culture | Growth at 7 days on Lowenstein-Jensen agar, incubated under aerobic conditions with $CO_2$ at 35°C |
| Gram stain | Delicate branching gram-positive rods |
| Acid-fast stain | Branching, filamentous, "partially" acid-fast bacterium |

These results are consistent with which of the following genera?

a.  *Nocardia*
b.  *Mycobacterium*
c.  *Actinomyces*
d.  *Streptomyces*


*399. Susceptibility testing performed on quality control organisms using a new media lot number yielded zone sizes that were too large for all antibiotics tested. The testing was repeated using media from a previously used lot number, and all zone sizes were acceptable. Which of the following best explains the unacceptable zone sizes?

a.  the antibiotic disks were not stored with the proper desiccant
b.  the depth of the media was too thick
c.  the depth of the media was too thin
d.  the antibiotic disks were not properly applied to the media


*400. The streptococci most likely to have a high MIC (minimum inhibitory concentration) with penicillin are:

a.  enterococci
b.  unable to grow in 6.5% NaCl solution
c.  typed as Lancefield group A streptococci
d.  susceptible to bacitracin

*401. A technologist repeatedly misses tubercle bacilli when examining stained smears for acid-fast bacilli. What plan of action should the supervisor FIRST take to correct this problem?

   a. Issue a written warning.
   b. Send the employee to a workshop to improve his/her knowledge.
   c. Review the diagnostic criteria with the employee and monitor progress.
   d. Reassign the employee to another part of the laboratory.

*402. The quickest and most direct sensitive antigen detection test for *Haemophilus influenzae* in body fluids is:

   a. countercurrent immunoelectrophoresis
   b. microtiter indirect immunofluorescence
   c. latex agglutination test
   d. fluorescent-antibody test

*403. In reviewing the number of *Mycobacterium* isolates for the current year, it was noted that there were 76% fewer isolates than the previous year (115 vs 28). The technologist in charge of the area has documented that the quality control of media, reagents, and stains has been acceptable and there has been no gross contamination of the cultures noted. The most appropriate course of action to pursue would be:

   a. stop use of commercial media and produce in-house
   b. change to different formulations of egg- and agar-based media
   c. change over to the Bactec™ system for isolation of *Mycobacterium*
   d. review the digestion and decontamination procedure

*404. After proficiency in performing disk diffusion susceptibility tests is demonstrated, the frequency of quality control can be reduced from daily to:

   a. twice a week
   b. every week
   c. every other week
   d. every month

*405. The lab has been using a latex agglutination assay to detect *Clostridium difficile* in stools, which probably identifies a nontoxin cell wall antigen. You are considering adoption of an EIA method that detects *Clostridium difficile* toxin A. Which of the following would provide the best comparison?

   a. latex agglutination vs culture on cycloserine cefoxitin-egg-fructose agar
   b. latex agglutination vs EIA vs cell culture cytotoxin assay
   c. EIA vs culture on cycloserine cefoxitin-egg-fructose agar
   d. EIA vs cell culture cytotoxin assay

*406. Enterococcal isolates from a patient with a case of endocarditis should be tested for routine susceptibility and:

a. screened for high-level aminoglycoside resistance
b. checked for tolerance
c. assayed for serum antimicrobial activity
d. routinely speciated


*407. A *Staphylococcus aureus* isolate has an intermediate MIC of 4 μg/mL to oxacillin. There is uncertainty whether this represents an oxacillin (heteroresistant) resistant strain or a hyper-producer of β-lactamase. If the strain is heteroresistant the expected results for the oxacillin (OXA) and the ampicillin-clavulanic (AMP-CLAV) acid would be:

| | OXA | AMP-CLAV |
|------|-----|----------|
| a. | S | S |
| b. | S | R |
| c. | R | S |
| d. | R | R |


*408. To quality control the autoclave, a vial of *Bacillus stearothemophilus* is autoclaved and should then be:

a. inoculated to blood agar
b. incubated at 37°C
c. inoculated to chocolate agar
d. incubated at 56°C


*409. When grown in the dark, yellow to orange pigmentation of the colonies is usually demonstrated by:

a. *Mycobacterium tuberculosis*
b. *Mycobacterium kansasii*
c. Battey strains
d. scotochromogens


*410. The mycobacteria that produce a deep yellow or orange pigment in both the dark and light are:

a. photochromogens
b. scotochromogens
c. nonphotochromogens
d. rapid growers

*411. *Candida albicans* differs from other *Candida* species in that *Candida albicans*:

    a. is not pathogenic to man
    b. shows budding
    c. ferments carbohydrates
    d. produces chlamydospores on cornmeal agar

*412. A sputum specimen received at 8 AM for an AFB smear reveals acid-fast bacilli. An additional sputum is submitted that afternoon. This specimen was concentrated by the NALC-sodium hydroxide method, inoculated on two Lowenstein-Jensen slants, and held for 8 weeks at 35°C in 5%-10% $CO_2$. No growth occurs. The best explanation is that:

    a. the hypochlorite technique is a better concentration procedure
    b. an improper specimen was submitted for culture
    c. improper media was used for culture
    d. cultures were held for an insufficient period of time

*413. Which of the following procedures should be performed to confirm that an unknown mold is one of the pathogenic dimorphic fungi?

    a. animal inoculation
    b. culture conversion to yeast form
    c. demonstration of sexual and asexual reproduction
    d. serological studies

*414. The best method to detect infections due to rubella, Epstein-Barr, and human immunodeficiency viruses is:

    a. antigen detection by EIA
    b. cell culture
    c. antigen detection by Western blot
    d. antibody detection by EIA

*415. Safe handling and disposal of laboratory generated infectious wastes require:

    a. disinfection of all waste
    b. thorough mixing of infectious and noninfectious wastes
    c. separation of infectious and noninfectious wastes
    d. incineration of all waste

*416. The proper blood-to-broth ratio for blood cultures to reduce the antibacterial effect of serum in adults is:

    a. 1:2
    b. 1:3
    c. 1:10
    d. 1:30

*417. The major features by which molds are routinely identified are:

    a. mode of sporulation, morphology and arrangement of spores
    b. biochemical reactions and mycelial morphology
    c. mycelial morphology and selective media
    d. specialized sexual reproductive structures

*418. Which organism fails to grow on artificial media or in cell cultures?

    a. *Chlamydia trachomatis*
    b. *Neisseria gonorrhoeae*
    c. *Treponema pallidum*
    d. herpes simplex virus

*419. An unusual number of *Mycobacteria gordonae* have been isolated. This organism is reported as a "probable contaminant." The MOST likely source is:

    a. an outbreak of infections due to *Mycobacteria gordonae*
    b. contamination by water organisms
    c. contamination of commercial Lowenstein-Jensen tubes
    d. contamination of the specimen collection containers

*420. The presence of *Haemophilus influenzae* in CSF can be rapidly detected by:

    a. differential staining
    b. bacterial antigen testing
    c. processing in the Bactec™
    d. cytocentrifugation

# Microbiology Answer Key

| | | | | |
|---|---|---|---|---|
| 1. b | 42. a | 83. c | 124. c | 165. c |
| 2. d | 43. a | 84. d | 125. d | 166. a |
| 3. d | 44. d | 85. a | 126. a | 167. c |
| 4. b | 45. c | 86. b | 127. a | 168. b |
| 5. b | 46. d | 87. b | 128. a | 169. c |
| 6. d | 47. c | 88. d | 129. c | 170. d |
| 7. d | 48. c | 89. d | 130. a | 171. b |
| 8. d | 49. a | 90. b | 131. a | 172. a |
| 9. b | 50. c | 91. c | 132. b | 173. d |
| 10. d | 51. c | 92. d | 133. b | 174. d |
| 11. a | 52. c | 93. d | 134. d | 175. d |
| 12. c | 53. d | 94. b | 135. a | 176. d |
| 13. d | 54. c | 95. c | 136. a | 177. c |
| 14. d | 55. a | 96. c | 137. c | 178. b |
| 15. a | 56. a | 97. c | 138. d | 179. b |
| 16. c | 57. d | 98. a | 139. d | 180. b |
| 17. d | 58. b | 99. d | 140. b | 181. c |
| 18. d | 59. b | 100. d | 141. a | 182. d |
| 19. c | 60. c | 101. b | 142. a | 183. d |
| 20. d | 61. d | 102. c | 143. b | 184. b |
| 21. b | 62. c | 103. d | 144. c | 185. b |
| 22. a | 63. a | 104. c | 145. c | 186. d |
| 23. b | 64. d | 105. c | 146. b | 187. d |
| 24. d | 65. b | 106. c | 147. b | 188. a |
| 25. b | 66. a | 107. d | 148. b | 189. c |
| 26. b | 67. b | 108. d | 149. c | 190. b |
| 27. a | 68. d | 109. c | 150. d | 191. d |
| 28. d | 69. a | 110. b | 151. b | 192. d |
| 29. a | 70. c | 111. b | 152. c | 193. d |
| 30. c | 71. b | 112. b | 153. a | 194. a |
| 31. c | 72. c | 113. b | 154. a | 195. d |
| 32. a | 73. b | 114. a | 155. b | 196. b |
| 33. a | 74. d | 115. c | 156. a | 197. a |
| 34. a | 75. a | 116. a | 157. a | 198. a |
| 35. a | 76. a | 117. d | 158. b | 199. b |
| 36. d | 77. c | 118. c | 159. d | 200. d |
| 37. d | 78. a | 119. b | 160. c | 201. b |
| 38. c | 79. d | 120. b | 161. c | 202. c |
| 39. c | 80. d | 121. b | 162. c | 203. b |
| 40. b | 81. c | 122. d | 163. c | 204. c |
| 41. a | 82. b | 123. d | 164. d | 205. d |

| | | | | |
|---|---|---|---|---|
| 206. d | 249. d | 292. b | 335. d | 378. c |
| 207. a | 250. d | 293. d | 336. c | 379. a |
| 208. b | 251. d | 294. a | 337. c | 380. a |
| 209. d | 252. d | 295. b | 338. c | 381. b |
| 210. a | 253. d | 296. c | 339. c | 382. d |
| 211. c | 254. d | 297. c | 340. a | 383. d |
| 212. d | 255. a | 298. d | 341. d | 384. a |
| 213. a | 256. b | 299. b | 342. c | 385. d |
| 214. b | 257. d | 300. c | 343. b | 386. c |
| 215. c | 258. a | 301. c | 344. d | 387. c |
| 216. a | 259. b | 302. a | 345. c | 388. b |
| 217. a | 260. b | 303. d | 346. d | 389. d |
| 218. b | 261. d | 304. b | 347. d | 390. b |
| 219. a | 262. c | 305. b | 348. d | 391. b |
| 220. c | 263. b | 306. d | 349. d | 392. b |
| 221. b | 264. a | 307. d | 350. c | 393. b |
| 222. d | 265. a | 308. c | 351. d | 394. c |
| 223. c | 266. d | 309. b | 352. a | 395. c |
| 224. d | 267. a | 310. b | 353. d | 396. b |
| 225. a | 268. c | 311. a | 354. d | 397. d |
| 226. a | 269. b | 312. c | 355. c | 398. a |
| 227. a | 270. a | 313. a | 356. d | 399. c |
| 228. b | 271. d | 314. d | 357. b | 400. a |
| 229. b | 272. b | 315. c | 358. a | 401. c |
| 230. b | 273. c | 316. a | 359. b | 402. c |
| 231. d | 274. d | 317. d | 360. c | 403. d |
| 232. a | 275. c | 318. d | 361. c | 404. b |
| 233. c | 276. d | 319. c | 362. c | 405. b |
| 234. b | 277. b | 320. c | 363. d | 406. a |
| 235. d | 278. a | 321. c | 364. c | 407. d |
| 236. d | 279. d | 322. d | 365. c | 408. d |
| 237. c | 280. a | 323. b | 366. b | 409. d |
| 238. a | 281. a | 324. a | 367. a | 410. b |
| 239. d | 282. a | 325. d | 368. c | 411. d |
| 240. d | 283. a | 326. d | 369. b | 412. b |
| 241. c | 284. d | 327. d | 370. b | 413. b |
| 242. c | 285. d | 328. d | 371. c | 414. d |
| 243. d | 286. a | 329. d | 372. d | 415. c |
| 244. b | 287. b | 330. b | 373. a | 416. c |
| 245. c | 288. b | 331. b | 374. d | 417. a |
| 246. c | 289. d | 332. b | 375. b | 418. c |
| 247. d | 290. c | 333. d | 376. c | 419. b |
| 248. b | 291. c | 334. a | 377. a | 420. b |

# CHAPTER 15

## *Urinalysis and Body Fluids*

*The following items have been identified as appropriate for both entry level medical technologists and medical laboratory technicians.*

1. Which of the following would be affected by allowing a urine specimen to remain at room temperature for three hours before analysis?

   a. occult blood
   b. specific gravity
   c. pH
   d. protein

2. A technologist performed a stat microscopic urinalysis and reported the following:

| | |
|---|---|
| WBCs | 10 to 13 |
| RBCs | 2 to 6 |
| Hyaline casts | 5 to 7 |
| Bacteria | 1+ |

The centrifuge tube was not discarded and the urine sediment was reevaluated microscopically 5 hours after the above results were reported. A second technologist reported the same results, except 2+ bacteria and no hyaline casts were found. The most probable explanation for the second technologist's findings is:

   a. sediment was not agitated before preparing the microscope slide
   b. casts dissolved due to decrease in urine pH
   c. casts dissolved due to increase in urine pH
   d. casts were never present in this specimen

3. Which of the following urinary parameters are measured during the course of concentration and dilution tests to assess renal tubular function?

   a. urea, nitrogen, and creatinine
   b. osmolality and specific gravity
   c. sodium and chloride
   d. sodium and osmolality

Questions 4-5 refer to the following illustration:

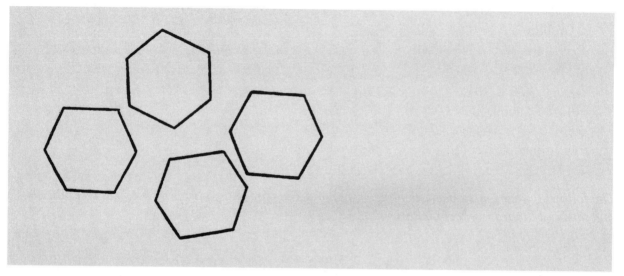

4. Colorless crystals, such as those depicted above, were seen in a urine specimen. This patient is most likely to have which of the following clinical conditions?

   a. gout
   b. renal damage
   c. bilirubinuria
   d. cystinuria

5. The colorless crystals depicted above would be found in a urine which has a(n):

   a. acid pH
   b. alkaline pH
   c. neutral pH
   d. variable pH

6. The part of the kidney in which there is selective retention and excretion of various substances and in which the concentration of urine occurs is the:

   a. glomerulus
   b. papilla
   c. tubule
   d. ureter

7. A urinalysis performed on a 27-year-old woman yields the following results:

Specific gravity = 1.008
pH = 5.0
Protein = 2+
Glucose = negative
Ketones = negative
Bilirubin = negative
Blood = 3+
Nitrite = negative
Leukocytes = positive
Urobilinogen = 0.1 EU/dL

Microscopic:
WBC/HPF = 20-30
RBC/HPF = 30-55
Casts/LPF
  Hyaline = 5-7
  RBC = 2-5
  Coarse granular = 2-3
  Waxy = 1-3
Uric acid crystals = moderate

The above data are MOST consistent with:

a. yeast infections
b. pyelonephritis
c. bacterial cystitis
d. glomerulonephritis

8. A urinalysis performed on a 27-year-old woman yields the following results:

Specific gravity = 1.008
pH = 5.0
Protein = 2+
Glucose = negative
Ketones = negative
Bilirubin = negative
Blood = 3+
Nitrite = negative
Leukocytes = positive
Urobilinogen = 0.1 EU/dL

Microscopic:
WBC/HPF = 20-30
RBC/HPF = 30-55
Casts/LPF
  Hyaline = 5-7
  Epithelial = 1-3
  Coarse granular = 2-3
  Waxy = 1-3
Uric acid crystals = moderate

The above data are consistent with:

a. nephrotic syndrome
b. gout
c. biliary obstruction
d. chronic renal disease

9. Which of the following urine results is most apt to be changed by prolonged exposure to light?

a. pH
b. protein
c. ketones
d. bilirubin

10. A urine specimen comes to the laboratory 7 hours after it is obtained. It is acceptable for culture only if the specimen has been stored:

    a. at room temperature
    b. at 4°C-7°C
    c. frozen
    d. with a preservative additive

11. While performing a urinalysis, a technologist notices that the urine specimen has a fruity odor. This patient's urine most likely contains:

    a. acetone
    b. bilirubin
    c. coliform bacilli
    d. porphyrin

12. The pH of a urine specimen measures the:

    a. free sodium ions
    b. free hydrogen ions
    c. total acid excretion
    d. volatile acids

13. Some regional and public health laboratories carry out mass screening tests on the urine of newborns for a genetic disorder involving metabolism of:

    a. fructose
    b. galactose
    c. glucose
    d. lactose

14. A test area of a urine reagent strip is impregnated with only sodium nitroprusside. This section will react with:

    a. acetoacetic (diacetic) acid
    b. leukocyte esterase
    c. beta-hydroxybutyric acid
    d. ferric chloride

15. Myoglobinuria is MOST likely to be noted in urine specimens from patients with which of the following disorders?

    a. hemolytic anemias
    b. lower urinary tract infections
    c. myocardial infarctions
    d. paroxysmal nocturnal hemoglobinuria

16. The method of choice for performing a specific gravity measurement of urine following administration of x-ray contrast dyes is:

   a. reagent strip
   b. refractometer
   c. urinometer
   d. densitometer


17. All casts typically contain:

   a. albumin
   b. globulin
   c. immunoglobulins G and M
   d. Tamm-Horsfall glycoprotein


18. The presence of leukocytes in urine is known as:

   a. chyluria
   b. hematuria
   c. leukocytosis
   d. pyuria


19. The amber yellow color of urine is primarily due to:

   a. urochrome pigment
   b. methemoglobin
   c. bilirubin
   d. homogentisic acid


20. Urine reagent strips should be stored in a(n):

   a. refrigerator (4°C-7°C)
   b. incubator (37°C)
   c. cool dry area
   d. open jar exposed to air


21. An ammonia-like odor is characteristically associated with urine from patients who:

   a. are diabetic
   b. have hepatitis
   c. have an infection with *Proteus* sp
   d. have a yeast infection

22. Routine screening of urine samples for glycosuria is performed primarily to detect:

    a. glucose
    b. galactose
    c. bilirubin
    d. ketones

23. Which of the following factors will NOT interfere with the reagent strip test for leukocytes?

    a. ascorbic acid
    b. formaldehyde
    c. nitrite
    d. urinary protein level of 500 mg/dL

24. Hyaline casts are usually found:

    a. in the center of the coverslip
    b. under subdued light
    c. under very bright light
    d. in the supernatant

25. A technologist is having trouble differentiating between red blood cells, oil droplets, and yeast cells on a urine microscopy. Acetic acid should be added to the sediment to:

    a. lyse the yeast cells
    b. lyse the red blood cells
    c. dissolve the oil droplets
    d. crenate the red blood cells

26. A patient's urinalysis revealed a positive bilirubin and a decreased urobilinogen level. These results are associated with:

    a. hemolytic disease
    b. biliary obstruction
    c. hepatic disease
    d. urinary tract infection

27. Red colored urine may be due to:

    a. bilirubin
    b. excess urobilin
    c. myoglobin
    d. homogentisic acid

28. A microscopic examination of a urine sediment reveals ghost cells. These red blood cells were most likely lysed due to:

    a. greater than 2% glucose concentrations
    b. specific gravity less than 1.007
    c. large amounts of ketone bodies
    d. neutral pH

29. A urine specimen is analyzed for glucose by a glucose oxidase reagent strip and a copper reduction test. If both results are positive, which of the following interpretations is correct?

    a. Galactose is present.
    b. Glucose is present.
    c. Lactose is not present.
    d. Sucrose is not present.

30. False results in urobilinogen testing may occur if the urine specimen is:

    a. exposed to light
    b. adjusted to a neutral pH
    c. cooled to room temperature
    d. collected in a nonsterile container

31. Using polarized light microscopy, which of the following urinary elements are birefringent?

    a. cholesterol
    b. triglycerides
    c. fatty acids
    d. neutral fats

32. An antidiuretic hormone deficiency is associated with a:

    a. specific gravity around 1.031
    b. low specific gravity
    c. high specific gravity
    d. variable specific gravity

33. Which of the following casts is characteristically associated with acute pyelonephritis?

    a. red cell
    b. white cell
    c. waxy
    d. fatty

34. The type of urinary cast that is most characteristically associated with glomerular injury is a(n):

   a. epithelial cell
   b. white cell
   c. red cell
   d. fatty


35. Glitter cells are a microscopic finding of:

   a. red blood cells in hypertonic urine
   b. red blood cells in hypotonic urine
   c. white blood cells in hypertonic urine
   d. white blood cells in hypotonic urine


36. Bilirubinuria may be associated with:

   a. strenuous exercise
   b. increased destruction of platelets
   c. viral hepatitis
   d. hemolytic anemia


37. A reagent strip test for hemoglobin has been reported positive. Microscopic examination fails to yield red blood cells. This patient's condition can be called:

   a. hematuria
   b. hemoglobinuria
   c. oliguria
   d. hemosiderinuria


38. Polyuria is usually correlated with:

   a. acute glomerulonephritis
   b. diabetes mellitus
   c. hepatitis
   d. tubular damage


39. A urine's specific gravity is directly proportional to its:

   a. turbidity
   b. dissolved solids
   c. salt content
   d. sugar content

40. Which of the following inorganic substances are excreted in the urine in the largest amount?

    a. urea and NaCl
    b. creatine and NaCl
    c. creatine and ammonia
    d. urea and glucose

41. The confirmatory test for a positive protein result by the reagent strip method uses:

    a. Ehrlich's reagent
    b. a diazo reaction
    c. sulfosalicylic acid
    d. a copper reduction tablet

42. Which of the following casts is most likely to be found in healthy people?

    a. hyaline
    b. red blood cell
    c. waxy
    d. white blood cell

43. Waxy casts are most easily differentiated from hyaline casts by their:

    a. color
    b. size
    c. granules
    d. refractivity

44. A milky colored urine from a 24-year-old woman would most likely contain:

    a. spermatozoa
    b. many white blood cells
    c. red blood cells
    d. bilirubin

45. When performing a routine urinalysis, the technologist notes a 2+ protein result. He should:

    a. request another specimen
    b. confirm with the acid precipitation test
    c. test for Bence Jones protein
    d. report the result obtained without further testing

46. When using the sulfosalicylic acid test, false-positive protein results may occur in the presence of:

    a. ketones
    b. alkali
    c. glucose
    d. radiographic contrast media

47. The clarity of a urine sample should be determined:

    a. using glass tubes only, never plastic
    b. following thorough mixing of the specimen
    c. after addition of sulfosalicylic acid
    d. after the specimen cools to room temperature

48. When employing the urine reagent strip method, a false-positive protein result may occur in the presence of:

    a. large amounts of glucose
    b. x-ray contrast media
    c. Bence Jones protein
    d. highly alkaline urine

49. A patient with uncontrolled diabetes mellitus will most likely have:

    a. pale urine with a high specific gravity
    b. concentrated urine with a high specific gravity
    c. pale urine with a low specific gravity
    d. dark urine with a high specific gravity

50. Which of the following is the average volume of urine excreted by an adult in 24 hours?

    a. 750 mL
    b. 1000 mL
    c. 1500 mL
    d. 2000 mL

51. The normal pH value for a healthy adult's urine is:

    a. 4.5
    b. 5.0
    c. 6.0
    d. 8.0

52. Normal urine primarily consists of:

    a. water, protein, and sodium
    b. water, urea, and protein
    c. water, urea, and sodium chloride
    d. water, urea, and bilirubin

53. Patients with diabetes mellitus have urine with:

    a. decreased volume and decreased specific gravity
    b. decreased volume and increased specific gravity
    c. increased volume and decreased specific gravity
    d. increased volume and increased specific gravity

54. Cessation of urine flow is defined as:

    a. azotemia
    b. dysuria
    c. diuresis
    d. anuria

55. Upon standing at room temperature a urine pH typically:

    a. decreases
    b. increases
    c. remains the same
    d. changes depending on bacterial concentration

56. Antidiuretic hormone regulates the reabsorption of:

    a. water
    b. glucose
    c. potassium
    d. calcium

57. Calibration of refractometers is done by measuring the specific gravity of:

    a. distilled water and protein
    b. distilled water and glucose
    c. distilled water and sodium chloride
    d. distilled water and urea

58. A 17-year-old girl decided to go on a starvation diet. After 1 week of starving herself, what substance would most likely be found in her urine?

a. protein
b. ketones
c. glucose
d. blood

59. Which of the following crystals may be found in acidic urine?

a. calcium carbonate
b. calcium oxalate
c. calcium phosphate
d. triple phosphate

60. Which of the following reagents is used to react with ketones in the urine?

a. sodium nitroprusside
b. acetoacetic acid
c. acetone
d. beta-hydroxybutyric acid

61. A woman in her ninth month of pregnancy has a urine sugar that is negative with the urine reagent strip but gives a positive reaction with the copper reduction method. The sugar most likely responsible for these results is:

a. maltose
b. galactose
c. glucose
d. lactose

62. Which of the following casts is most indicative of severe renal disease?

a. hemoglobin
b. granular
c. cellular
d. waxy

63. Which of the following is the primary reagent in the copper reduction tablet?

a. sodium carbonate
b. copper sulfate
c. glucose oxidase
d. polymerized diazonium salt

64. Which of the following is an abnormal crystal described as a hexagonal plate?

   a. cystine
   b. tyrosine
   c. leucine
   d. cholesterol


65. Which of the following cells is the largest?

   a. glitter
   b. WBC
   c. transitional epithelial
   d. renal epithelial


66. What cell is MOST commonly associated with vaginal contamination?

   a. white
   b. transitional
   c. squamous
   d. glitter


67. Urinary calculi most often consist of:

   a. calcium
   b. uric acid
   c. leucine
   d. cystine


68. Small round objects found in a urine sediment that dissolve after addition of dilute acetic acid and do not polarize most likely are:

   a. air bubbles
   b. calcium oxalate
   c. red blood cells
   d. yeast cells


69. Tiny colorless, dumbbell-shaped crystals were found in an alkaline urine sediment. They most likely are:

   a. calcium oxalate
   b. calcium carbonate
   c. calcium phosphate
   d. amorphous phosphate

70. A 24-year-old obese diabetic woman had the following blood and urine test results from specimens obtained at the same time:

pH = 7.5
Protein = 30 mg/dL
Glucose = negative
Ketones = 15 mg/dL
Bilirubin = negative
Blood = negative
Nitrite = negative
Urobilinogen = 1 EU/dL
Specific gravity = 1.008

Microscopic:
Epithelial cells = 3-5
Bacteria = many
Yeast = many
Amorphous = moderate

Blood sugar = 195 mg/dL

Which of the following is the MOST likely explanation for the negative urine glucose finding?

a. There is a false-negative glucose due to oxidizing contaminants.
b. There is a false-negative glucose due to the alkaline pH.
c. The specimen is probably old and the bacteria and yeast have consumed the glucose.
d. Glucose would not be present in the urine specimen since the blood sugar was normal.

71. A patient has two separate urinalysis reports that contain the following data:

| | Report A | Report B |
|---|---|---|
| Specific gravity | 1.004 | 1.017 |
| pH 5.5 | 7.0 | |
| Protein | Negative | Trace |
| Glucose | Negative | Trace |
| Blood | Negative | Negative |
| Microscopic | Rare epithelial cells | Occasional granular cast |
| | | Rare hyaline cast |
| | | Moderate epithelial cells |

Which of the following statements best explains these results?

a. The protein, glucose, and microscopic findings of A are falsely negative because of the specific gravity.
b. The protein and glucose are falsely positive in B due to the specific gravity.
c. The microscopic findings of A is falsely negative because of the pH.
d. The microscopic findings of B is falsely positive because of the pH.

72. A clean-catch urine sample is submitted to the laboratory for routine urinalysis and culture. The routine urinalysis is done first, and the specimen is then sent to microbiology for culture. The specimen should:

a. be centrifuged and the supernatant cultured
b. be rejected due to possible contamination from routine urinalysis
c. not be cultured if no bacteria are seen
d. be immediately processed for culture regardless of urinalysis results

73. A 52-year-old man has urine glucose measurements performed as part of a 3-hour glucose tolerance test. The test results are as follows:

| Time | Serum Glucose | Urine Glucose |
|------|---------------|---------------|
| Fasting | 82 mg/dL | Negative |
| 1/2 hour | 120 mg/dL | Negative |
| 1 hour | 190 mg/dL | Negative |
| 2 hours | 115 mg/dL | 1+ |
| 3 hours | 95 mg/dL | Trace |

The best explanation for these findings is that the:

a. serum level must exceed the threshold level before glucose is filtered by the renal glomeruli
b. serum level must exceed the threshold level before reabsorption of glucose is exceeded
c. tested patient probably has renal glucosuria
d. tested patient probably has diabetes mellitus

74. A 24-hour urine from a man who had no evidence of kidney impairment was sent to the laboratory for hormone determination. The volume was 600 mL, but there was some question as to the completeness of the 24-hour collection. The next step would be to:

a. perform the hormone determination, since 600 mL is a normal urine 24-hour volume
b. check the creatinine level; if it is less than 1 g do the procedure
c. report the hormone determination in milligrams per deciliter in case the specimen was incomplete
d. check the creatinine level; if it is greater than 1 g do the procedure

75. The following urine results were obtained on a 25-year-old female:

Color = amber
Appearance = cloudy
Specific gravity = 1.015
pH = 5.0
Protein = 1+
Glucose = negative
Blood = small

Microscopic:
Bacteria = many
WBC casts = few
WBC/HPF = 30-40

These results are most compatible with:

a. glomerulonephritis
b. renal calculus
c. vaginitis
d. pyelonephritis

76. Urine samples should be examined within 1 hour of voiding because:

    a. red blood cells, leukocytes, and casts agglutinate after standing for several hours at room temperature
    b. urobilinogen increases and bilirubin decreases after prolonged exposure to light
    c. bacterial contamination will cause alkalinization of the urine
    d. ketones will increase due to bacterial and cellular metabolism


77. The results of a urinalysis on a first-morning specimen are:

| Specific gravity | 1.024 |
| pH | 8.5 |
| Protein | Negative |
| Glucose | Negative |
| Microscopic | Uric acid crystals |

The next step is to repeat the:

    a. microscopic examination
    b. protein and glucose
    c. specific gravity
    d. pH and microscopic examination


78. The principle of the reagent strip test for urine protein depends on:

    a. an enzyme reaction
    b. protein error of indicators
    c. copper reduction
    d. the toluidine reaction


79. After receiving a 24-hour urine sample for quantitative total protein analysis, the technician must first:

    a. subculture the urine for bacteria
    b. add the appropriate preservative
    c. screen for albumin using a dipstick
    d. measure the total volume


80. Which of the following is the best guide to consistent centrifugation?

    a. potentiometer setting
    b. armature settings
    c. tachometer readings
    d. rheostat readings

81. In addition to the sperm count in a fertility study, analysis of seminal fluid should also include:

    a. time of liquefaction, estimation of motility, morphology
    b. motility, morphology, test for alkaline phosphatase
    c. time of liquefaction, test for acid phosphatase, qualitative test for hemoglobin
    d. time of liquefaction, qualitative test for hemoglobin and motility

82. A physician attempts to aspirate a knee joint and obtains 0.1 mL of slightly bloody fluid. Addition of acetic acid results in turbidity and a clot. This indicates that:

    a. the fluid is synovial fluid
    b. plasma was obtained
    c. red blood cells caused a false-positive reaction
    d. the specimen is not adequate

83. A sperm count is diluted 1:20 and 50 sperm are counted in two large squares of the Neubauer counting chamber. The sperm count in mLs is:

    a. 5000
    b. 50,000
    c. 500,000
    d. 5,000,000

84. Ammonium sulfate was added to red urine. The urine had a positive reaction for blood, but no RBCs were seen on microscopic examination. After centrifugation the supernatant fluid is red. The abnormal color is caused by:

    a. Pyridium
    b. hemoglobin
    c. porphyrins
    d. myoglobin

85. Urine from a 50-year-old man was noted to turn dark red on standing. This change is caused by:

    a. glucose
    b. porphyrins
    c. urochrome
    d. creatinine

86. The principal mucin in synovial fluid is:

    a. hyaluronate
    b. albumin
    c. orosomucoid
    d. pepsin

87. A turbid cerebrospinal fluid is most commonly caused by:

    a. increased white blood cells
    b. increased protein
    c. increased glucose
    d. increased bacterial organisms

88. The synovial fluid easily forms small drops from the aspirating syringe. This viscosity is:

    a. normal
    b. increased
    c. associated with inflammation
    d. associated with hypothyroidism

89. Pleural transudates differ from pleural exudates in that transudates have:

    a. protein values of > 4 g/100 mL
    b. specific gravity values of > 1.020
    c. LD values of > 200 U/L
    d. relatively low cell counts

90. A urine tested with Clinitest exhibits a pass through reaction and is diluted by adding 2 drops of urine to 10 drops water. This is a dilution of:

    a. 1 to 4
    b. 1 to 5
    c. 1 to 6
    d. 1 to 8

91. The normal renal threshold for glucose in the adult is approximately:

    a. 50 mg/dL
    b. 100 mg/dL
    c. 160 mg/dL
    d. 300 mg/dL

92. Urine osmolality is related to:

    a. pH
    b. filtration
    c. specific gravity
    d. volume

93. A micropipet graduated to the tip and calibrated to contain should:

    a. be drained
    b. be rinsed
    c. not be blown out
    d. not be rinsed

94. The primary constituent of hyaline casts is:

    a. fat
    b. cells
    c. protein
    d. mucus

95. The knob between the eyepieces on a binocular microscope is used to:

    a. correct for optical differences between the right and left eyes
    b. adjust for distances between one's eyes
    c. change the magnification of the oculars
    d. improve the equivalent focus of the microscope

96. Urine that develops a port wine color after standing may contain:

    a. melanin
    b. porphyrins
    c. bilirubin
    d. urobilinogen

97. To avoid falsely elevated spinal fluid cell counts:

    a. use an aliquot from the first tube collected
    b. use only those specimens showing no turbidity
    c. centrifuge all specimens before counting
    d. select an aliquot from the last tube collected

98. The volume of urine excreted in a 24-hour period by an adult patient was 500 mL. This condition would be termed:

    a. anuria
    b. oliguria
    c. polyuria
    d. dysuria

99. Which of the following can give a false-negative urine protein reading?

    a. contamination with vaginal discharge
    b. heavy mucus
    c. presence of blood
    d. very dilute urine


100. An acid urine that contains hemoglobin will darken on standing due to the formation of:

    a. myoglobin
    b. sulfhemoglobin
    c. methemoglobin
    d. red blood cells


101. A centrifuge head has a diameter of 60 cm and spins at 3000 rpm. What is the maximum achievable $g$ force ($g = 0.00001$ x radius in cm x rpm$^2$)?

    a. 1.8$g$
    b. 2700$g$
    c. 27,000$g$
    d. 90,000$g$


102. Osmolality is a measure of:

    a. dissolved particles, including ions
    b. undissociated molecules only
    c. total salt concentration
    d. molecule size


103. A urine with an increased protein has a high specific gravity. Which of the following would be a more accurate measure of urine concentration?

    a. osmolality
    b. ketones
    c. refractive index
    d. pH


104. A 59-year-old man is evaluated for back pain. Urine studies (urinalysis by multiple reagent strip) include:

| Urinalysis | |
| --- | --- |
| Specific gravity | 1.017 |
| pH | 6.5 |
| Protein | Negative |
| Glucose | Negative |
| Blood | Negative |
| Microscopic | Rare epithelial cells |

Which of the following statements best explains these results?

a. The urine protein is falsely negative due to the specific gravity.
b. The urine protein is falsely negative because the method is not sensitive for Bence Jones protein.
c. The microscopic examination is falsely negative due to the specific gravity.
d. The electrophoresis is incorrect and should be repeated.

105. In most compound light microscopes, the ocular lens has a magnification of:

   a. 10x
   b. 40x
   c. 50x
   d. 100x

106. A positive result for bilirubin on a reagent strip should be followed up by:

   a. notifying the physician
   b. requesting a new specimen
   c. performing an Ictotest™
   d. performing a urobilinogen

107. Which parts of a microscope magnify the images observed?

   a. ocular and condenser
   b. objective and ocular
   c. aperture and objective
   d. diaphragm and condenser

108. The sequence of light through a microscope is:

   a. condenser, stage, objective
   b. iris diaphragm, condenser, ocular
   c. stage, condenser, iris, objective, ocular
   d. diaphragm, condenser, objective, ocular

109. The normal glomerular filtration rate is:

   a. 1 mL/min
   b. 120 mL/min
   c. 660 mL/min
   d. 1200 mL/min

110. Following the addition of acid, white precipitate in a cloudy urine sample dissolves. This most likely indicates the presence of:

    a. amorphous urates
    b. WBCs
    c. amorphous phosphates
    d. bacteria

*The remaining questions (\*) have been identified as more appropriate for the entry level medical technologist.*

*111. On bright-light microscopic examination of a urinary sediment, round refractile globules are noted in cells encapsulated within a hyaline matrix. A polarized-light microscopic examination of the urinary structure showed the globules to be birefringent in the shape of Maltese crosses. These urinary structures can be identified as:

    a. waxy casts associated with advanced tubular atrophy
    b. granular casts containing plasma protein aggregates
    c. crystal casts associated with obstruction due to tubular damage
    d. fatty casts containing lipid-laden renal tubular cells

*112. The following results were obtained on a urine specimen at 8 AM:

| | |
|---|---|
| pH | 5.5 |
| Protein | 2+ |
| Glucose | 3+ |
| Ketones | 3+ |
| Blood | Negative |
| Bilirubin | Positive |
| Nitrite | Positive |

If this urine specimen was stored uncapped at 5°C without preservation and retested at 2 PM, which of the following test results would be changed due to these storage conditions?

    a. glucose
    b. ketones
    c. protein
    d. nitrite

*113. Ketones in urine are due to:

    a. complete utilization of fatty acids
    b. incomplete fat metabolism
    c. high carbohydrate diets
    d. renal tubular dysfunction

*114. A reagent strip area impregnated with stabilized, diazotized 2,4-dichloroaniline will yield a positive reaction with:

a. bilirubin
b. hemoglobin
c. ketones
d. urobilinogen

*115. Round refractile globules noted on bright-light microscopy of a urinary sediment were birefringent with polarized-light and appeared as perfect Maltese crosses. These globules are most likely:

a. neutral fats
b. starch
c. triglycerides
d. cholesterol

*116. An urinalysis performed on a 2-week-old infant with diarrhea shows a negative reaction with the glucose oxidase reagent strip. A copper reduction tablet test should be performed to check the urine sample for the presence of:

a. glucose
b. galactose
c. bilirubin
d. ketones

*117. While performing an analysis of a baby's urine, the technologist notices the specimen to have a "mousy" odor. Of the following substances that may be excreted in urine, the one that MOST characteristically produces this odor is:

a. phenylpyruvic acid
b. acetone
c. coliform bacilli
d. porphyrin

*118. Isosthenuria is associated with a specific gravity, which is usually:

a. variable between 1.001 and 1.008
b. variable between 1.015 and 1.022
c. fixed around 1.010
d. fixed around 1.020

*119. Glycosuria may be due to:

    a. hypoglycemia
    b. increased renal threshold
    c. renal tubular dysfunction
    d. increased glomerular filtration rate

*120. Broad waxy casts are LEAST likely to be associated with:

    a. advanced tubular atrophy
    b. end-stage renal disease
    c. fatty degeneration tubular disease
    d. formation in a pathologically dilated tubule

*121. Use of a refractometer over a urinometer is preferred due to the fact that the refractometer uses a:

    a. large volume of urine and compensates for temperature
    b. small volume of urine and compensates for glucose
    c. small volume of urine and compensates for temperature
    d. small volume of urine and compensates for protein

*122. The protein section of the urine reagent strip is MOST sensitive to:

    a. albumin
    b. mucoprotein
    c. Bence Jones protein
    d. globulin

*123. A brown-black colored urine would most likely contain:

    a. bile pigment
    b. porphyrins
    c. melanin
    d. blood cells

*124. An abdominal fluid is submitted from surgery. The physician wants to determine if this fluid could be urine. The technologist should:

    a. perform a culture
    b. smell the fluid
    c. test for urea, creatinine, sodium, and chloride
    d. test for protein, glucose, and pH

*125. Microscopic analysis of a urine specimen yields a moderate amount of red blood cells in spite of a negative result for occult blood using a reagent strip. The technologist should determine if this patient has taken:

a. vitamin C
b. a diuretic
c. high blood pressure medicine
d. antibiotics

*126. A urine specimen collected from an apparently healthy 25-year-old man shortly after he finished eating lunch was cloudy but showed normal results on a multiple reagent strip analysis. The most likely cause of the turbidity is:

a. fat
b. white blood cells
c. urates
d. phosphates

*127. The fluid leaving the glomerulus normally has a specific gravity of:

a. 1.001
b. 1.010
c. 1.020
d. 1.030

*128. Refractive index is a comparison of:

a. light velocity in solutions with light velocity in solids
b. light velocity in air with light velocity in solutions
c. light scattering by air with light scattering by solutions
d. light scattering by particles in solution

*129. Oval fat bodies are defined as:

a. squamous epithelial cells that contain lipids
b. renal tubular epithelial cells that contain lipids
c. free-floating fat droplets
d. white blood cells with phagocytized lipids

*130. Which of the following ketone bodies is excreted in the largest amount in ketonuria?

a. acetone
b. acetoacetic acid
c. cholesterol
d. beta-hydroxybutyric acid

*131. White blood cell casts are most likely to indicate disease of the:

    a. bladder
    b. ureter
    c. urethra
    d. kidney

*132. Which of the following components is/are present in serum but NOT present in the glomerular filtrate?

    a. glucose
    b. amino acids
    c. urea
    d. large molecular weight proteins

*133. A patient with renal tubular acidosis would most likely excrete a urine with a:

    a. low pH
    b. high pH
    c. neutral pH
    d. variable pH

*134. A 21-year-old woman had glucose in her urine with a normal blood sugar. These findings are most consistent with:

    a. renal glycosuria
    b. diabetes insipidus
    c. diabetes mellitus
    d. alkaline tide

*135. Which of the following crystals appear as fine, silky needles?

    a. cholesterol
    b. leucine
    c. hemosiderin
    d. tyrosine

*136. Excess urine on the reagent test strip can turn a normal pH result into a falsely acidic pH when which of the following reagents runs into the pH pad?

    a. tetrabromphenol blue
    b. citrate buffer
    c. glucose oxidase
    d. alkaline copper sulfate

*137. A component seen during a microscopic urinalysis stains positively with Sudan III stain but does not polarize. This most likely is a:

    a. cholesterol ester
    b. neutral fat
    c. lipid
    d. leucine


*138. In which of the following metabolic diseases will urine turn dark brown to black upon standing?

    a. phenylketonuria
    b. alkaptonuria
    c. maple syrup disease
    d. aminoaciduria


*139. A urine specimen with an elevated urobilinogen and a negative bilirubin may indicate:

    a. obstruction of the biliary tract
    b. viral hepatitis
    c. hemolytic jaundice
    d. cirrhosis


*140. A 27-year-old woman with severe lower back pain has the following urinalysis test results:

| | |
|---|---|
| pH | 5.5 |
| Protein | Trace |
| Glucose | Negative |
| Ketones | Negative |
| Blood | Negative |
| Bilirubin | Negative |
| Nitrite | Negative |
| Urobilinogen | 0.1 EU/dL |
| Specific gravity | 1.018 |
| Sulfosalicylic acid for protein | 20 mg/dL |
| Microscopic: | |
| WBC | 3 to 5 |
| RBC | 25 to 50 |
| Epithelial cells | 3 to 5 |
| Mucous strands | Moderate |

Which of the following is the MOST likely explanation for the discrepancy in the blood portion of the urine reagent strip and the microscopic RBC finding?

    a. Oxidizing contaminants are causing a false-negative blood on the urine reagent strip.
    b. More red blood cells must be present in order for the blood portion to react.
    c. The red blood cells reported may actually be the round form of calcium oxalate crystals.
    d. The urine reagent strip is more sensitive to red blood cells than to hemoglobin.

*141. A 62-year-old patient with hyperlipoproteinemia has a large amount of protein in his urine. Microscopic analysis yields moderate to many fatty, waxy, granular, and cellular casts. Many oval fat bodies are also noted. This is most consistent with:

a. nephrotic syndrome
b. viral infection
c. acute pyelonephritis
d. acute glomerulonephritis

*142. A 42-year-old man is admitted to the emergency room with multiple abrasions, several broken bones, a fractured pelvis, and a crushed femur. The following urinalysis results are obtained:

| | |
|---|---|
| Clarity | Hazy |
| Color | Red-brown |
| Specific gravity | 1.026 |
| pH | 6.0 |
| Protein | 300 mg/dL |
| Glucose | Negative |
| Ketones | Negative |
| Blood | 4+ |
| Bilirubin | Negative |
| Nitrite | Negative |
| Urobilinogen | 0.1 EU/dL |
| Microscopic: | |
| Hemoglobin granular casts | 3-5 |

What is the MOST likely explanation for the discrepancy between the 4+ blood result, hemoglobin granular casts, and the complete absence of red cells on the microscopic?

a. There is a false-positive reaction for blood on the urine strip due to the large amount of protein.
b. The blood portion of the urine reagent strip is more sensitive to hemoglobin than intact red cells.
c. Red blood cells have been lysed due to the pH and the specific gravity.
d. The hemoglobin granular casts which were reported may actually be white blood cell casts.

*143. The following urinalysis results were obtained from an 18-year-old woman in labor:

| | |
|---|---|
| pH | 6.5 |
| Protein | 30 mg/dL |
| Glucose | 250 mg/dL |
| Ketones | Negative |
| Bilirubin | Small (color slightly abnormal) |
| Blood | Negative |

| | |
|---|---|
| Nitrite | Negative |
| Urobilinogen | 0.1 EU/dL |
| Specific gravity | 1.025 |
| Copper reduction test | 1.0 g/dL |
| Sulfosalicylic acid test for protein | 30 mg/dL |

Which of the following is the MOST likely explanation for the patient's positive copper reduction test?

a. Only glucose is present.
b. Only lactose is present.
c. Glucose and possibly other reducing substances/sugars are present.
d. Results are false positive due to the presence of protein.

*144. A 2-year-old child had a positive urine ketone. This would most likely be caused by:

a. vomiting
b. anemia
c. hypoglycemia
d. biliary tract obstruction

*145. After warming to 60°C, a cloudy urine clears. This is due to the presence of:

a. urates
b. phosphates
c. WBCs
d. bacteria

*146. The following lab values were obtained on a body fluid sample:

| | |
|---|---|
| Protein | 3 g/dL |
| Albumin | 2.1 g/dL |
| Hyaluronate | 0.4 g/dL |
| Glucose | 80 mg/dL |
| Lactate | 10 mg/dL |

The sample is:

a. pleural fluid
b. synovial fluid
c. urine
d. cerebrospinal fluid

*147. Synovial fluid is analyzed with a polarizing microscope. Strongly birefringent needles are seen. This most likely indicates:

    a. monosodium urate crystals
    b. calcium pyrophosphate crystals
    c. corticosteroid crystals
    d. talc crystals


*148. Pleural fluid from a patient with congestive heart failure would be expected to:

    a. contain bacteria
    b. have a high protein content
    c. be purulent
    d. appear clear and pale yellow


*149. Urine specific gravity is an index of the ability of the kidney to:

    a. filter the plasma
    b. concentrate the urine
    c. alter the hydrogen ion concentration
    d. reabsorb sodium ions


*150. To prepare a solution appropriate for quality control of the refractometer, a technician should use:

    a. urea with a specific gravity of 1.040
    b. water with a specific gravity of 1.005
    c. sodium chloride with a specific gravity of 1.022
    d. calcium chloride with an osmolarity of 460


*151. To prepare the reagent used in confirmatory protein testing, a technician would:

    a. dissolve 3 g sulfosalicylic acid in 100 mL of water
    b. dissolve 5 g trichloracetic acid in 100 mL of water
    c. combine 3 mL of hydrochloric acid and 97 mL of water
    d. combine 5 mL of glacial acetic acid and 95 mL of water


*152. To prepare the reagent used for mucin clot determination of synovial fluid, water is mixed with:

    a. hydrochloric acid
    b. sodium hydroxide
    c. trichloroacetic acid
    d. glacial acetic acid

*153. A patient has glucosuria, hyperglycemia, and polyuria. These findings would be associated with:

    a. renal glucosuria
    b. diabetes mellitus
    c. emotional stress
    d. eating a heavy meal

# *Urinalysis and Body Fluids* **Answer Key**

| | | | | |
|---|---|---|---|---|
| 1. c | 32. b | 63. b | 94. c | 125. a |
| 2. c | 33. b | 64. a | 95. b | 126. d |
| 3. b | 34. c | 65. c | 96. b | 127. b |
| 4. d | 35. d | 66. c | 97. d | 128. b |
| 5. a | 36. c | 67. a | 98. b | 129. b |
| 6. c | 37. b | 68. c | 99. d | 130. d |
| 7. d | 38. a | 69. b | 100. c | 131. d |
| 8. d | 39. b | 70. c | 101. b | 132. d |
| 9. d | 40. a | 71. a | 102. a | 133. b |
| 10. b | 41. c | 72. b | 103. a | 134. a |
| 11. a | 42. a | 73. b | 104. b | 135. d |
| 12. b | 43. d | 74. d | 105. a | 136. b |
| 13. b | 44. b | 75. d | 106. c | 137. b |
| 14. a | 45. b | 76. c | 107. b | 138. b |
| 15. c | 46. d | 77. d | 108. d | 139. c |
| 16. a | 47. b | 78. b | 109. b | 140. c |
| 17. d | 48. d | 79. d | 110. c | 141. a |
| 18. d | 49. a | 80. c | 111. d | 142. b |
| 19. a | 50. c | 81. a | 112. b | 143. c |
| 20. c | 51. c | 82. a | 113. b | 144. a |
| 21. c | 52. c | 83. d | 114. a | 145. a |
| 22. a | 53. d | 84. d | 115. d | 146. b |
| 23. c | 54. d | 85. b | 116. b | 147. a |
| 24. b | 55. b | 86. a | 117. a | 148. d |
| 25. b | 56. a | 87. a | 118. c | 149. b |
| 26. b | 57. c | 88. c | 119. c | 150. c |
| 27. c | 58. b | 89. d | 120. c | 151. a |
| 28. b | 59. b | 90. c | 121. c | 152. d |
| 29. b | 60. a | 91. c | 122. a | 153. b |
| 30. a | 61. d | 92. c | 123. c | |
| 31. a | 62. d | 93. b | 124. c | |

# CHAPTER 16

## Computer Practice Tests

The computer program is designed to simulate the Board of Registry's computerized adaptive test. There are approximately 2000 items in the Study Guide program. The program will administer many different practice tests, each consisting of 50 questions. New tests will be presented until all of the items have been used. You will be notified when the program has used all questions once and is beginning to reuse questions. The distribution of the questions across content areas is comparable to the MT or MLT content guidelines (see Chapter 7).

The computerized practice tests have three phases. First, 50 items are presented, then the program automatically enters the review phase. While reviewing, all 50 questions may be seen again, and the answers may be changed. The third phase is feedback. In the feedback phase, the program displays each question on your practice exam with the answer you selected and the correct answer.

When taking a practice test, you must answer each question before moving to the next question. Illustrations will appear on the screen with the questions. Each test will run for a maximum of 2 hours. After 2 hours, the test will automatically stop.

*Individuals should use the same ID number each time the program is used. Using the same ID number enables the program to keep track of questions seen by each individual.*

### Suggestions for Taking a Computer-Administered Test

1. Read the instructions carefully before beginning.
2. Read the questions carefully, looking for words such as *best, most likely,* and *not.*
3. Read all the responses before answering. Sometimes what appears initially to be a correct answer may not be the best answer.
4. Try to stay relaxed and think clearly and logically through the problems presented.
5. You must answer each question to the best of your ability when it is presented. Take as much time as you feel is necessary (within reason) to answer the question correctly.
6. When using the computer mouse, always use the left mouse button.

# Directions for Installing the Study Guide Program

Your system must be IBM compatible, 386 or higher with a:

- 3.5-inch disk drive
- hard disk drive with at least 13 MB free disk space
- Super VGA monitor
- Super VGA video card with 256 colors
- 4 MB RAM (minimum)
- Windows 3.1, 3.11, or Windows95

Faster machines will permit the program to run faster and more efficiently.

1. **Turn on the computer.**
   *Windows 3.1 or 3.11:*
   Bring up the Program Manager Window in the WINDOWS operating system.
   *Windows95:*
   Click the Start button to display the menu.

2. **Place disk 1 into the 3.5" drive (usually A).**
   *Windows 3.1 or 3.11:*
   a. Click on File, then click on Run (in the File drop-down menu).
   b. In the box under Command line, type A:\SETUP and then press the ENTER key.
   *Windows95:*
   a. Click on Run.
   b. In the box next to Open, type A:\SETUP, then click on OK.

3. **A window labeled Introduction will appear.**

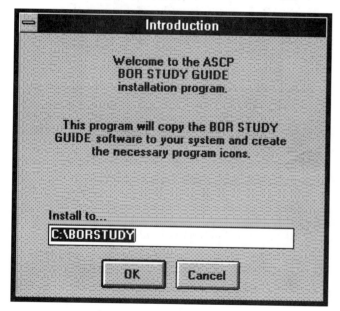

The Study Guide program will create a directory called BORSTUDY on the hard drive. All of the required files are placed in that directory.

  a. If you wish to install the program on a different directory and/or drive, type the directory name and/or drive in the box.

  b. Click on OK to begin the installation.

  c. Insert disks 2 and 3 following the on-screen directions.

  d. A window labeled Setup will appear.

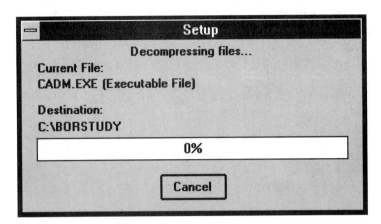

4. **After all disks have been installed, a window labeled Program Group will appear with the messages:**

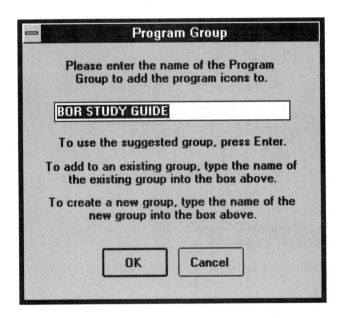

The program will automatically name the group BOR Study Guide unless otherwise specified. If you do not want to create the BOR Study Guide Group and instead wish to add the study guide program to an existing group, type the name of the existing group in the box. To create a new group, type the new name in the box.

**5. A window labeled Conclusion will appear. Click on OK.**

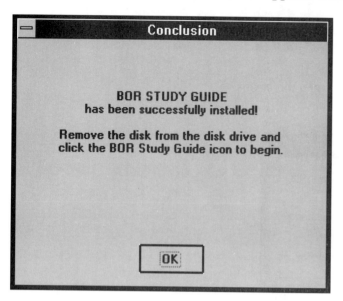

The installation process needs to be done only once. Remove the disk from the floppy drive, then follow the instructions for taking MT or MLT level tests.

## Directions for Beginning the Study Guide Program

1. **Windows 3.1 or 3.11:**
   a. Access the Program Manager window.
   b. Double-click on the STUDY GUIDE icon. If this icon is not available, double-click on the BOR Study Guide group icon. The BOR Study Guide icon will now appear.

**Group Icon**          **Icon**

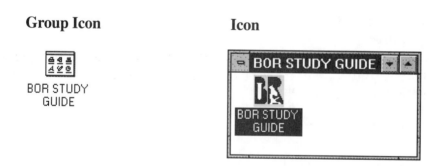

   **Windows95:**
   a. Click on the Start button, and click on BOR Study Guide.

**2. A window labeled Pick Battery will appear.**

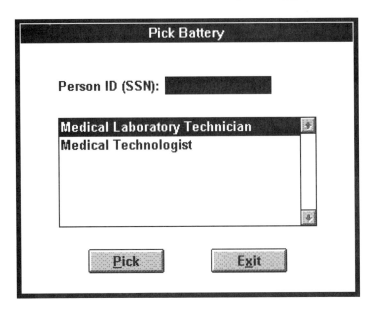

a. Use the keyboard to enter an ID number (each student should use his or her own ID number).
b. Click on Medical Laboratory Technician or Medical Technologist.
c. Click on the Pick button.

**3. A window labeled Confirmation Screen will appear. Click on Confirm.**

**4. The instructions for taking the test will appear on the screen.**

**5. The study guide questions will appear after the test instructions. There will be 50 items on each practice exam.**

## Using the Study Guide Program

**1. You may use the mouse and/or the keyboard with this program. To use the mouse, point then click with the left mouse button. If you prefer to use the keyboard you will use the TAB, ENTER, and the number (1,2,3,4) keys.**

**2. Select your answers by doing either of the following:**
a. Use the mouse to click on the gray and white bubble next to your selected answer.
or
b. Use the keyboard to press the number of the answer you selected.

3. **Record your answers by:**
   a. Clicking on the NEXT button.
   or
   b. Using the TAB key to move the highlight (dashed-line square) to the NEXT button, then pressing the ENTER key to record your answer.

| Answer not selected | Answer selected | Next button without highlight | Next button with highlight |
|---|---|---|---|

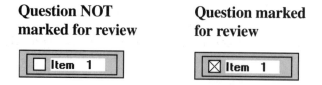

4. **You may change your answer as many times as you wish before moving to the next question. You must answer each question before the program will allow you to move to the next question.**

5. **To use the row of buttons at the bottom of the screen, use the mouse to click on the appropriate button, or use the TAB key to move the highlight to the desired button, then press ENTER. You may use the HELP and TIME functions at any time. The PREVIOUS and REVIEW buttons will activate after 50 questions have been seen.**

6. **To mark questions for review:**
   a. Move the highlight to the ITEM number button, then press the ENTER key.
   or
   b. Click on the white square in the ITEM number button.

An X appearing in the white square means the question has been marked for review. Students have access to all questions while reviewing. Marked questions are signified with an X in the review table to remind the student which questions they would particularly like to review.

| Question NOT marked for review | Question marked for review |
|---|---|
| ☐ Item 1 | ☒ Item 1 |

7. **To end the program before seeing all 50 questions, use the STOP button.**

8. **After you have answered 50 questions, the program will automatically enter the review mode. At this time, you will be able to review all questions and your answers.**

# Reviewing Your Answers

Our research has shown that changing responses does not necessarily improve test performance. The purpose of review is to correct any entry errors or obviously incorrect responses. When the REVIEW button is used the following Review window will appear.

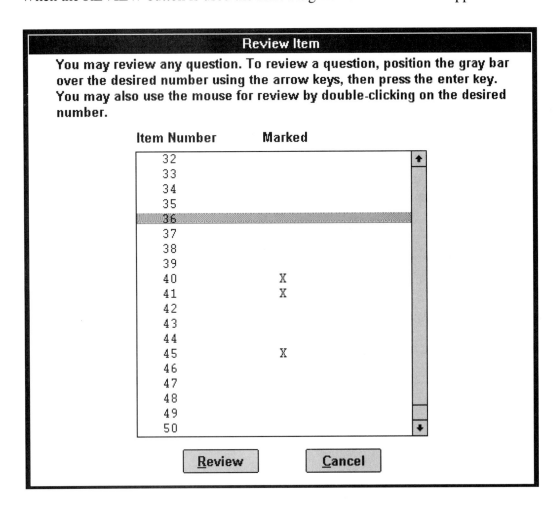

Items marked for review will have an X in the marked column. Position the gray bar over the question number you would like to review, then press enter or click on the review button.

1. **The gray bar may be moved by using the arrow keys on the keyboard or clicking on the question number with the mouse.**

2. **When reviewing a question, the answer you recorded is indicated. You may change your answer if you wish. The last answer entered will be recorded for the feedback phase.**

3. **To change your answer, click on a different response.**

4. **To move through the questions, use the NEXT, PREVIOUS, or REVIEW buttons.**

5. The HELP and TIME screens are available throughout the review mode by using the appropriate buttons.

6. To end review and enter the feedback phase, use the STOP button.

## Feedback on Your Answers

After you have finished reviewing, the program will enter the feedback mode. This enables you to assess your performance on the practice test.

1. In the feedback mode, each question is presented with your response highlighted. An information window will appear on the screen and display the correct answer.

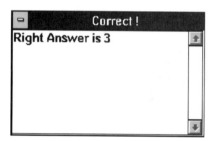
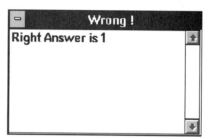

2. You may see all questions on your exam. Move to any question by using the NEXT, PRE-VIOUS, or REVIEW buttons.

3. To end the performance review, use the STOP button.

## Troubleshooting

*Installation Problems*
1. **Problem:** System Error—Cannot read from drive E.
   **Solution:** *None. The program is not compatible with some laptop computers. Try installing the program on a different system.*

**2. Problem:** The following screen appears:

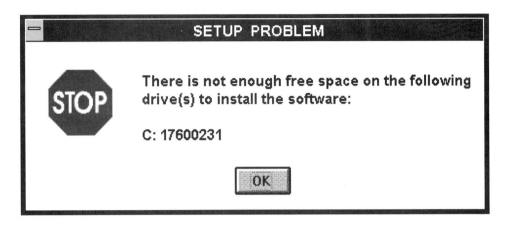

> **Solution:** *There is insufficient disk space. Back up files, then erase existing files until 13 MB of disk space is available.*

**3. Problem:** The following screen appears:

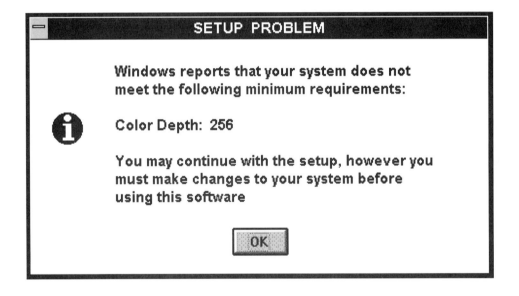

This screen appears because the computer does not have a Super VGA monitor and/or a Super VGA video card, or the Windows display settings are not set up for 256 colors.

> **Solution:** *The resolution must be set to 640 x 480, 256 colors.*

*(Note: Write down the current display settings in the event you need to reset your system.)*

CONSULT YOUR OWNER'S MANUAL TO ENSURE YOU HAVE A SUPER VGA CARD BEFORE PROCEEDING! **DO NOT** CHANGE YOUR RESOLUTION IF YOU DO NOT HAVE A SUPER VGA CARD!

**Windows 3.1 or 3.11:**
- Access the Main group.
- Double-click on Windows Setup icon.
- Click on Options, and choose Change System Settings from the drop-down menu.
- Click on the Display bar and choose 640 x 480, 256 colors.

**Windows95**
- Click on Settings.
- Go to Control Panel.
- Choose the Display icon.
- Access Settings.
- Change the Desktop Area to 640 x 480, 256 colors.

If you have changed your settings, and the screen is unreadable, this probably indicates that you do not have a Super VGA monitor and/or card. Press the ALT and F4 keys simultaneously or reboot your system. From the DOS prompt, type setup and reset your original settings. You will not be able to run this program.

4. **Problem:** System Error—Cannot read from drive A.
   **Solution:** *Click on Retry. If installation does not continue then click on cancel. Reboot the system if the error does not disappear. The disk could be defective. You may return disks to ASCP for a replacement set.*

*Program Usage Problems*
1. **Problem:** Program is reusing questions on sequential tests taken by the same person.
   **Solution:** *Use the same ID number each time you use the program.*

2. **Problem:** The Task bar of Windows95 covers the study guide program's function buttons.
   **Solution:** *You may hide the task bar by doing the following:*

   - Click on the Start button and click on Settings.
   - Point to Task bar and click.
   - Click in the white box next to the Auto hide, so a ✔ appears in the box.

3. **Problem:** Color photographs will not appear.
   **Solution:** *A Super VGA card and monitor are needed to view the color photographs.*

4. **Problem:** The testing screen does not use the entire screen.
   **Solution:** *The resolution must be set to 640 x 480, 256 colors.*

*(Note: Write down the current display settings in the event you need to reset your system.)*

CONSULT YOUR OWNER'S MANUAL TO ENSURE YOU HAVE A SUPER VGA CARD BEFORE PROCEEDING! **DO NOT** CHANGE YOUR RESOLUTION IF YOU DO NOT HAVE A SUPER VGA CARD!

**Windows 3.1 or 3.11:**
- Access the Main group.
- Double-click on Windows Setup icon.
- Click on Options, and choose Change System Settings from the drop-down menu.
- Click on the Display bar and choose 640 x 480, 256 colors.

**Windows95**
- Click on Settings.
- Go to Control Panel.
- Choose the Display icon.
- Access Settings.
- Change the Desktop Area to 640 x 480, 256 colors.

# Reading Lists

*This list is intended only as a partial reference source. Its distribution does not indicate endorsement by the Board of Registry or the American Society of Clinical Pathologists, nor does the Society wish to imply that the content of the examination will be drawn from these publications.*

## General, Education, and Laboratory Operations

Cembrowski GS, Carey RN. *Laboratory Quality Management: QC & QA*. Chicago, IL: American Society of Clinical Pathologists; 1989.

Henry JB, ed. *Todd-Sanford-Davidsohn: Clinical Diagnosis and Management by Laboratory Methods*. 19th ed. 2 vol. Philadelphia, PA: WB Saunders; 1996.

Howanitz PJ, Howanitz JH. *Laboratory Quality Assurance*, New York, NY: McGraw-Hill; 1987.

## Hematology

Brown B. *Hematology, Principles and Practice*. 6th ed. Philadelphia, PA: Lea & Febiger; 1993.

Beutler E, Erslev AJ, Williams WJ, et al, eds. *Hematology*. 5th ed. New York, NY: McGraw-Hill; 1995.

Harmening-Pittiglio D. *Clinical Hematology and Fundamentals of Hemostasis*. 3rd ed. Philadelphia, PA: FA Davis; 1996.

Kapff CT, Jandl JH. *Blood: Atlas & Sourcebook of Hematology*. 2nd ed. Boston, MA: Little, Brown & Company; 1991.

Lee GR, et al. *Wintrobe's Clinical Hematology*. 9th ed. Philadelphia, PA: Lea & Febiger; 1993.

McKenzie SB. *Textbook of Hematology*. 2nd ed. Philadelphia, PA: Lea & Febiger; 1996.

National Committee on Clinical Laboratory Standards. *Collection Transport and Preparation of Blood Specimens for Coagulation Testing and Performance of Coagulation Assays: Approved Guideline*. Villanova, PA: National Committee on Clinical Laboratory Standards; 1991.

## Immunology

Roitt I. *Essential Immunology*. 8th ed. Oxford, England: Blackwell Scientific; 1994.

Rose NR, Friedman H, Fahey JL, eds. *Manual of Clinical Laboratory Immunology*. 4th ed. Washington, DC: American Society for Microbiology; 1992.

Sheehan C. *Clinical Immunology, Principles and Laboratory Diagnosis*. Philadelphia, PA: JB Lippincott; 1990.

## Microbiology

Ash L, Orihel T. *Atlas of Human Parasitology*. 3rd ed. Chicago, IL: American Society of Clinical Pathologists; 1990.

Baron EJ, Finegold SM. *Bailey and Scott's Diagnostic Microbiology*. 9th ed. St. Louis, MO: CV Mosby; 1994.

Howard BJ, Klaas J, Rubin SJ, Weissfeld AS, Tilton R. *Clinical and Pathogenic Microbiology*. 2nd ed. St. Louis, MO: CV Mosby; 1993.

Koneman EW, Allen SD, Dowell VR, et al. *Color Atlas and Textbook of Diagnostic Microbiology*. 4th ed. Philadelphia, PA: JB Lippincott; 1992.

Lennette EH, Balows A, Hausler WJ Jr, et al, eds. *Manual of Clinical Microbiology*. 6th ed. Washington, DC: American Society for Microbiology; 1995.

McGinnis MR. *Laboratory Handbook of Medical Mycology*. New York, NY: Academic Press; 1981.

Neva FA. *Basic Clinical Parasitology*. 6th ed. Norwalk, CT: Appleton & Lange; 1994.